BRIDGING THE TRANSITION TO HOUSING

This book presents a detailed exploration of the Bridging the Transition framework, an approach designed to guide practitioners, researchers, policymakers, and advocates on strategies for preventing and ending homelessness.

Taking a functional and participation approach to homelessness prevention, chapters describe the processes of leaving homelessness, strategies that can be used at individual, community, and population levels for supporting function and participation in daily life, and guiding principles for practice, research, and policy. This book advances an argument that effective, evidence-based approaches for preventing and ending homelessness are known, yet mobilizing and implementing this knowledge remains a barrier to addressing the growing problem of homelessness and housing precarity in our communities.

An ideal resource for a range of health and social care practitioners, researchers, and policymakers who wish to advance homelessness prevention efforts, this book may also be of specific interest to occupational therapists, psychologists, physicians, social workers, peer support specialists, and as a reference text for students in health and social care or research programmes.

Carrie Anne Marshall is a tenured associate professor in the School of Occupational Therapy at Western University, Director of the Social Justice in Mental Health Research Lab, and a Western Research Chair in Homelessness Prevention and Mental Health Equity at Western University in London, Ontario, Canada. She has a PhD in Rehabilitation Science from Queen's University (Kingston, Ontario, Canada) and is a registered occupational therapist in Ontario, Canada.

Rebecca Gewurtz is a tenured associate professor at the School of Rehabilitation Science in the Faculty of Health Sciences at McMaster University in Hamilton, Ontario, Canada. She has a PhD from the University of Toronto (Toronto, Ontario, Canada) and is a registered occupational therapist in Ontario, Canada.

Skye Barbic is a tenured associate professor in the Department of Occupational Science and Occupational Therapy (Vancouver, British Columbia, Canada) and is the Canada Research Chair (Tier 2) in integrated youth services. She has completed a PhD in Rehabilitation Science at McGill University in Montreal, Quebec, Canada. She is a registered occupational therapist in British Columbia, Canada.

BRIDGING THE TRANSITION TO HOUSING

A Homelessness Prevention Framework

Edited by Carrie Anne Marshall, Rebecca Gewurtz and Skye Barbic

Routledge
Taylor & Francis Group
NEW YORK AND LONDON

Designed cover image: Carrie Anne Marshall

First published 2026
by Routledge
605 Third Avenue, New York, NY 10158

and by Routledge
4 Park Square, Milton Park, Abingdon, Oxon, OX14 4RN

Routledge is an imprint of the Taylor & Francis Group, an informa business

ISBN: 978-1-032-89134-7 (hbk)
ISBN: 978-1-032-88298-7 (pbk)
ISBN: 978-1-003-54133-2 (ebk)

DOI: 10.4324/9781003541332

Typeset in Times New Roman
by SPi Technologies India Pvt Ltd (Straive)

We dedicate this book to all of the people and communities who are denied basic human rights – to housing, food, and a meaningful life. Your experiences matter. Your voices deserve to be heard. We are committed to doing more.

CONTENTS

CONTRIBUTORS

Tim Aubry, PhD, CPsych Emeritus Professor of Psychology, Senior Researcher, Centre for Research on Educational and Community Services, University of Ottawa

Oyedeji Ayonrinde, MBBS, MSc, FRCPsych, MBA, Professor, Department of Psychiatry, Queen's University. Division Chair and Clinical Director, Community Psychiatry, Providence Care, Kingston, Ontario, Canada

Skye Barbic, PhD, OT Reg. (BC), Canada Research Chair in Integrated Youth Services, Associate Professor, Faculty of Medicine, University of British Columbia, Vancouver, British Columbia, Canada

Leonie Boland, PhD., BScOT, Clinical Specialist Occupational Therapist, Programme for the Homeless, HSE Dublin North City Mental Health Services, Ireland; Honorary Lecturer, Occupational Therapy, University of Plymouth, UK; Adjunct Assistant Professor, Discipline of Occupational Therapy, Trinity College Dublin, Ireland

Chiue Bute, Co-researcher, Wilfred Laurier University, Ontario, Canada

Ana Carolina da Silva Almeida Prado, OT (Brazil), PhD Candidate, Postgraduate Program in Occupational Therapy, Metuia Network - Social Occupational Therapy, Federal University of São Carlos, Brazil

Erin Dej, PhD., Wilfrid Laurier University, Brantford, Ontario, Canada

John Ecker, PhD, Adjunct Scientist, MAP Centre for Urban Health Solutions, St. Michael's Hospital, Unity Health Toronto

Regina Celia Fiorati, PhD., Professor and Researcher in the Undergraduate Course in Occupational Therapy, Department of Health Sciences, University of São Paulo, Ribeirão Preto, Brazil

Rebecca Gewurtz, PhD., OT Reg.(Ont.), Associate Professor, McMaster University, Hamilton, Ontario, Canada

Jeff Karabanow, PhD., RSW, Professor, Dalhousie University, Halifax, Ontario, Canada

Nick Kerman, PhD, CPsych, Scientific Associate, Centre for Addiction and Mental Health, Toronto, Ontario, Canada

Andrea LeFlore, OTD, OTR/L, Director of Programs, ReVive Center for Housing and Healing, Chicago, Illinois, USA

Jayne Malenfant, PhD., Assistant Professor, McGill University, Montréal, Québec, Canada

Ana Paula Serrata Malfitano, PhD., OT (Brazil), Professor, Postgraduate Program in Occupational Therapy, Occupational Therapy Department, Metuia Network - Social Occupational Therapy, Federal University of São Carlos, Brazil

Carrie Anne Marshall, PhD, OT Reg.(Ont.), Associate Professor, Western Research Chair in Homelessness Prevention and Mental Health Equity, Director of the Social Justice in Mental Health Research Lab, Western University, London, Ontario, Canada

Abe Oudshoorn, RN, PhD., Associate Professor and Assistant Dean, Western University, London, Ontario, Canada

Holly Petersen, Co-researcher, Carleton University, Ottawa, Ontario, Canada

Tom Regehr, Executive Director, CAST Canada, McMaster University, Hamilton, Ontario, Canada

Laurence Roy, PhD., Erg., Associate Professor, School of Rehabilitation, Université de Montréal

Brenna Schmitt, MScOT, OT Reg. (Ont.), Altum Health, Stoney Creek, Ontario, Canada

Kaitlin Schwan, PhD., Associate Professor of Family Medicine, Keck School of Medicine, University of Southern California, Los Angeles, California, United States

Carla Regina Silva, Associate Professor and Researcher in the Occupational Therapy Department, Federal University of São Carlos, Brazil

Charlotte Smith, Co-researcher, Wilfred Laurier University, Brantford, Ontario, Canada

Tracy Smith-Carrier, PhD., RSW, Royal Roads University, Victoria, British Columbia, Canada

Victoria Smye, PhD., RN, FCAN, Western University, London, Ontario, Canada

Larissa Soares de Melo, Occupational Therapist, former Coordinator of the Specialized Reference Center for the Homeless Population and former Head of the High-Complexity Services Management Division at the Municipal Secretariat of Social Assistance of Ribeirão Preto, São Paulo, Brazil

Andrea Titterness, MA, PhD, Wholetherapy, Dartmouth, NS

Bhavana Varma, OOnt, Former President and CEO United Way KFL&A, Kingston, Ontario, Canada

Nadine Wathen, PhD., FCAHS, Western University, London, Ontario, Canada

Lee Ann Westover, MS, PP-OTD, OTR/L Rehabilitation and Regenerative Medicine, Columbia University Vagelos College of Physicians and Surgeons, New York, NY, United States

Julia Woodhall-Melnik, PhD., Associate Professor & Canada Research Chair in Resilient Communities, Co-Director of the Housing, Mobilization & Engagement Research Lab (HOME-RL), University of New Brunswick, Saint John, New Brunswick, Canada

FOREWORD

Despite the development of numerous evidence-based strategies that prevent and end homelessness, it is increasingly being perceived by the public and politicians as an intractable problem in Western countries, including in Canada. Efforts to protect people who were unhoused during the COVID pandemic by moving them out of crowded shelters into temporary accommodations seem to have contributed to increasing unsheltered homelessness with many people choosing to live in encampments instead of returning to shelters.

In this context, Carrie Anne Marshall, Rebecca Gewurtz, Skye Barbic, Laurence Roy, Abrial Cooke, and Rosemary Lysaght, prominent Canadian occupational therapists, developed the Bridging the Transition to Housing Framework. This conceptual framework provides comprehensive guidance for practitioners aiming to address homelessness among individuals who are unhoused and supports their reintegration into the community.

The framework includes guiding principles that are central in health and social services for people who are unhoused, notably associated with intersectionality, trauma- and violence-informed care, harm reduction, recovery, Housing First, and social justice. A focus on function and participation in daily life is a particularly unique feature of the framework. These are considered integral elements in applying these guiding principles to prevent and end homelessness.

Three of the co-authors of the framework, Carrie Anne Marshall, Rebecca Gewurtz, and Skye Barbic, who are accomplished Canadian community mental health researchers, have undertaken an ambitious task as editors of this interdisciplinary book. They have gathered an international line-up of prominent homelessness researchers and practitioners from multiple disciplines to contribute chapters that use the Bridging the Transition Framework to organize their content.

Contributors to the book describe in detail in the early chapters the framework and how its central features of function and participation in daily life can be applied to prevent homelessness and facilitate social inclusion for people who have experienced homelessness. The book is practical in its content, with chapters on strategies for supporting function and participation in daily life at the individual, community, and population levels. They also provide chapters on each of the guiding principles of the framework and how they can be applied at each of these levels.

The last section of the book presents reviews of research on causes of homelessness and evidence-based strategies for specific under researched populations, notably women and gender diverse people, 2SLGBTQ2IA+, racialized persons, and youth. The authors of these chapters also draw from the Bridging the Transition Framework to organize its content.

The visibility and exacerbation of homelessness over the last 30 years throughout North America and Europe have spawned multiple books on the topic. However, the book *Bridging the Transition to Housing: A Homelessness Prevention Framework* is unique in that its content will be valued-added for both researchers and practitioners who work in the area. The framework around which the book is organized provides coherence and direction to research on and strategies that can ultimately prevent and end homelessness.

As a researcher focused on community mental health services, homelessness, and Housing First, this book represents my initial encounter with the Bridging the Transition to Housing Framework. I am struck by how comprehensively this book demonstrates its applicability and utility in guiding our efforts to end homelessness and achieve social inclusion for the most marginalized individuals among us. It is an invaluable read for both newcomers to the field and seasoned professionals who have dedicated their careers to addressing homelessness.

Tim Aubry, PhD, CPsych
Emeritus Professor of Psychology,
Senior Researcher,
Centre for Research on Educational and
Community Services,
University of Ottawa

PREFACE

Carrie Anne Marshall, Rebecca Gewurtz and Skye Barbic

We are living in a time of growing inequality, where few enjoy vast wealth and an unacceptably large and increasing mass of people are struggling to meet their basic needs for food, shelter, and safety. These economic developments, however, are full of contradictions as they are occurring during a time of unprecedented wealth across the globe. Most countries, including those that have adequate resources for all, are struggling to manage a housing and homelessness crisis where billions of people are left without access to suitable, safe, or affordable housing. The growth of homelessness and income inequality in recent decades is the direct consequence of policy decisions that have led to increasing housing costs, while neglecting the needs of people living on the lowest incomes of our society. Effectively addressing this problem requires intentional and targeted homelessness prevention efforts, which are critical for mitigating further growth of this seemingly intractable social problem.

In this book, we present a framework for homelessness prevention that places function and participation in daily life at the centre of efforts to prevent and end homelessness. The Bridging the Transition Framework was originally developed to guide health professionals, specifically occupational therapists, as they supported individuals across the trajectory of unhoused to housing. We developed this framework based on empirical research exploring experiences of functioning and participating in daily life across the trajectory of unhoused to housing. We then refined this framework with the input of a group of international occupational therapy researchers and practitioners with expertise in homelessness. Since its initial release in 2020, this framework has attracted the attention of a range of health and social care providers, researchers, and policymakers, and in this book, we present this framework for the first time for an interdisciplinary audience.

Other frameworks focused on homelessness prevention have been developed and advanced in existing literature. These frameworks are informed by public health frameworks emphasizing primary, secondary, and tertiary prevention approaches. The Bridging the Transition Framework builds on these frameworks by focusing specifically on *tertiary prevention*. That is, preventing homelessness among people who have experienced homelessness in the past, and often repeatedly across the course of their lives. For this group, function and participation in daily life are critical to well-being, but are also at the core of ongoing challenges with homelessness. Central to the Bridging the Transition Framework is the belief that by improving function and participation in daily life, individuals and families who experience homelessness can move towards community integration and well-being and leave homelessness altogether.

Further to a focus on function and participation, we advance a perspective on homelessness prevention across the chapters in this book that is focused not solely on the individual person, but at the community and population level. We have taken this perspective because homelessness is not caused by the shortcomings of an individual person or family. It has deep roots in problematic structures in society that need to be addressed at those levels – across the communities in which people live, and especially in problematic policies that have been implemented across communities and countries. As such, health and social care providers, researchers, and policymakers are encouraged to focus their efforts on approaches beyond the individual level as a way of influencing meaningful and lasting changes for preventing and ending homelessness.

This book is structured in four key sections, prepared by leading practitioners, researchers, and advocates from across the globe. In Chapters 1–3, contributors provide a foundation for what a functional and participation approach is, and why it is a critical perspective for preventing and ending homelessness. In Chapters 4–14, contributors describe the various components of the Bridging the Transition Framework, drawing on evidence from a range of fields to illustrate each concept. In Chapters 15–17, contributors apply the framework at individual, community, and population levels. Finally, in Chapters 18–22, key social locations related to homelessness prevention are presented, focusing on gender, sexual orientation, race, youth homelessness, and homelessness in the Global South. We then conclude by reflecting on the framework, and how it has been explored and applied across all chapters in the book.

Homelessness prevention is more important than ever before. The fact that so many people across the globe are unable to secure and sustain adequate housing is an international human rights catastrophe that is increasingly being accepted as a "new normal." This is not the time for complacency – but rather action towards immediate societal changes that address the root causes of homelessness. The Bridging the Transition Framework is one such approach for structuring the efforts of practitioners, researchers, and policymakers towards a common goal of preventing and ending homelessness for individuals, communities, and populations.

Homelessness is a crisis and we need to treat it like one. We cannot, however, solve it alone. Through our collective action at individual, community, and population levels, it is possible to prevent ongoing homelessness and end it altogether.

SECTION 1

Function and Participation in Daily Activities as a Key Homelessness Prevention Strategy

1

INTRODUCTION TO THE ORIGINS AND COMPONENTS OF THE BRIDGING THE TRANSITION FRAMEWORK

Carrie Anne Marshall

As homelessness continues to grow internationally, prevention approaches are needed. This chapter provides an overview of the Bridging the Transition Framework, summarizes how it was developed, and describes its various components. This framework represents one of several homelessness prevention frameworks, yet it is unique in its focus on supporting function and participation across the trajectory of unhoused to housing at the individual, community, and population levels.

How this Chapter Guides Practice, Research, and Policy in Homelessness Prevention

The Bridging the Transition Framework was designed to guide health and social care practitioners, researchers, and policymakers to focus on finding ways of supporting individuals to function and participate in daily life in a way that supports well-being in the transition to housing following homelessness. The overall goal of this framework is to encourage practitioners, researchers, and policymakers to advance homelessness prevention by supporting individuals to function, participate, and integrate into their communities through securing and sustaining housing, developing social networks, and finding belonging in their communities.

Introduction

Homelessness is a serious social problem across the globe, with 1.6 billion individuals living in inadequate housing conditions and an additional 15

DOI: 10.4324/9781003541332-2

million forcefully evicted from their homes (United Nations, 2020). The presence and rapid growth of homelessness over the last several decades is indicative of growing inequities and wealth gaps in most countries worldwide, a problem that has disproportionately affected women, racialized persons, disabled individuals, and persons who identify as 2SLGBTQIA+ (Ecker et al., 2019; Yakubovich and Maki, 2022; Fowle, 2022; O'Donovan and Whittle, 2024). A rise in homelessness in recent decades is the direct consequence of a lack of political will to address this social problem in most countries. Policy failures, including inadequate investment in *deeply affordable* housing, coupled with poor availability of high-quality healthcare services for individuals living in poverty, have left communities struggling to support a growing number of individuals who experience homelessness. This rapid growth of homelessness internationally means that efforts aimed at preventing and ending homelessness are more crucial than ever before.

Homelessness Prevention

In this book, homelessness prevention is presented as a continuum of approaches that can be employed to prevent initial homelessness on one end, and ongoing homelessness among individuals who have been previously unhoused on the other end. Frameworks for guiding practitioners, researchers, and policymakers towards homelessness prevention have been developed in recent years and are primarily informed by public health approaches. These approaches emphasize a comprehensive series of strategies designed for primary prevention (i.e. preventing a first episode of homelessness), secondary prevention (i.e. preventing homelessness among individuals at immediate risk of homelessness), and tertiary prevention (i.e. preventing ongoing homelessness among individuals who have previously been unhoused) (Fitzpatrick et al., 2021; Gaetz and Dej, 2017; Montgomery et al., 2013). The typology of homelessness prevention advanced by Gaetz and Dej (2017) includes a range of strategies for preventing and ending homelessness that build on this public health approach. These strategies include: (1) structural prevention, (2) systems prevention, (3) early intervention, (4) evictions prevention, and (5) housing stability. Structural prevention includes strategies aimed at shifting policies and legislation to promote social inclusion and equality. Systems prevention includes addressing institutional and systemic problems that lead to homelessness. Early intervention pertains to approaches aimed at supporting individuals at imminent risk of homelessness by preventing tenancy loss. Evictions prevention includes approaches that seek to prevent homelessness from occurring by preventing tenancy loss for people who are currently housed. Finally, housing stability refers to the provision of person-centred supports to help a person to avoid homelessness once it has been experienced. A final domain, "empowerment," was added to this framework following its initial development (Oudshoorn et al., 2020). This domain emphasizes the need for providing services that preserve autonomy and acknowledge a person's fundamental need for personal choice.

While these public health-informed approaches emphasize a primary focus on preventing tenancy loss, the Bridging the Transition Framework is specifically focused on supporting health and well-being as a primary mode of homelessness prevention through a focus on function and participation in daily life. While consistent with existing frameworks for homelessness prevention, the Bridging the Transition Framework guides practitioners, researchers, and policymakers on specific strategies that can be used to prevent homelessness based on a person's current housing status and across the trajectory of unhoused to housing. Further, the Bridging the Transition Framework highlights the role of function and participation in daily life as crucial for supporting well-being across the trajectory of unhoused to housing, an objective that is essential for preventing ongoing homelessness in all communities, and something that has been highlighted by persons with experiences of homelessness in existing research.

The Bridging the Transition Framework and Its Development

Recognizing a gap in resources for an increasing number of occupational therapy practitioners, researchers, and policymakers working in the area of homelessness, the authors of the Bridging the Transition Framework designed this approach specifically for guiding occupational therapists in research and practice. The framework was developed from 2018 to 2020 by a group of Canadian researchers based on empirical research conducted on the transition to housing following homelessness (Marshall et al., 2022b) and input from occupational therapy researchers and practitioners with expertise in homelessness in the United States, Canada, Brazil, Ireland, and the United Kingdom (Marshall et al., 2023b). While delivering workshops on this framework, the authors quickly began to realize its relevance for a range of health and social care professionals when multiple attendees from a range of professions would attend workshops or request input on documentation on the framework (Marshall et al., 2023a; Marshall et al., 2020a). To respond, the authors adapted the second edition of the framework document published in 2023 for an interdisciplinary audience and have furthered this adaptation in the current book. As such, in this book, we present the Bridging the Transition Framework as an interdisciplinary framework relevant to a range of health and social care practitioners and researchers.

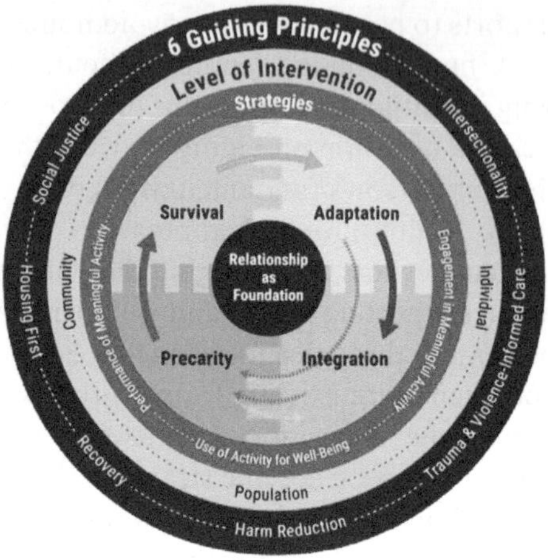

FIGURE 1.1 Bridging the Transition Framework.

What Is the Bridging the Transition Framework?

The Bridging the Transition Framework is an approach which emphasizes the importance of a functional and participation lens in supporting the well-being of individuals during and following homelessness using evidence-based strategies. In advancing this framework, the authors contend that supporting optimal function and participation in daily life is essential for supporting permanent transitions from homelessness. The authors further contend that such an approach has the potential to increase resilience to ongoing homelessness, thereby preventing its recurrence in the future. See Figure 1.1 for a graphic representation of the various components of the Bridging the Transition framework. These components are introduced in the following sections and expanded upon throughout the book.

Relationship as Foundation

At the core of the Bridging the Transition Framework is the relationship between persons experiencing homelessness, practitioners, researchers, and policymakers. In previous research, individuals have discussed the need for health and social care practitioners who demonstrate emotional consistency, authenticity, and reliability (Marshall et al., 2022b). Difficult past experiences with health and social care professionals, coupled with more prevalent histories of trauma among persons experiencing homelessness, mean that developing meaningful and trusting relationships with this population is critically important for the delivery of effective services (Wiewel and Hernandez, 2021; Marshall et al., 2022c). In the Bridging the Transition Framework, we emphasize the importance of developing meaningful and trusting relationships with individuals, communities, and populations before proceeding with any assessment or intervention approach designed to address their needs. This component of the framework is expanded upon further in Chapter 4.

From Survival to Integration: The Four Processes of Leaving Homelessness

In the Bridging the Transition Framework, the authors describe the experience of leaving homelessness as occurring across four distinct processes: Survival, Adaptation, Integration, and Precarity. In the Survival Process, a person is currently unhoused, depicted in orange in Figure 1.1. During this process, the greatest priority is housing and maintaining mental and social well-being. Once a person has secured housing, they are then considered to be in the Adaptation Process (depicted in light green in Figure 1.1), where they have recently become housed and are adapting to living in housing after leaving shelters, encampments, or the street. During this process, the priority is learning or re-learning skills that facilitate function and participation in daily life following homelessness. The Integration Process (depicted in darker green in Figure 1.1) is the time during which a person is building connections with their community and increasing resilience to ongoing homelessness. While in the Integration Process, priorities for preventing homelessness include solidifying community connections and supporting ongoing function and participation in daily life. After securing housing, some individuals may become at risk of tenancy loss. This is called the Precarity Process (depicted in red in Figure 1.1) in the Bridging the Transition Framework. During this period, the priority of health and social care practitioners, researchers, and policymakers should be to contribute to solutions aimed at helping to avoid tenancy loss. It should be mentioned that many individuals who experience homelessness may cycle through some or all four of these processes over the course of years, while others may only experience the precarity process. For example, a person might transition to housing, begin to integrate into their community, and then experience housing precarity several years after being housed. If that same person were to lose their housing, they would then enter into the survival process again, followed by the adaptation and integration processes. The Four Processes are discussed in detail in Chapter 5.

Strategies

Strategies emphasized in the Bridging the Transition Framework across the four processes of leaving homelessness are aimed at improving function and participation in daily life through the trajectory of unhoused to housing (presented in the blue ring in Figure 1.1). These strategies include supporting individuals with: (1) engagement in meaningful activity, (2) performance of meaningful activity, and (3) use of activity for well-being. Engagement in

Meaningful Activity refers to strategies aimed at promoting *participation* in activities that are meaningful. Existing evidence indicates that individuals who live in poverty and experience homelessness frequently lack opportunities to participate in meaningful activities, something that contributes positively to well-being (Marshall et al., 2024a). Performance of Meaningful Activity refers to strategies aimed at promoting *function* in meaningful activities. In the Bridging the Transition Framework, "function" refers to a person's ability to perform the tasks associated with a meaningful activity to a degree that enables completion of that activity in a way that is satisfying to the person who is performing it. Function is distinct from participation, as a person may have access to an activity, but may struggle to function in that activity effectively or to a degree that is satisfying. Research exploring function in daily activities for individuals who experience homelessness indicates that promoting function in daily life is essential for efforts designed for homelessness prevention (Marshall et al., 2021). Finally, the Use of Activity for Well-Being is emphasized as a key strategy across the trajectory of unhoused to housing. This is because meaningful activities have therapeutic value and are known to enhance well-being for individuals who experience homelessness. Further, meaningful activities provide important opportunities for connecting individuals to social networks in their community (Marshall et al., 2024b; Marshall et al., 2022a; Marshall et al., 2020b). Consistent with the definition advanced by the World Health Organization, "well-being" in the Bridging the Transition Framework is conceptualized as a "… positive state experienced by individuals and societies … [and] encompasses quality of life and the ability of people and societies to contribute to the world with a sense of meaning and purpose" (World Health Organization, , 2025). Meaningful activity is emphasized in this framework, as it is a primary mode of function and participation in daily life and has been identified as essential for the well-being of all persons, including individuals who experience homelessness (Marshall et al., 2020c; Marshall et al., 2018). Strategies that can be used to enhance function and participation of individuals at the individual, community, and population level are presented in Chapters 6–8. In Chapters 15–17, the authors apply strategies described in the framework with individuals, communities, and populations.

Level of Intervention

In the Bridging the Transition Framework, the authors emphasize intervention not only at the level of the individual but also at the community and population levels across the Four Processes of leaving homelessness. This is depicted as a light blue ring in Figure 1.1. At the Individual Level, the authors of the Bridging the Transition Framework emphasize the use of strategies that are focused on individuals, informed by their unique needs and strengths, and situated within their specific environmental contexts. At the Community Level, the authors encourage the use of strategies focused on how health and social care practitioners, researchers, and policymakers might work with communities to address the needs of persons experiencing homelessness. Communities, in this framework, do not refer to the development and implementation of therapeutic groups or groups of individuals in a single program, but rather groups of citizens that gather around common geography, interests, or goals. Population Level strategies include approaches delivered with population groups *across communities*. Such approaches include strategies meant to support persons experiencing homelessness regionally, nationally, or internationally, including a range of public health interventions and research initiatives. These levels of intervention are described in detail in Chapters 6–8. Specific case applications of these levels of intervention are presented in Chapters 15–17.

Six Guiding Principles

Six guiding principles for informing research, practice and policy in homelessness prevention are emphasized in the Bridging the Transition Framework: (1) Social Justice, (2) Housing First, (3) Recovery, (4) Harm Reduction, (5) Trauma and Violence-Informed Care, and (6) Intersectionality. These principles can be considered interrelated philosophies and/or interventions that can guide practitioners, researchers, and policymakers to adopt evidence-based and anti-oppressive approaches in their work.

Guiding Principle 1: Social Justice. Social justice is an interdisciplinary concept acknowledging the ways in which resources are distributed in society, with an interest in advancing the common well-being of all by seeking to distribute resources in a more equitable manner (Stronks et al., 2016). Social justice is fundamentally connected with human rights in that it aims to elevate the well-being of oppressed populations (Stronks et al., 2016). Homelessness is often the direct result of poverty (Gaetz et al., 2016) and is an issue for which a social justice lens is particularly useful. Many persons who experience homelessness live in situations of extreme deprivation in countries that have ample resources for all. As health and social care practitioners, researchers, and policymakers, we have a role in seeking to realize social justice for individuals who experience homelessness through our individual encounters and using community- and population-level approaches. The concept of social justice is discussed in detail in Chapter 9.

Guiding Principle 2: Housing First. Housing First is a person-centred philosophy which emphasizes that individuals are "housing ready" from the moment they are born and do not need to prove housing readiness prior to being offered permanent housing (Tsemberis, 2011). Housing First emerged from criticisms of the "treatment first" approach to homelessness services, which emphasized the treatment of mental health and substance use challenges before an individual could be regarded as "housing ready." These "treatment first" approaches emphasized the use of shelters and transitional housing and are often seen as inhumane because they prolong homelessness for individuals who already live with multiple health and social challenges. Health and social care practitioners using this framework should emphasize the primacy of permanent supportive housing in their support of persons experiencing homelessness over encouraging "housing readiness." Housing First is discussed further in Chapter 10.

Guiding Principle 3: Recovery. Rates of mental illness and substance use disorders are known to be high among persons who experience homelessness (Hossain et al., 2020). The recovery model posits that a person living with mental illness (including substance use disorder) can create a life of personal meaning in the face of challenges imposed by a diagnosis (Davidson and Roe, 2009; Deegan, 1988). Many individuals living with mental illness (including substance use disorder) experience symptoms episodically or chronically, meaning that they live with these challenges to a greater or lesser degree in the long term. Adopting a recovery-oriented approach to practice, research, and policy is particularly important, given that individuals may lose their housing in part due to functional challenges associated with mental illness, and these challenges are likely to persist across the trajectory of unhoused to housing. A recovery-oriented approach emphasizes hope and creating a meaningful life on one's own terms despite living with the symptoms of mental illness (including substance use disorder). Recovery is discussed in more detail in Chapter 11.

Guiding Principle 4: Harm Reduction. Harm reduction is a philosophy of practice that emphasizes the safety of individuals engaged in activities that have the potential to impose harm, such as substance use and sex work (Ashford et al., 2019; Levenson et al., 2023). Harm reduction approaches encourage the use of a range of practices, including the provision of clean and safe tools for administering substances or providing condoms and sexual health education. One common misconception is that harm reduction precludes discussions of reduction or abstinence from substances (Henwood et al., 2014). Health and social care practitioners, researchers, and policymakers may consider that the use of a harm reduction philosophy does not mean withholding support for reducing or abstaining from substances, but rather providing a range of options for reducing the harms of substance use, including services to reduce substance use should a person wish to do so. Harm Reduction is described in greater depth in Chapter 12.

Guiding Principle 5: Trauma and Violence-Informed Care. It is widely recognized that individuals who experience homelessness have endured physical, sexual, and emotional trauma both before and during homelessness (Gutwinski et al., 2021). Homelessness has been described as a form of trauma in that the denial of the right to housing can be experienced as deep exclusion and abandonment by one's community. Knowledge that trauma is more prevalent among persons who experience homelessness means that it is necessary to use approaches that acknowledge the presence of this trauma in the delivery of services. When using this framework, health and social care practitioners, researchers, and policymakers are encouraged to use a "universal precautions" approach to trauma. This means assuming that any person with experiences of homelessness or housing precarity may have experienced trauma. As such, practice, research, and policy should be conducted in a way that limits further activation of this prior trauma through the use of "Trauma and Violence-Informed Care." Trauma and violence-informed care is an approach that builds on "Trauma Informed Care" by acknowledging that individuals may experience trauma both from interpersonal experiences (i.e. physical and emotional abuse) and from the structural environments in which they are situated (Wathen et al., 2023). Trauma and violence-informed care is discussed in detail in Chapter 13.

Guiding Principle 6: Intersectionality. Intersectionality acknowledges the ways in which race, gender, ability, sexual orientation, and class intersect to influence social possibilities and health (Oexle and Corrigan, 2018). The fact that racialized persons, men, individuals identifying as 2SLGBTQIA+, Indigenous persons, and individuals living with disabilities are disproportionately represented in statistics on homelessness suggests that these social locations should be accounted for in practice, research, and policy. Often, these social locations may layer over one another to create deep degrees of discrimination and health and social inequities. Intersectionality and its implications for health and social care practitioners, researchers, and policymakers are explored further in Chapter 14.

Conclusion

Homelessness prevention is a pressing need in most countries internationally in the midst of a housing crisis that has been growing over the past several decades. Preventing and ending homelessness requires not only housing but supports for individuals to function and participate optimally in their daily lives to support well-being beyond tenancy sustainment alone (Ndayisenga et al., 2024). In this chapter, we have provided an overview of the Bridging the Transition Framework, its origins, and its various components. A focus on function and participation was identified as a unique contribution of this framework and will be expanded upon throughout the following chapters. Attending to the functional and participation needs of persons who experience homelessness is a key approach to homelessness prevention that needs to be incorporated in practice, research, and policy with individuals, communities, and populations.

References

Ashford, R. D., Brown, A. M., Dorney, G., Mcconnell, N., Kunzelman, J., Mcdaniel, J. & Curtis, B. (2019). Reducing harm and promoting recovery through community-based mutual aid: Characterizing those who engage in a hybrid peer recovery community organization. *Addictive Behaviors*, 98, 106037.

Davidson, L. & Roe, D. (2009). Recovery from versus recovery in serious mental illness: One strategy for lessening confusion plaguing recovery. *Journal of Mental Health*, 16, 459–470.

Deegan, P. E. (1988). Recovery: The lived experience of rehabilitation. *Psychosocial Rehabilitation Journal*, 11, 11–19.

Ecker, J., Aubry, T. & Sylvestre, J. (2019). A review of the literature on LGBTQ adults who experience homelessness. *Journal of Homosexuality*, 66, 297–323.

Fitzpatrick, S., Mackie, P. & Wood, J. (2021). Advancing a five-level typology of homelessness prevention. *International Journal on Homelessness*, 1, 79–97.

Fowle, M. Z. (2022). Racialized homelessness: A review of historical and contemporary causes of racial disparities in homelessness. *Housing Policy Debate*, 32, 940–967.

Gaetz, S. & Dej, E. (2017). A new direction: A framework for homelessness prevention. Available: https://www.homelesshub.ca/sites/default/files/attachments/COH PreventionFramework_1.pdf [Accessed March 13, 2024].

Gaetz, S., Dej, E., Richter, T. & Redman, M. (2016). *The State of Homelessness in Canada 2016*. Toronto: Canadian Observatory on Homelessness Press.

Gutwinski, S., Schreiter, S., Deutscher, K. & Fazel, S. 2021. The prevalence of mental disorders among homeless people in high-income countries: An updated systematic review and meta-regression analysis. *PLOS Medicine*, 18, e1003750.

Henwood, B. F., Padgett, D. K. & Tiderington, E. (2014). Provider views of harm reduction versus abstinence policies within homeless services for dually diagnosed adults. *Journal of Behavioral Health Services & Research*, 41, 80–9.

Hossain, M. M., Sultana, A., Tasnim, S., Fan, Q., Ma, P., Mckyer, E. L. J. & Purohit, N. (2020). Prevalence of mental disorders among people who are homeless: An umbrella review. *International Journal of Social Psychiatry*, 66, 528–541.

Levenson, J., Textor, L., Bluthenthal, R., Darby, A., Wahbi, R. & Clayton-Johnson, M. A. (2023). Abolition and harm reduction in the struggle for "Care, Not Cages". *International Journal of Drug Policy*, 121, 104163.

Marshall, C., Easton, C., Holmes, J., Javadizadeh, E., Phillips, B. & Isard, R. (2024a). Effectiveness of interventions for meaningful activity participationin homelessness: A systematic review. *Canadian Journal of Occupational Therapy*, 91(3), 256–271.

Marshall, C., Gewurtz, R., Barbic, S., Roy, L., Cooke, A. & Lysaght, R. (2023a). Bridging the transition to housing: A social justice framework to guide the practice of occupational therapists and other professionals who support individuals with experiences of homelessness. Available online at: https://www.sjmhlab.com/_files/ugd/fbaf23_99bc69b1d337487cabc709d27e6770c8.pdf

Marshall, C., Gewurtz, R., Barbic, S., Roy, L., Lysaght, R. C. R., Becker, A., Cooke, A. & Kirsh, B. (2020a). Bridging the transition from homeless to housed: A social justice framework to guide the practice of occupational therapists. Available online at: https://www.osot.on.ca/docs/practice_resources/Bridging_the_Transition_from_Homeless_to_Housed.pdf

Marshall, C., Holmes, J., Todd, E., Hall, M., Panter, G., Plett, P., Easton, C., Perez, S., Landry, T., Lambert, E., Collins, S., Greening, T., Ravnaas, C., O'Brien, A., Jastak, M., Ridge, R., Goldszmidt, R., Laliberte-Rudman, D., Carlsson, A., Kiwala, S. & Oudshoorn, A. (2024b). Co-designing the "Peer to Community (P2C) Model" for promoting community integration following homelessness: The transition from homelessness study. *International Journal of Homelessness*, 5(1), 208–230.

Marshall, C. A., Boland, L., Westover, L. A., Goldszmidt, R., Bengall, J., Aryobi, S., Isard, R., Easton, C. & Gewurtz, R. (2022a). Effectiveness of employment-based interventions for persons experiencing homelessness: A systematic review. *Health & Social Care in the Community*, 30, 2142–2169.

Marshall, C. A., Boland, L., Westover, L. A., Isard, R. & Gutman, S. A. (2021). A systematic review of occupational therapy interventions in the transition from homelessness. *Scandinavian Journal of Occupational Therapy*, 28, 171–187.

Marshall, C. A., Boland, L., Westover, L. A., Marcellus, B., Weil, S. & Wickett, S. (2020b). Effectiveness of interventions targeting community integration among individuals with lived experiences of homelessness: A systematic review. *Health & Social Care in the Community*, 28, 1843–1862.

Marshall, C. A., Boland, L., Westover, L. A., Wickett, S., Roy, L., Mace, J., Gewurtz, R., Barbic, S. & Kirsh, B. (2020c). Occupational experiences of homelessness: A systematic review and meta-aggregation. *Scandinavian Journal of Occupational Therapy*, 27, 394–407.

Marshall, C. A., Cooke, A., Gewurtz, R., Barbic, S., Roy, L., Ross, C., Becker, A., Lysaght, R. & Kirsh, B. (2023b). Bridging the transition from homelessness: Developing an occupational therapy framework. *Scandinavian Journal of Occupational Therapy*, 30, 953–969.

Marshall, C. A., Gewurtz, R., Ross, C., Becker, A., Cooke, A., Roy, L., Barbic, S., Lysaght, R. & Kirsh, B. (2022b). Beyond Securing a tenancy: Using the capabilities approach to identify the daily living needs of individuals during and following homelessness. *Journal of Social Distress and Homelessness*, 33, 81–95.

Marshall, C. A., Lysaght, R. & Krupa, T. (2018). Occupational transition in the process of becoming housed following chronic homelessness: La transition occupationnelle liee au processus d'obtention d'un logement a la suite d'une itinerance chronique. *Canadian Journal of Occupational Therapy*, 85, 33–45.

Marshall, C. A., Phillips, B., Holmes, J., Todd, E., Hill, R., Panter, G., Easton, C., Landry, T., Collins, S., Greening, T., O'Brien, A., Jastak, M., Ridge, R., Goldszmidt, R., Shanoff, C., Laliberte Rudman, D., Carlsson, A., Aryobi, S., Perez, S. & Oudshoorn, A. (2022c). 'We stick people in a house and say okay, you're housed. The problem is solved': A qualitative study of service provider and organisational leader perspectives on thriving following homelessness. *Health & Social Care in the Community*, 30, e6018–e6029.

Montgomery, A. E., Metraux, S. & Culhane, D. (2013). Rethinking homelessness prevention among persons with serious mental illness. *Social Issues and Policy Review*, 7, 58–82.

Ndayisenga, J. P., Oudshoorn, A., Marshall, C. A., Barbic, S. P., Kidd, S. A. & Gaetz, S. A. (2024). Thriving after homelessness: A concept analysis. *International Journal on Homelessness*, 4, 281–295.

O'Donovan, M. & Whittle, E. L. (2024). Housing, homelessness and disability: The commodification of a core human right and breach of this right for people with disability. *Advances in Neurodevelopmental Disorders*, 8, 141–150.

Oexle, N. & Corrigan, P. W. (2018). Understanding mental illness stigma toward persons with multiple stigmatized conditions: Implications of intersectionality theory. *Psychiatric Services*, 69, 587–589.

Oudshoorn, A., Dej, E., Parsons, C. & Gaetz, S. (2020). Evolving an evidence-based model for homelessness prevention. *Health & Social Care in the Community*, 28, 1754–1763.

Stronks, K., Toebes, B., Hendriks, A., Ikram, U. & Venkatapuram, S. (2016). Social justice and human rights as a framework for addressing social determinants of health. *Final Report of the Task Group on Equity, Equality and Human Rights*. Available: https://www.euro.who.int/__data/assets/pdf_file/0006/334356/HR-task-report.pdf

Tsemberis, S. (2011). Housing first: The pathways model to end homelessness for people with mental illness and addiction manual. *European Journal of Homelessness*, 5.
United Nations (2020). *First-ever United Nations Resolution on Homelessness*[Online]. New York: United Nations. Available: https://www.un.org/development/desa/dspd/2020/03/resolution-homelessness/
Wathen, C. N., Schmitt, B. & Macgregor, J. C. D. (2023). Measuring trauma-(and violence-) informed care: A scoping review. *Trauma Violence Abuse*, 24, 261–277.
Wiewel, B. & Hernandez, L. (2021). Traumatic stress and homelessness: A review of the literature for practitioners. *Clinical Social Work Journal*, 50, 218–230.
World Health Organization (2025). *Promoting well-being* [Online]. WHO. Available: https://www.who.int/activities/promoting-well-being [Accessed January 13 2025].
Yakubovich, A. R. & Maki, K. (2022). Preventing gender-based homelessness in Canada during the COVID-19 pandemic and beyond: The need to account for violence against women. *Violence Against Women*, 28, 2587–2599.

2

FUNCTION AND PARTICIPATION IN DAILY LIFE ACTIVITIES AS A KEY COMPONENT OF RESEARCH AND PRACTICE IN HOMELESSNESS PREVENTION

Laurence Roy

Individuals at risk of or experiencing homelessness may present with complex health and social profiles that impact the level and type of supports they need to obtain, maintain, and thrive into housing. Disability, housing, and homelessness practitioners and researchers have suggested that understanding and acting on the functional and participation impacts of health issues and disability is an essential component of homelessness prevention. In this chapter, we explore how a function and participation approach to homelessness prevention can be framed, building on key concepts from the Bridging the Transition Framework presented in Chapter 1. We then examine the current state of knowledge regarding how function and participation challenges impact housing outcomes and risk of first-time or repeated homelessness. Finally, we explore the practical and research implications of taking a function and participation approach to homelessness prevention for health and social care practitioners.

How this Chapter Guides Practice and Research in Homelessness Prevention

This chapter builds on concepts described in the Bridging the Transition Framework to identify how a function and participation lens can be used to prevent homelessness with individuals, communities, and populations. The chapter will allow readers to understand the complexity of securing, sustaining, and thriving into housing when confronted with participation and function challenges such as social isolation, boredom, lack of opportunities for meaningful activity engagement, financial issues, interpersonal conflicts, and difficulties

DOI: 10.4324/9781003541332-3

with self-advocacy. The chapter also offers guidance to health and social care practitioners and researchers to assess and address functional and participation challenges during the survival, adaptation, integration, and precarity processes of leaving homelessness. Finally, the chapter builds on the Framework's principles of social justice and intersectionality by framing homelessness as a disability rights issue to advance housing practice, research, and policy.

Introduction

Liam is a 21-year-old man living with two roommates in a three-bedroom apartment of a large Canadian urban center. He has moved to the city from a remote small town one year ago, fleeing long-standing conflicts with his parents and brothers over Liam's sexual orientation. Liam struggled with school and was diagnosed with a learning disability at age 13. He dropped out of school in grade 10 and worked at a grocery store in his hometown. Liam now works evening shifts in a coffee shop and spends most nights going out to bars and dancing with his roommates and colleagues. One evening, Liam leaves a club and falls down a flight of stairs, hitting his head on the pavement. Liam is transported unconscious to the nearest hospital, where he is diagnosed with a broken clavicle and a moderate traumatic brain injury. He is discharged from the hospital five days later with a referral for outpatient rehabilitation services. The services do not start immediately, and Liam is sent home. Liam goes back to his apartment, where he struggles with severe headaches, fatigue, and drowsiness. He is mostly alone at home as his roommates are busy with work and nightlife. While his friends initially attempt to show Liam some comfort, he becomes estranged from the group. The discomfort associated with his fracture impacts his sleep and mood. Three weeks after the injury, Liam attempts to go back to work, but he cannot finish his shift as his headaches increase with the loud music and the pace of the work. He makes other attempts to resume work or clubbing and gets increasingly frustrated and isolated. He finally decides to quit his job at the coffee shop. While knowing that he needs to fill in documentation for unemployment benefits, he delays them and spends most of his days sleeping or looking at friends' posts on social media. Two months after the injury, his roommates initiate a conversation, noting that Liam is late on rent. They also raise the question of whether Liam still fits in their "roommate culture". Liam, feeling hurt and rejected, collects most of his belongings, yells at his roommates, and decides to take the next bus to his hometown. At the bus station, he calls his mother, announcing that he is coming back, but she replies that his cousin is now staying in his former room and that they have no place for him.

Liam's story illuminates many of the features that complexify intervention and prevention approaches with people experiencing homelessness. First, it exemplifies the notion of Relationships as Foundation, as disruptions in meaningful and trusting relationships with one's family, social networks, and communities are at the core of the experience of homelessness. Second, it illustrates how several people experiencing or at risk of homelessness live with disabilities that impact their ability to function and participate in activities that are meaningful and necessary in their daily lives (Marshall et al., 2019a). Meta-analyses and systematic reviews indicate that people experiencing homelessness are much more likely than the general population to live with acquired brain injuries, mental illness, substance use disorders, musculoskeletal disabilities, and chronic pain, among other health conditions (Anastas et al., 2023; Guillén, Panadero, & Vázquez, 2021; Gutwinski et al., 2021; Stubbs et al., 2020). Multiple and interrelated disabilities seem to be the norm rather than the exception, with people experiencing homelessness presenting with complex health profiles that impact function and participation (Omerov et al., 2020). Situations of violence that lead many people into homelessness and that continue to happen during episodes of homelessness create physical and psychological injuries that contribute to, precipitate, and exacerbate disability (Calvo et al., 2021). Violence can also contribute to relational losses and disruptions, further eroding one's support system and protective network against homelessness (Samuels, Curry, & Cerven, 2021).

This chapter will explore how taking a function and participation approach is an essential perspective in homelessness prevention across the four stages of leaving homelessness. First, we will define the key concepts of function and participation, grounding them in an understanding of homelessness and housing precarity as social and occupational justice issues. Second, we will examine the current state of knowledge regarding how function and participation challenges impact housing outcomes and risk of housing precarity. Finally, we will explore the implications of taking a function and participation approach to homelessness prevention across the four processes of leaving homelessness: Survival, Adaptation, Integration, and Precarity.

Key Concepts of Function and Participation

In this chapter, we draw on foundational knowledge, mostly from the occupational therapy and occupational science literature, of two complementary approaches to daily life activities. First, we are interested in *what* people do in their everyday life, and how patterns of activities are linked to housing (in) stability. This is termed participation, or occupational participation, when we are specifically interested in activities that are deemed culturally and personally meaningful (Egan & Restall, 2022). For instance, in the Adaptation process, individuals to housing may experience a lack of opportunities to meet and connect with other people, and a profound sense of boredom (Marshall et al., 2019b). Over time, these experiences may lead people to feel out of place in their housing and to revert to homelessness to regain a sense of connection and engagement (Marshall et al., 2019c).

Second, we are interested in *how* people do their everyday life activities, or their level of performance in daily tasks such as household management, work, community navigation, leisure, or financial management. This is what we refer to as function, a complex concept located at the intersection of personal abilities, environmental features, and characteristics of the activity or task itself (Baum, Bass, & Christiansen, 2021). For instance, to maintain one's housing over time, financial management is a key expectation, and failure to pay rent and other bills in a timely and effective fashion may contribute to conflicts with landlords and eviction. Participation and function are closely interrelated, and, together, can act as protective or risk factors for housing loss. Activity and participation needs may differ substantially across stages of leaving homelessness and should be assessed and acted on with the stage-specific priority in mind.

Participation, Housing, and Homelessness

Liam's story illustrates the complex interaction between disability, participation, and risk of homelessness. Many people who experience a sudden decrease in income, are living in poverty or are adapting to a new housing situation after an episode of homelessness, may have limited financial means to engage in desired activities (Cantor et al., 2022; Jacobsen et al., 2024), resulting in diminished participation. Sub-optimal spaces or poor material conditions of daily living can also negatively impact possibilities for participation (Nubani et al., 2022). Stigma and discriminatory processes exclude people labeled as disabled or living with mental illness, cognitive impairment, or substance use, from spaces of occupational participation (Cantor et al., 2022). These processes of exclusion based on disability or health can intersect with stigma associated with other social identifies such as Indigeneity, ethnoracial status, sexuality, and/or gender. Physical and sensory symptoms such as pain, diminished endurance, and sensitivity to loud noises, combined with cognitive and affective symptoms such as reduced attention and irritability, interfered with Liam's engagement in activities that were previously meaningful for him, such as working, clubbing, and dancing. This complex interplay of personal and environmental factors either fosters or limits occupational participation (Egan & Restall, 2022). In previous studies among people transitioning from homelessness to housing, cognitive and mobility limitations and mental health challenges have been identified as important correlates of community participation (Chang et al., 2015; Czechowski et al., 2022).

Liam's difficulty to engage in valued activities resulted in decreased participation, which is known to negatively affect one's health and well-being (Bejerholm & Eklund, 2007; Egan & Restall, 2022). Lack of engagement and occupational opportunities may also lead to a sense of boredom, which has been shown to drive substance use (Marshall et al., 2019a) and may contribute to relational conflicts. Challenges with participation can occur and should be considered at each of the Framework's level of intervention. At the level of the individual, decreased participation in social activities can erode one's social ties and support network (Roy et al., 2024). At the level of the community, previous studies have linked participation in activities that foster a sense of belonging in one's community to sustaining one's tenancy (Boland, 2018). For individuals transitioning into housing after an episode of homelessness, the shift from communal living in homelessness-specific services to living by oneself in an apartment can also come with a decrease in participation in social activities and a sense of isolation that can jeopardize housing tenure (Boland, Yarwood, & Bannigan, 2023; Jacobsen et al., 2024). Conversely, the ability and opportunity to establish routines or consistent activity patterns after a transition from homelessness to housing is associated with tenancy sustainment (Boland, Yarwood, & Bannigan, 2023). At the level of the population, legal and public safety practices may exclude local homeless populations from engaging in meaningful or survival occupations through regulation of specific spaces (Pizarro et al., 2018).

Function, Housing, and Homelessness

Functional challenges in many domains of daily activities may increase one's vulnerability to adverse housing outcomes. Here, we focus on three specific domains that have been shown to be particularly challenging for individuals at risk of homelessness (Gabrielian et al., 2019): financial management, interpersonal relationships, and self-advocacy. Other domains of daily activities that could be affected and increase risk of homelessness across the four processes of leaving homelessness include household management, community navigation, health and substance use management, and performance in work and education (Gutman & Raphael-Greenfield, 2017; Marshall et al., 2020).

Financial Management

Financial difficulties have been shown to contribute to risk of homelessness (Thornhill IV, Black, & Rosen, 2018; Valdes, Lunsford, & Castelli, 2022). For people with acquired brain injuries, substance use disorders, and/or severe mental illness, previous studies have identified how cognitive difficulties in areas such as short-term memory, attention, and executive functioning can impair the ability to perform financial management tasks essential for housing stability (Adshead, Norman, & Holloway, 2019; Andersen et al., 2014; Engel et al., 2024). These tasks can include planning and managing a budget, navigating banking services, paying rent and bills, filling in forms, making financial choices, and getting finance-related help (Engel et al., 2024). Affective difficulties such as impulse control, emotional regulation, and stress management can also play a role in financial capability, such as the ability to resist the urge to buy unplanned items (Rosen et al., 2009). Lack of accessibility of financial institutions or organizations providing financial help, including online, can also decrease financial capability of individuals with disabilities (Omerov et al., 2020; Wentz et al., 2019). These difficulties are compounded by the inherent challenge of planning and managing a budget while living on a very low income and within a banking and financial system that is increasingly managerial, bureaucratic, and complex to navigate (Engel et al., 2024; Koller et al., 2016). Foregrounding the Framework's key principle of social justice, this analysis needs to consider the broader environmental context of social policies and a rental market that entrench many individuals and households in poverty(Czechowski et al., 2022).

Social Interactions in and around Living Environments

Risk of homelessness increases when interpersonal conflicts with cohabiting family members, roommates, neighbors, or landlords emerge and persist (Backer & Howard, 2007; Czechowski et al., 2022; Gabrielian et al., 2016). Conversely, positive social interactions contribute to housing tenure and can strengthen one's support system (Boland, Yarwood, & Bannigan, 2023). A functional analysis of interpersonal conflicts and social interactions requires one to examine personal factors, environmental dimensions, and activity components. Persons living with various disabilities may display challenges with social skills, such as the ability to communicate emotions and thoughts effectively, understand others' expectations, make requests, negotiate in interpersonal relationships, problem-solve interpersonal conflicts, and assert oneself (Gabrielian et al., 2019). Psychological factors such as anxiety, stress, or low self-efficacy can lead individuals to avoid social interactions that are important to secure and maintain their tenure, such as reporting a need for repair or other issues with their housing (Gabrielian et al., 2024). Various attributes of the social environment in which interpersonal interactions take place can negatively affect function. Those attributes include discriminatory attitudes, statements or actions toward individuals living with mental illness or substance use issues, or with a history of homelessness, as well as safety threats and violence (Czechowski et al., 2022).

Self-advocacy and Upholding One's Rights as Tenant and Citizen

People living in poverty or integrating into housing after an episode of homelessness may be eligible for but not receiving various social benefits (Marshall et al., 2023). The complexity and technology requirements of access to benefits may act as a barrier to seeking and receiving them, particularly for individuals living with psychiatric or cognitive disabilities (Engel et al., 2024). Personal factors such as low educational level and low literacy, lack of familiarity with administrative processes, limited tolerance for wait times and frustration, among others, may prevent persons at risk of homelessness from seeking and receiving benefits that might improve their financial situations and protect them from housing loss. The same functional analysis may apply to other rights, such as knowledge of and self-advocacy regarding rights as tenant, for instance when one is threatened with eviction. In those cases, the burden is often placed on the individual, and failure to uphold one's rights may be blamed on the individual. The Framework ensures that the needs of the individuals are considered, while putting the onus on the necessary population and community factors that need to be in place to support recovery and social justice.

Implications for Homelessness Prevention

The previous sections have reiterated the relevance of applying a transactional view of participation and function as affected by personal factors, environmental features, and characteristics of the activity itself. In this final section, we argue that a participation and function lens can well be integrated into a broader view of homelessness prevention as defined in the Bridging the Transition Framework. Here, we provide examples of evidence-informed strategies for preventing homelessness at the individual, community, and population levels, while acknowledging that these strategies can be creatively applied to the four processes of survival, adaptation, integration, and precarity.

Population-Level Homelessness Prevention Strategies

This level of prevention includes strategies meant to support persons experiencing homelessness regionally, nationally, or internationally, particularly through evidence-informed public and social policy development in areas such as poverty reduction, public health, income support, or affordable housing supply. One key example of integrating a function and participation approach to structural prevention would be situating homelessness as a disability rights violation (Marshall et al., 2019b) and integrating this vision into housing and homelessness policy (Sperrin, 2023). One approach to enacting the social justice, recovery, and intersectionality principles of the Framework includes efforts to improve the social and physical accessibility of housing, financial, social, and health services needed by persons experiencing or at risk of homelessness.

Community-Level Homelessness Prevention Strategies

This level of prevention focuses on how health and social care practitioners, researchers, and policymakers work with communities to address the needs of persons experiencing homelessness. Within this broader group of interventions, systems prevention (Oudshoorn et al., 2020) targets efforts at improving transitions from and between institutions to avoid discharges into homelessness. This domain of homelessness prevention appears to be particularly amenable to implementation of a function and participation approach. Occupational therapists in settings such as inpatient psychiatric, neurological, geriatric, or substance use units already contribute to orient decisions regarding discharge planning through functional assessments and intervention plans. A more widespread use of this approach could be implemented in settings where occupational therapists are less present, such as correctional or youth protection facilities. Cross-sector work between health and social care institutions and the housing and community sector is also warranted to better expand a function and participation approach (Vitopoulos et al., 2018).

A vital step to better prevent homelessness at the level of communities includes the implementation of processes to systematically screen for risk of homelessness with health, rehabilitation, correctional, or youth protection institutions to improve transitions. As highlighted in Liam's story, risk of homelessness might not be readily identified when individuals are discharged from these institutions (Doran et al., 2022).

Individual-Level Homelessness Prevention Strategies

Several approaches have already been developed to support individuals across the four processes of leaving homelessness. A function and participation approach can be integrated into existing models of care delivery for people leaving or at risk of homelessness, such as Housing First, Assertive Community Treatment, or Intensive Case Management (Woellenstein et al., 2023). These models of care may or may not foreground function and participation, and as such have been criticized for their lack of effect on community integration outcomes (Marshall et al., 2020). Some studies have evaluated the implementation of occupational therapy interventions within HF, ACT, or ICM models. Those interventions generally focus on functional challenges in areas such as financial management, interpersonal relationships, and household management, with promising results (Chapleau et al., 2012; Gutman & Raphael-Greenfield, 2017; Helfrich & Fogg, 2007). Interventions foregrounding participation during housing stabilization after episodes of homelessness have been identified as relevant for homelessness prevention (Marshall et al., 2023), although implementation and evaluation studies remain scarce.

At the stage of precarity, eviction prevention has been recognized as a promising but least developed approach to homelessness prevention (Oudshoorn et al., 2020). Landlords may be particularly receptive to mitigation interventions when a tenant's situation is explained through the lens of functional challenges. One promising approach to developing a participation and function lens into eviction prevention could be the integration of occupational therapy expertise in social housing or primary health and social care where tenants at risk of eviction are likely to seek services.

Finally, in line with the notion of Relationships as Foundation in the Framework, empowerment has been identified as a cross-cutting theme in homelessness prevention, and relies on the notion that agency, choice, and control should be foregrounded in housing research and services (Oudshoorn et al., 2020). This appears to be a powerful point of convergence between homelessness prevention and occupational participation. The very notion of occupational participation entails that engagement in activity should not be imposed or prescribed, but rather personally and culturally meaningful. Future homelessness prevention research and practice could foreground empowerment and occupational participation by ensuring that people with lived and living experiences of homelessness and housing precarity are supported as peer researchers and workers.

Conclusion

Preventing homelessness is a complex endeavor that calls for involvement and accountability of all sectors of society. Traditionally, the homelessness and disability sectors have operated in silos. This chapter has outlined how the function and participation approach typical of practice, service, and research in the disability sector can play a crucial role in homelessness prevention. Understanding homelessness as a disability rights issue can create momentum for increased communication and collaboration across sectors to improve housing outcomes, health, and well-being for people at risk of or experiencing homelessness.

References

Adshead, C. D., Norman, A., & Holloway, M. (2019). The inter-relationship between acquired brain injury, substance use and homelessness; the impact of adverse childhood experiences: An interpretative phenomenological analysis study. *Disability and Rehabilitation*, *43*(17), 2411–2423. https://doi.org/10.1080/09638288.2019.1700565

Anastas, T. M., Stewart, J. C., Rand, K. L., & Hirsh, A. T. (2023). Pain in people experiencing homelessness: A scoping review. *Annals of Behavioral Medicine*, *57*(4), 288–300. https://doi.org/10.1093/abm/kaac060

Andersen, J., Kot, N., Ennis, N., Colantonio, A., Ouchterlony, D., Cusimano, M. D., & Topolovec-Vranic, J. (2014). Traumatic brain injury and cognitive impairment in men who are homeless. *Disability and Rehabilitation*, *36*(26), 2210–2215. https://doi.org/10.3109/09638288.2014.895870

Backer, T. E., & Howard, E. A. (2007). Cognitive impairments and the prevention of homelessness: Research and practice review. *The Journal of Primary Prevention*, *28*(3–4), 375–388.

Baum, C. M., Bass, J. D., & Christiansen, C. H. (2021). The person-environment-occupation-performance model. In *Foundations for Practice in Occupational Therapy*, edited by E. A. S. Duncan (sixth edition). Elsevier.

Bejerholm, U., & Eklund, M. (2007). Occupational engagement in persons with schizophrenia: Relationships to self-related variables, psychopathology, and quality of life. *The American Journal of Occupational Therapy*, *61*, 21–32. https://doi.org/10.5014/ajot.61.1.21

Boland, L. (2018). *Transitioning from Homelessness into a Sustained Tenancy: What Enables Successful Tenancy Sustainment? (The Moving on Project)*. University of Plymouth.

Boland, L., Yarwood, R., & Bannigan, K. (2023). 'Making a home': An occupational perspective on sustaining tenancies following homelessness. *Housing Studies*, *38*(7), 1239–1259. https://doi.org/10.1080/02673037.2021.1935757

Calvo, F., Watts, B., Panadero, S., Giralt, C., Rived-Ocaña, M., & Carbonell, X. (2021). The prevalence and nature of violence against women experiencing homelessness: A quantitative study. *Violence against Women*, *28*(6–7), 1464–1482. https://doi.org/10.1177/10778012211022780

Cantor, P., Polakowska, M., Proietti, A., Tran, V., Lebire, J., & Roy, L. (2022). Leisure possibilities of adults experiencing poverty: A community-based participatory study. *Canadian Journal of Occupational Therapy*, *89*(2), 103–114. https://doi.org/10.1177/00084174211073266

Chang, F.-H., Helfrich, C. A., Coster, W. J., & Rogers, E. S. (2015). Factors associated with community participation among individuals who have experienced homelessness. *International Journal of Environmental Research and Public Health*, *12*(9), 11364–11378.

Chapleau, A., Seroczynski, A. D., Meyers, S., Lamb, K., & Buchino, S. (2012). The effectiveness of a consultation model in community mental health. *Occupational Therapy in Mental Health*, *28*(4), 379–395. https://doi.org/10.1080/0164212X.2012.708609

Czechowski, K., Sylvestre, J., Gogosis, E., Agha, A., Kerman, N., Polillo, A., Palepu, A., & Hwang, S. W. (2022). Cycles of instability: Proximal and distal influences on residential instability among people with histories of homelessness in three Canadian cities. *Journal of Community Psychology*, *50*(8), 3402–3420. https://doi.org/10.1002/jcop.22843

Doran, K. M., Johns, E., Zuiderveen, S., Shinn, M., Dinan, K., Schretzman, M., Gelberg, L., Culhane, D., Shelley, D., & Mijanovich, T. (2022). Development of a homelessness risk screening tool for emergency department patients. *Health Services Research*, *57*(2), 285–293. https://doi.org/10.1111/1475-6773.13886

Egan, M., & Restall, G. (2022). *Promoting Occupational Participation: Collaborative Relationship-Focused Occupational Therapy*. Canadian Association of Occupational Therapists.

Engel, L., Arowolo, I., Ewesesan, R., Khan, M. N., Ripat, J., Bottari, C., Hunt, A., Poncet, F., & Karpa, J. (2024). Contextual factors of financial capability and financial well-being for adults living with brain injury: A qualitative photovoice study. *Brain Injury*, *38*(4), 273–281. https://doi.org/10.1080/02699052.2024.2310210

Gabrielian, S., Burns, A. V., Nanda, N., Hellemann, G., Kane, V., & Young, A. S. (2016). Factors associated with premature exits from supported housing. *Psychiatric Services*, *67*(1), 86–93. https://doi.org/10.1176/appi.ps.201400311

Gabrielian, S., Hamilton, A. B., Gelberg, L., Koosis, E. R., Hoffmann, L., Carlson, D. M., & Young, A. S. (2024). Testing an implementation package in a housing skills training pilot for homeless-experienced persons with serious mental illness. *Implementation Research and Practice*, *5*. https://doi.org/10.1177/26334895241236679

Gabrielian, S., Hamilton, A. B., Gelberg, L., Koosis, E. R., Johnson, A., & Young, A. S. (2019). Identifying social skills that support housing attainment and retention among homeless persons with serious mental illness. *Psychiatric Services*, *70*(5), 374–380. https://doi.org/10.1176/appi.ps.201800508

Guillén, A. I., Panadero, S., & Vázquez, J. J. (2021). Disability, health, and quality of life among homeless women: A follow-up study. *American Journal of Orthopsychiatry*, *91*(4), 569–577. https://doi.org/10.1037/ort0000559

Gutman, S. A., & Raphael-Greenfield, E. I. (2017). Effectiveness of a supportive housing program for homeless adults with mental illness and substance use: A two-group controlled trial. *British Journal of Occupational Therapy*, *80*(5), 286–293. https://doi.org/10.1177/0308022616680368

Gutwinski, S., Schreiter, S., Deutscher, K., & Fazel, S. (2021). The prevalence of mental disorders among homeless people in high-income countries: An updated systematic review and meta-regression analysis. *PLOS Medicine*, *18*(8), e1003750.

Helfrich, C. A., & Fogg, L. F. (2007). Outcomes of a life skills intervention for homeless adults with mental illness. *Journal of Primary Prevention*, *28*(3–4), 313–326. http://ovidsp.ovid.com/ovidweb.cgi?T=JS&CSC=Y&NEWS=N&PAGE=fulltext&D=med5&AN=17541828http://mcgill.on.worldcat.org/atoztitles/link?sid=OVID:medline&id=pmid:17541828&id=doi:&issn=0278-095X&isbn=&volume=28&issue=3&spage=313&pages=313-26&date=2007&title=Journa+l+of+Primary+Prevention&atitle=Outcomes+of+a+life+skills+intervention+for+homeless+adults+with+menta+l+illness.&aulast=Helfrich

Jacobsen, K., Roy, L., Seto, V., Marshall, C. A., & Perreault, M. (2024). "I Always Have my Key in my Hand": A photovoice exploration with women in post-shelter transition. *International Journal on Homelessness*, *4*(2), 256–280.

Koller, K., Woods, L., Engel, L., Bottari, C., Dawson, D. R., & Nalder, E. (2016). Loss of financial management independence after brain injury: Survivors' experiences. *American Journal of Occupational Therapy*, *70*(3), 1–8. https://doi.org/10.5014/ajot.2016.020198

Marshall, C., Gewurtz, R., Barbic, S., Roy, L., Cooke, A., & Lysaght, R. (2023). *Bridging the Transition to Housing: A Social Justice Framework to Guide the Practice of Occupational Therapists and other Professionals Who Support Individuals with Experiences of Homelessness* (2nd Edition). Accessed at https://www.sjmhlab.com/publications

Marshall, C. A., Boland, L., Westover, L. A., Isard, R., & Gutman, S. A. (2020). A systematic review of occupational therapy interventions in the transition from homelessness. *Scandinavian Journal of Occupational Therapy*, *28*(3), 171–187. https://doi.org/10.1080/11038128.2020.1764094

Marshall, C. A., Boland, L., Westover, L. A., Wickett, S., Roy, L., Mace, J., Gewurtz, R., Barbic, S., & Kirsh, B. (2019a). Occupational experiences of homelessness: A systematic review and meta-aggregation. *Scandinavian Journal of Occupational Therapy*, *27*(6), 394–407. https://doi.org/10.1080/11038128.2019.1689292

Marshall, C. A., Davidson, L., Li, A., Gewurtz, R., Roy, L., Barbic, S., Kirsh, B., & Lysaght, R. (2019b). Boredom and meaningful activity in adults experiencing homelessness: A mixed-methods study. *Canadian Journal of Occupational Therapy*, *86*(5), 357–370. https://doi.org/10.1177/0008417419833402

Marshall, C. A., Roy, L., Becker, A., Nguyen, M., Barbic, S., Tjörnstrand, C., Gewurtz, R., & Wickett, S. (2019c). Boredom and homelessness: A scoping review. *Journal of Occupational Science*, 1–18. https://doi.org/10.1080/14427591.2019.1595095

Nubani, L., De Biasi, A., Ruemenapp, M. A., Tams, L. D., & Boyle, R. (2022). The impact of living in an un- or under-furnished house on individuals who transitioned from homelessness. *Journal of Community Psychology*, *50*(8), 3681–3699. https://doi.org/10.1002/jcop.22865

Omerov, P., Craftman, Å. G., Mattsson, E., & Klarare, A. (2020). Homeless persons' experiences of health- and social care: A systematic integrative review. *Health & Social Care in the Community*, *28*(1), 1–11. https://doi.org/10.1111/hsc.12857

Oudshoorn, A., Dej, E., Parsons, C., & Gaetz, S. (2020). Evolving an evidence-based model for homelessness prevention. *Health & Social Care in the Community*, *28*(5), 1754–1763. https://doi.org/10.1111/hsc.13000

Pizarro, E., Silvana, E., Fernanda, F., Francisca, H., Claudia, P., & Whiteford, G. (2018). Understanding occupational justice from the concept of territory: A proposal for occupational science. *Journal of Occupational Science*, *25*(4), 463–473. https://doi.org/10.1080/14427591.2018.1487261

Rosen, M. I., Carroll, K. M., Stefanovics, E., & Rosenheck, R. A. (2009). A randomized controlled trial of a money management-based substance use intervention. *Psychiatric Services*, *60*(4), 498–504. https://doi.org/10.1176/ps.2009.60.4.498

Roy, L., Leclair, M., Crocker, A. G., Abdel-Baki, A., de Benedictis, L., Bérubé, F.-A., Thibeault, E., Latimer, E., & Roy, M.-A. (2024). Risk factors for homelessness and housing instability in the first episode of mental illness: Initial findings from the AMONT study. *Early Intervention in Psychiatry*, *18*(7), 561–570. https://doi.org/10.1111/eip.13495

Samuels, G. E. M., Curry, S. R., & Cerven, C. (2021). Theorizing a social ecology of displacement: Structural-, relational-, and individual-level conditions of homelessness among young people. *Social Service Review*, *95*(4), 561–615. https://doi.org/10.1086/717434

Sperrin, Á. (2023). A disability rights approach to a constitutional right to housing. *The International Journal of Disability and Social Justice*, *3*(1), 80–95. https://www.jstor.org/stable/48724368

Stubbs, J. L., Thornton, A. E., Sevick, J. M., Silverberg, N. D., Barr, A. M., Honer, W. G., & Panenka, W. J. (2020). Traumatic brain injury in homeless and marginally housed individuals: A systematic review and meta-analysis. *The Lancet Public Health*, *5*(1), e19–e32. https://doi.org/10.1016/S2468-2667(19)30188-4

Thornhill IV, T. A., Black, A. C., & Rosen, M. I. (2018). Financial capability: Clinicians' assessment of beneficiaries with dual diagnoses. *Journal of Dual Diagnosis*, *14*(2), 130–136. https://doi.org/10.1080/15504263.2018.1436732

Valdes, K., Lunsford, D., & Castelli, J. (2022). Financial acumen improves after financial literacy training in individuals with substance use disorder. *OTJR: Occupational Therapy Journal of Research*, *43*(2), 296–302. https://doi.org/10.1177/15394492221101846

Vitopoulos, N. A., Frederick, T. J., Leon, S., Daley, M., McDonald, C., Morales, S., Cerswell Kielburger, L., Cohen, S., Eacott, K., Howes, C., Gutierrez, R., McGavin, K., Peters, K., Vanderheul, J., McKenzie, K., & Kidd, S. A. (2018). Development of a complex tertiary prevention intervention for the transition out of youth homelessness. *Children and Youth Services Review*, *94*, 579–588. https://doi.org/10.1016/j.childyouth.2018.08.038

Wentz, B., Pham, D., Feaser, E., Smith, D., Smith, J., & Wilson, A. (2019). Documenting the accessibility of 100 US bank and finance websites. *Universal Access in the Information Society*, *18*(4), 871–880. https://doi.org/10.1007/s10209-018-0616-6

Woellenstein, L., Cuthill, F., Manrai, R., & Henderson, D. (2023). Homelessness prevention interventions for single adults at risk of or experiencing MEH: A systematic review on their effectiveness. *International Journal on Homelessness*, *3*(2), 1–67.

3

SOCIAL INCLUSION AND ITS RELEVANCE TO HOMELESSNESS PREVENTION AND TRANSITIONING OUT OF HOMELESSNESS

Erin Dej, Charlotte Smith, Holly Petersen, Chiue Bute, Kaitlin Schwan and Jayne Malenfant

The Canadian homelessness sector has begun to embrace prevention, shifting efforts towards stopping homelessness before it begins. While there is significant emphasis on housing, social inclusion is integral to maintaining housing stability and a key aspect of process of leaving homelessness. Research demonstrates that for youth, a sense of belonging enhances their health, stability, and well-being. Social inclusion is a critical pillar of homelessness prevention, where a connection to neighbourhoods, broader communities, and people is essential to ensuring housing stability and preventing homelessness (re)occurrence. In this chapter, we use findings from a study of young women and gender-diverse youths' transitions from homelessness to housing as an example of the prevention process. Through this multi-phase, participatory action research project, we add to the existing evidence-base on the efficacy of prevention efforts by identifying key systemic, early intervention, and housing stabilization prevention strategies that illustrate the centrality of social inclusion within homelessness prevention.

How this Chapter Guides Practice and Research in Homelessness Prevention

This chapter uses the framework for homelessness prevention (Gaetz & Dej, 2017; Gaetz et al., 2018) to identify how social inclusion underscores each of the elements of the typology. By highlighting the need for social integration as key to preventing homelessness, especially for people who have previously experienced homelessness, this chapter demonstrates the complementary

DOI: 10.4324/9781003541332-4

nature between the homelessness prevention framework and the Bridging the Transition framework, as outlined in Chapter 1. The process of leaving homelessness is not linear, and as such, a range of prevention strategies are necessary that focus on people's well-being and sense of belonging. Using key findings from a study with young women and gender-diverse youth transitioning from homelessness to housing as an example, this chapter explores the issues of safety, housing, the unique needs of newcomers, young parents, and accessing formal and informal support acts as key issues to consider when people are navigating the process of leaving homelessness. The chapter offers guidance on how to apply three types of prevention strategies to each of these themes: systemic prevention, early intervention prevention, and housing stability. Using the voices of young women and gender-diverse youth with lived experience of homelessness as our anchor, readers will have a strong understanding of why social inclusion should be central to all efforts to prevent homelessness and to support those transitioning out of homeless.

Introduction

In the past decade, the homelessness sector has begun shifting from an emergency response to adopting principles and practices to stop homelessness before it starts. In 2017, Gaetz and Dej added to the emerging scholarship on homelessness prevention (Browne Gott, Mackie, & England, 2021; Mackie, Thomas, & Bibbings, 2017) by creating a framework that defines homelessness prevention as:

> Policies, practices, and interventions that reduce the likelihood that someone will experience homelessness. It also means providing those who have been homeless with the necessary resources and supports to stabilize their housing, enhance integration and social inclusion, and ultimately reduce the risk of the recurrence of homelessness.
>
> *(Gaetz & Dej, 2017, p. 35)*

This chapter focuses on tertiary prevention, which is concerned with preventing the recurrence of homelessness through housing stability supports, enhanced integration, and creating social inclusion (Gaetz & Dej, 2017). The framework identifies five kinds of homelessness prevention, three of which we unpack here: structural prevention through legislation, policies, and investments; early intervention that provides rapid supports to people who are at imminent risk or who have just become homeless; and housing stability to support people to maintain housing. The Bridging the Transition framework complements the homelessness prevention framework, especially as it relates to tertiary prevention. The former outlines the process to achieve housing stabilization through individual, community, and population-level strategies (Marshall, 2025). Specifically, the Bridging the Transition framework highlights how more than housing alone, efforts to achieve well-being are headmost in securing and maintaining permanent housing.

Homelessness prevention looks different for young people, defined as people between the ages of 13–24 experiencing homelessness independent of their family, whose causes and experiences of homelessness are unique from the adult population (Gaetz et al., 2018), and for young women and gender-diverse youth specifically (Schwan et al., 2021). Schwan et al. (2018) outline factors that youth identified to prevent their homelessness, such as upstream responses, mechanisms for youth to signal abuse or precarity, and eliminating stigma in social systems. Youth homelessness prevention requires a holistic approach to meet young people's cognitive, emotional, and physical needs (MacDonald et al., 2023). Once housed, many youth become mired in the precarity process outlined in the Bridging the Transition Framework, as they continue to face extreme precarity in terms of poverty, mental health and substance use challenges (Kidd et al., 2016), and an ongoing "fog of exclusion" (Thulien et al., 2023, p. 900). As identified in the Bridging the Transition Framework, a strong support network and sense of connection increases newly housed youths' resilience, self-esteem, and ability to access and benefit from services (Oliver & Cheff, 2012). Well-being supports ensure that people move from survival and precarity to the integration process, where connections with community and a strong self-identity allow people to weather the ups and downs of life (Marshall, 2025).

While housing is key to preventing homelessness, we cannot ignore the importance of fostering social inclusion through community building. Young people at risk of or experiencing homelessness often face high levels of social exclusion, including challenges staying in school; feeling unwelcome at community activities; or feeling unsafe, stigmatized, or discriminated against, including by adults in authority and peers (Gaetz et al., 2018; Oliver & Cheff, 2012). In this chapter, we contend that social inclusion is integral to homelessness prevention efforts, especially for young women and gender-diverse youth. The Bridging the Transition Framework provides a range of strategies to increase social integration, especially around actively participating in activities that are meaningful.

Understanding Belonging and Social Inclusion as Homelessness Prevention

Youth homelessness is often caused by family breakdown, experiences of abuse, involvement with child protection services, as well as certain groups being at higher risk of homelessness, such as 2SLGBTQIA+ youth and Indigenous youth, due to ongoing experiences of colonialism, racism, and a lack of culturally appropriate services and research (Ansloos, Wager, & Dunn, 2022; Gaetz et al., 2016). Youth homelessness practice and research often focuses on young people ages 13–24; this is a key developmental age where social belonging is vital to health and well-being (Nichols et al., 2017). A lack of social inclusion in this age group can lead to poor physical and mental health outcomes, unstable housing, low educational and employment outcomes, and victimization during this critical developmental period (Calsyn & Winter, 2002; DiGuiseppi et al., 2021).

Young women and gender-diverse youth feel this sense of disconnection distinctly, as they are more likely to experience homelessness at a younger age than cis men, encounter more violence, and navigate greater mental health challenges (Gaetz et al., 2016; Kidd et al., 2021; Nelson, Malenfant, & Schwan, 2023; Schwan et al., 2021). Housing-insecure young women and gender-diverse youth commonly experience challenges with safety, parenting, and violence/exploitation, negatively impacting their social inclusion, and ultimately their housing stability (Nichols et al., 2017; Perron, Cleverley, & Kidd, 2014).

We add to the existing research on social inclusion by focusing on young women and gender-diverse youths' transitions from homelessness to housing. We are a team of academic and lived-expert researchers who came together to carry out this participatory action research. Data collection included four phases: 22 semi-structured interviews about loneliness during the transition to housing with young women and gender-diverse from across Ontario, with an average age of 21; 20 of those participants participated in a week-long journaling exercise, followed by a second interview; interviews with 12 formal and informal support people; and 8 peer-designed and led member-checking virtual workshops, where 58 participants (17 unique youth) discussed loneliness, housing, safety, substance use, parenting, newcomer experiences, the impact of COVID-19, and solutions-building. The research received ethical approval from Wilfrid Laurier University, and all participants received cash honorariums, food gift cards, and a 'care bundle,' containing items such as a journal, colourful pens, stickers, a bookmark, and soap leaves, to thank them for their time and knowledge.

In this chapter, we situate the research findings within the youth homelessness prevention and Bridging the Transition frameworks. We identified five themes that impacted young women and gender-diverse youth's transition to housing, each of which has interventions for social inclusion at their core. For each theme, we explore how systemic, early intervention, and housing stabilization prevention strategies can improve social inclusion, well-being, and housing trajectory. By doing so, we elucidate how to apply the Bridging the Transition framework in action, making the case for meaningfully integrating social inclusion into prevention efforts.

Safety

A sense of safety is central to people's feelings of well-being and stability in their homes, with young women and gender-diverse youth's sense of safety intimately tied to a home free of violence and a place of privacy (Mayock, Bretherton, & Baptista, 2016; Schwan et al., 2020). Youth who had recently transitioned into housing described a multitude of ways they felt unsafe in their new homes, compromising their housing and ability to connect with others. They described dangers in their neighbourhood, building, and in their unit. To protect themselves, some participants carried safety tools like mace or weapons, risking criminalization. Others used buddy systems by checking in with friends or leaving home in pairs, though this was not an option for youth with limited social networks, leading to isolation. Below, we outline issues and solutions for incorporating social inclusion into various forms of homelessness prevention when people are transitioning into housing.

Systemic Prevention

Being newly housed does not eliminate risks or feelings of unsafety, identified in the Bridging the Transition framework as the precarity process. Addressing gender-based violence will improve young women and gender-diverse youths' safety and in turn, their ability to participate in activities and build their social network (Schwan et al., 2020).

> I wouldn't recommend just walking around like going for a jog if you're like a girl.
>
> —*Darika, interview participant*

Early Intervention Prevention

Many spaces geared towards people who are homeless are designed for men or are co-ed, where many young women and gender-diverse youth feel unsafe (Schwan et al., 2020). Given how central similarly situated peers are for young women and gender-diverse youth to maintain safety, feel understood, and create friendships (Oliver & Cheff, 2012), having a dedicated space to connect can create valuable bonds for mutual aid and provide a sense of belonging once housed.

> Having women and safe spaces, women only and safe spaces to go to are really important right now.
>
> —*Christina, interview participant*

Housing Stability

The youth in this study were housed at the time of the research, yet as highlighted in the Bridging the Transition framework, many people in the precarity process continue to feel unsafe. Many participants in this study described their housing unit as unsafe, often because of cis male neighbours. Given that at least 75% of women and gender-diverse people experiencing homelessness in Canada report being survivors of abuse (Schwan et al., 2021), ensuring they feel safe in their housing is paramount for long-term stability. Participants from our study who felt unsafe reported that they often isolated themselves and were reluctant to leave their unit.

> It's just like this young lady downstairs, unable to move how she wants to or live how she wants to because there's guys counter-stepping her movement and making her feel uncomfortable. It's sad because she wouldn't even go out from the front door because she's on the first floor... Like, she would crawl out her window to go take her dog for a walk or go to the store.
>
> —*Aaliyah, interview participant*

Housing

The adaptation and integration processes in the Bridging the Transition framework situate meaningful participation in daily life as contingent on housing (Marshall, 2025); however, housing after exiting homelessness is rarely stable or adequate (Kidd et al., 2016), with young women and gender-diverse youth in this study describing units in disrepair, with mould or infestations, unsafe living conditions, or impermanent housing arrangements. Most participants were staying with friends or family without clear terms, in short-term sublets, or in transitional housing with time and age-out limits. These conditions left many participants in an ongoing state of transience as explored through the precarity process (Marshall, 2025), unable to set down roots and build community.

Systemic Prevention

There are limited housing options available for young people that are permanent, safe, and truly affordable (Dada et al., 2022). While there are calls for all orders of government to properly invest in social and deeply affordable housing, special attention needs to be paid to housing that responds to the unique needs of youth and women and gender-diverse people (Schwan et al., 2020). Young people need access and choice in their housing, and be able to secure housing quickly, without having to be mired in homelessness to be eligible (Gaetz et al., 2018).

> Housing is only for people in shelters. If you are there, they try their best to get you housing. If you aren't and you are struggling somewhere, they do not help you. I think they should have another way for people to receive housing other than a shelter.
>
> —*Workshop participant*

Early Intervention Prevention

Understanding and being able to assert their tenancy rights, including around eviction processes, is a key prevention strategy for many people, specifically youth, to retain their housing and ensure it is kept in good repair. Youth in this study identified numerous instances where their tenancy rights were violated, especially racialized participants (Canadian Centre for Housing Rights, 2022). Accessible knowledge about tenants' rights and access to free legal support are essential for youth to retain their housing and gain stability.

> I've been to three shelters now. I moved in with a friend for a while, and housing was bad. We found a place, but it was full of roaches. Even in the winter, they didn't turn on the heater … it hasn't been good to be honest.
>
> —*Sade, interview participant*

Housing Stability

True to the Bridging the Transition framework, many young women and gender-diverse youth in our study reported that they require ongoing support regarding participation in daily life and their overall well-being to maintain their housing. Youth who have experienced homelessness are expected to have a high level of independence and responsibility that does not align with their developmental stage, and despite having often missed out on life skills training (Nichols et al., 2017). After-care supports can allow youth to stay stably housed and build roots in their community.

> But even with the subsidies, programs like the youth job connect programs should be more available. There should be like a program that you offer when kids are in school… At least they have their worker's rights, and their tenant's rights. They know how to budget and stuff like that. So they can get a job and everything.
>
> —*Josie, interview participant*

Newcomer Experiences

Newcomers who experience housing precarity face unique challenges with regard to housing in terms of the cost, barriers to navigating bureaucratic systems, unfamiliarity with cultural norms, and distrust in social services (de la Calzada-Calugay & Hanley, 2024; Walsh et al., 2016). They also traverse through the Bridges to Transition framework in particular ways, in terms of finding community and increasing social integration to support them in daily life (Kohlbacher, 2020). The nature and depth of loneliness was felt most strongly among the 45% (n=10) of youth in the study who identified as newcomers to Canada. Many described severe isolation, struggling with detachment from family, language, and culture. They encountered racism and discrimination, affecting their housing access, services, and relationships.

Systemic Prevention

Systemic racism among landlords is pervasive and disproportionately affects racialized women and women with children (Canadian Centre for Housing Rights, 2022). Creating anti-racism policies and providing newcomer youth with the resources to protect themselves from landlords who take advantage of them will contribute to equitable access to housing.

> It is difficult because you have a lot of people helping but when you get there the landlords say they don't take coloured people or these people … they are being racist.
>
> —*Brianna, interview participant*

Early Intervention Prevention

Supports specifically for newcomer youth allow them to connect with education, employment, and other spaces where they can achieve their goals and also connect with other young women and gender-diverse youth. The Bridging the Transition framework identifies community-level interventions to address the needs of people facing housing precarity or transitioning to housing. In the case of newcomers, creating and activating municipalities as sanctuary cities can act as a key community intervention (Bauder, 2017).

> In my situation [as a refugee] I had to wait 7 years before I got a hearing, and in that 7 years there wasn't many services I could access. In that 7 year period I could have achieved more if I had been given access to colleges and universities. They need to implement better rules to help us as refugees, rather than waiting for us to be permanent residents.
>
> —*Workshop participant*

Housing Stability

In our study, newcomer youth were among the most vocal about feeling lonely and looking to build friendships and find community. Many sought connections beyond the shelter system, to others who share a similar culture, religion, and/or background. Creating space in communities to welcome newcomer youth who are living independent of their families will foster social inclusion and well-being.

> So they [other youth in shelter] were bullying me because of how I speak. They say, 'oh you don't know how to speak English perfectly'. 'Look at your accent' and stuff. And, 'you're so ugly.' They said that. 'You don't do things, you are not cool'. And I was … feeling so hopeless that I would go to my room and start crying.
>
> —*Sahini, interview participant*

Parenting

Young women and gender-diverse youth who experience homelessness have a higher rate of pregnancy than their stably housed counterparts (Krahn et al., 2018), requiring unique social integration interventions. As Benbow et al. (2019) note, parents experiencing homelessness face social exclusion in two primary domains—exclusion from feelings of safety and being surveilled and judged. As the authors assert, for mothers, "exclusion from safety was experienced before, after, and during homelessness" (p. 207). This study complements Benbow et al.'s findings, with careful attention to how social exclusion is expressly felt for young people who are parents. Participants in this research described the challenges of securing housing, along with profound feelings of isolation and stigma. While some participants had access to services and family support, others faced parenthood alone, with few spaces where they felt free from judgement. Parenting is often a barrier to social inclusion, but can also act as an opportunity to connect with other young parents in similar circumstances.

Systemic Prevention

As described above, racialized mothers are the group most discriminated against by landlords (Canadian Centre for Housing Rights, 2022). Access to housing that meets the needs of the family composition and is truly affordable is extremely challenging to find. Young parents described needing housing and childcare that fit their budget so they could attend school or work.

> The place is like $1,400 or $1,600 a month, right. And when they see you as a single mother on maternity leave. They're like, 'how are you gonna be paying that?'… So the worker would come and … explain they would be sending the money directly to them not to me, right. So even with all that. I don't know. They just thought that I either couldn't pay my rent.
>
> —*Serena, interview participant*

Early Intervention Prevention

Young parents without strong support systems struggle to participate in education and work, often juggling these with childcare. This limits their ability to build connections, impacting their future opportunities and income. Conversely, young parents who have community (i.e. family, friends, dedicated programmes, connections through their children) can access immediate support to help avoid crisis.

> The schooling community, teachers and staff, it's all helpful. Say if something is being donated to the school, the secretary lets me know 'cause they know my situation. The school wants to help me, the community is caring and helpful.
>
> —*Workshop participant*

Housing Stability

Young people who have been homeless or precariously housed face significant isolation after becoming parents. Many youth drift away from friends who are at different life stages and struggle to find spaces that welcome them and their children. Young parents described wanting strong relationships but limiting who they spend time with to protect their children. Creating judgement-free, safe spaces for young parents to feel a sense of belonging is integral to their and their children's long-term well-being.

> To maintain relationships, you have to be truthful, honest, caring, kind, respectful. I have some friends; I keep my space small cause I don't wanna get hurt or have my kids hurt. The few I have I try to be close with and show love to them.
>
> —*Workshop participant*

Supports

Providing the right kinds of supports at the right time is key to homelessness prevention (de Vet et al., 2017). Echoing guiding principle 6 of the Bridges to Transition framework, these supports are accessed intersectionally, with young women and gender-diverse youth requiring different kinds of supports to meet their needs. The findings from this study show that youth are calling for supports at crucial times in their lives, especially during the adaptation and integration processes, to stabilize their housing and enhance their well-being. A range of holistic supports should be offered at all stages so that young people have support on their healing journey and can also provide lived experts with meaningful work options.

Systemic Prevention

No experience of homelessness is the same, and young women and gender-diverse youth wanted to access different styles of support in diverse ways. Following the shifts that took place during the pandemic, service providers have become adept at connecting with youth at risk of or experiencing homelessness in ways that work for them (Noble et al., 2022). The young people in this study were clear that providing targeted supports during the adaptation and precarity processes is key to prevention; experiencing the trauma of homelessness should not be an eligibility requirement.

> I think there definitely needs to be like some sort of counselling offers like online... It needs to be offered openly 'cause if they are offering it, I haven't heard of it and I think it would help a lot of people. I also think there should be more supports for young people who live on their own and have enough food to get by right now... The only wish I had was to get a little bit easier access to free counselling for like PTSD and all that stuff ... stuff like that should be more widely available.
>
> —*Anna, interview participant*

Early Intervention Prevention

With more capacity and resources, formal and informal support people are keen to foster social inclusion for young women and gender-diverse youth transitioning out of homelessness. As the Bridges to Transition Framework highlights, meaningful and trusting relationships are foundational for effective interventions (Marshall, 2025). Adequately resourcing programmes for housed youth so that there is immediate support available if their housing becomes at risk provides a key sense of strength for young women and gender-diverse youth.

> I'm glad that I'm able to provide that support and that they are able to approach me without me even approaching them. They usually give me a shout and we end up talking and figuring things out. So for me it's a good sign and very humbling to know that they have that type of support with me. 'Cause trust is a huge issue for vulnerable populations. And I know that myself, coming from a vulnerable population too.
>
> —*Anjali, support person*

Housing Stability

Maintaining housing is easier with community. A strong community promotes health, social care, and well-being (Marshall, 2025). For young women and gender-diverse youth who have experienced homelessness and/or housing precarity, being safely and securely housed includes having people, both formal and informal, who can provide support as they navigate independence, integration, and future challenges that risk housing precarity. Our study revealed that mutual aid and service provision are critical for creating social inclusion and providing the tools and resources for young people to stay stably housed.

> I think society needs to wake up, like we are all in this together, we need to help each other. That's not charity. People give and take. It's mutual aid. Which is really awesome. Awesome way to help people. Put it back into their hands, right? I think too, given that, one of the things that does help BIPOC youth and queer youth, is trying to build up their self-esteem. I think it's really paramount in getting them to a place where they are able to find services. And able to get themselves off the street.
>
> —*Blayke, support person*

Conclusion

Homelessness prevention reduces the likelihood that people face homelessness at all, or ever experience it again. While housing is key to homelessness prevention, social inclusion is fundamental to accessing and maintaining housing over time. For young women and gender-diverse youth, barriers like a lack of safety, inaccessible support, stigma, and a lack of community can make their housing further precarious. Social inclusion is crucial to preventing homelessness, where finding community can support lasting stability and well-being.

References

Ansloos, J.P., Wager, A.C. and Dunn, N.S. (2022). Preventing Indigenous youth homelessness in Canada: A qualitative study on structural challenges and upstream prevention in education. *Journal of Community Psychology*, 50(4), pp.1918–1934.

Bauder, H., (2017). Sanctuary cities: Policies and practices in international perspective. *International Migration*, 55(2), pp.174–187.

Benbow, S., Forchuk, C., Berman, H., Gorlick, C. and Ward-Griffin, C. (2019). Spaces of exclusion: Safety, stigma, and surveillance of mothers experiencing homelessness. *Canadian Journal of Nursing Research*, 51(3), pp.202–213.

Browne Gott, H., Mackie, P.K. and England, E. (2021). Housing rights, homelessness prevention and a paradox of bureaucracy? *Housing Studies*, 38(2), pp.250–268.

Calsyn, R.J. and Winter, J.P. (2002). Social support, psychiatric symptoms, and housing: A causal analysis. *Journal of Community Psychology*, 30(3), pp.247–259.

Canadian Centre for Housing Rights (2022). "*Sorry, It's Rented*": Measuring discrimination against newcomers in Toronto's rental housing market. *Canadian Centre for Housing Rights*. Available at: https://housingrightscanada.com/wp-content/uploads/2022/11/CCHR-Sorry-its-rented-Discrimination-Audit-2022.pdf [Accessed 2 May 2025].

Dada, O., de Pass, T., John, J.R., Lund, J. and Kidd, S. (2022). Identification of housing stabilization models for youth exiting homelessness: A grey literature review. *International Journal on Homelessness*, 2(2), pp.251–274.

de la Calzada-Calugay, R. and Hanley, J. (2024). Homelessness and housing insecurity among im/migrants in Canada: A scoping review. *Canadian Journal of Urban Research*, 33(1), pp.43–59.

De Vet, R., Beijersbergen, M. D., Jonker, I. E., Lako, D. A. M., van Hemert, A. M., Herman, D. B., & Wolf, J. R. L. M. (2017). Critical time intervention for homeless people making the transition to community living: A randomized controlled trial. *American Journal of Community Psychology*, *60*(1–2), 175–186. https://doi.org/10.1002/ajcp.12150

DiGuiseppi, G., Clomax, A., Rampton Dodge, J. and Rice, E. (2021). Social network correlates of education and employment service use among youth experiencing homelessness: A longitudinal study. *Child and Youth Services Review*, 106212.

Gaetz, S. and Dej, E. (2017). *A New Direction: A Framework for Homelessness Prevention*. Canadian Observatory on Homelessness Press.

Gaetz, S., O'Grady, B., Kidd, S.A. and Schwan, K. (2016). *Without a Home: The National Youth Homelessness Survey*. Canadian Observatory on Homelessness Press.

Gaetz, S., Schwan, K., Redman, M., French, D. and Dej, E. (2018). *The Roadmap for the Prevention of Youth Homelessness*. Canadian Observatory on Homelessness Press.

Kidd, S.A., Frederick, T., Karabanow, J., Hughes, J., Naylor, T. and Barbic, S. (2016). A mixed methods study of recently homeless youth efforts to sustain housing and stability. *Child and Adolescent Social Work Journal*, 33(3), pp.207–218.

Kidd, S.A., Gaetz, S., O'Grady, B., Schwan, K., Zhao, H., Lopes, K. and Wang, W. (2021). The second national Canadian homeless youth survey: Mental health and addiction findings. *The Canadian Journal of Psychiatry*, 66(10), pp.897–905.

Kohlbacher, J. (2020). Frustrating beginnings: How social ties compensate housing integration barriers for Afghan refugees in Vienna. *Urban Planning*, 5(3), pp.127–137.

Krahn, J., Caine, V., Chaw-Kant, J. and Singh, A.E. (2018). Housing interventions for homeless, pregnant/parenting women with addictions: A systematic review. *Journal of Social Distress and Homelessness*, 27(1), pp.75–88.

MacDonald, C., Sohn, J., Bonakdar, A. and Traher, C. (2023). A roof over your head is not a home: Youth homelessness in Canada. In *The Routledge International Handbook of Child and Adolescent Grief in Contemporary Contexts*, edited by C. Traher and L.J. Breen, Routledge, pp.180–191.

Mackie, P.K., Thomas, I. and Bibbings, J. (2017). Homelessness prevention: Reflecting on a year of pioneering Welsh legislation in practice. *European Journal of Homelessness*, 11(1), pp.81–107.

Marshall, C.A. (2025). Introduction to the origins and components of the bridging the transition framework. In *Bridging the Transition to Housing: A Homelessness Prevention Framework*, edited by C.A. Marshall, R. Gewurtz and S. Barbic, Routledge, pp.3–14.

Mayock, P., Bretherton, J. and Baptista, J. (2016). Women's homelessness and domestic violence: (In)visible interactions. In *Women's Homelessness in Europe*, edited by P. Mayock and J. Bretherton, Palgrave Macmillan, pp.127–154.

Nelson, A., Malenfant, J. and Schwan, K. (2023). *Housing Need & Homelessness amongst Gender-Diverse People in Canada*. Office of the Federal Housing Advocate, Canadian Human Rights Commission. Available at: https://womenshomelessness.ca/wp-content/uploads/Research-Brief-on-Housing-Need-Homelessness-amongst-Gender-Diverse-Persons.pdf [Accessed 2 May 2025].

Nichols, N., Schwan, K., Gaetz, S., Redman, M., French, D., Kidd, S. and O'Grady, B. (2017). *Child Welfare and Youth Homelessness in Canada: A Proposal for Action*. Canadian Observatory on Homelessness Press.

Noble, A., Thulien, N. S., Owens, B., Suleiman, A., Loganathan, M., Ali, D., Coplan, I., Neal, J., Baja, E., & Ramkissoon, K. (2022). *The Impact of COVID-19 on Youth Experiencing Homelessness: Shifting to a Collaborative, Prevention-Focused Response in a Large Urban Area*. Canadian Observatory on Homelessness Press.

Oliver, V. and Cheff, R. (2012). The social network: Homeless young women, social capital, and the health implications of belonging outside the nuclear family. *Youth & Society*, 46(5), pp.642–662.

Perron, J.L., Cleverley, K. and Kidd, S.A. (2014). Resilience, loneliness, and psychological distress among homeless youth. *Archives of Psychiatric Nursing*, 28(4), pp.226–229.

Schwan, K., Gaetz, S., French, D., Redman, M., Thistle, J. and Dej, E. (2018). *What Would it Take? Youth across Canada Speak out on Youth Homelessness Prevention*. Canadian Observatory on Homelessness Press.

Schwan, K., Vaccaro, M.-E., Reid, L., Ali, N. and Baig, K. (2021). *The Pan-Canadian Women's Housing & Homelessness Survey*. Canadian Observatory on Homelessness Press. Available at: https://womenshomelessness.ca/wp-content/uploads/EN-Pan-Canadian-Womens-Housing-Homelessness-Survey-FINAL-28-Sept-2021.pdf [Accessed 2 May 2025].

Schwan, K., Versteegh, A., Perri, M., Caplan, R., Baig, K., Dej, E., Jenkinson, J., Brais, H., Eiboff, F. and Pahlevan Chaleshtari, T. (2020). *The State of Women's Housing Need & Homelessness in Canada: Literature Review*. Canadian Observatory on Homelessness Press.

Thulien, N.S., Hwang, S.W., Kozloff, N., Nisenbaum, R., Akdikmen, A., Fambegbe, O., Feraday, R., Mathewson, C., Mutamiri, M., Roglich, J., Wang, A., Zagala, M. and Amiri, A. (2023). "When I think about my future, I just see darkness": How youth exiting homelessness navigate the hazy, liminal space between socioeconomic exclusion and inclusion. *Canadian Journal of Public Health*, 114(6), pp.893–905.

Walsh, C.A., Hanley, J., Ives, N. and Hordyk, S.R. (2016). Exploring the experiences of newcomer women with insecure housing in Montréal, Canada. *Journal of International Migration and Integration*, 17(3), pp.887–904

SECTION 2

The Bridging the Transition Framework and Its Various Components

4

RELATIONSHIP AS FOUNDATION

Nick Kerman

Homelessness is a period of profound instability and deprivation that can have a range of deleterious impacts, including on relationships. This chapter outlines the important role of working relationships with service providers during homelessness experiences and transitions. The relational needs of people experiencing homelessness in service contexts – to be seen, heard, and respected by service providers – are discussed along with the consequences when this occurs and does not occur. Transitions to housing also can disrupt social networks and connections, with strong working relationships with service providers again being important for promoting positive housing and health outcomes following exits from homelessness. The role of relationships for service providers who work with people experiencing homelessness is also discussed.

Component of the Bridging the Transition Framework Addressed in this Chapter

This chapter provides an overview on how relationships shape homelessness experiences, with a focus on how service providers can use the Bridging the Transition Framework to foster meaningful and helpful working relationships with people experiencing and leaving homelessness. The chapter is centered on the "Relationship as Foundation" component of the Bridging the Transition Framework (see Figure 4.1).

DOI: 10.4324/9781003541332-6

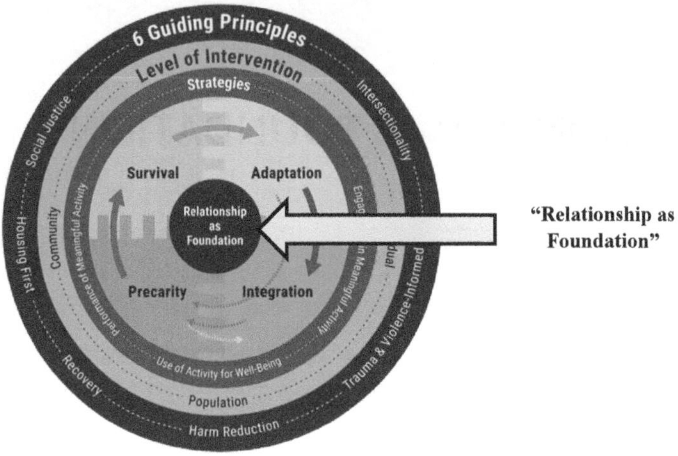

FIGURE 4.1 Relationship as Foundation.

How this Chapter Guides Practice and Research in Homelessness Prevention

Health and social service providers have instrumental roles in helping people to survive and leave homelessness. This chapter outlines how service providers – the individuals working and delivering supports in health and social service settings – can meaningfully respond to the upheaval in social networks and connections when people experience homelessness. Drawing extensively from qualitative research of the experiences and perceptions of individuals with histories of homelessness, the importance of service providers using a respectful and nonjudgmental approach is discussed, as are other considerations for forming safe and trustworthy working relationships with service users – the individuals with histories of homelessness who are accessing health and social services. This creates a strong and stable support foundation that can promote service continuation and potentially yield opportunities to facilitate exits from homelessness. The last part of the chapter discusses the impacts of relationships between service users and providers following exits from homelessness, highlighting how strong working alliances can be a protective factor against housing instability, especially during transitions to housing.

Introduction

> *I hate to be corny but you can feel love. You know? They ask me how I'm doing, mentally, physically. They don't just give me the equipment I need, they give me support that I need as well. You know, even if it's just, 'How's your day going? How's this? How's that?' You know? It's nice to know that someone cares and shows interest.*

> *You can tell when someone really does care about their job and people who are just doing a job. It's just attitude. It's just the way they talk to you. The way they try to shuffle you off as quickly as possible. You know, I'm gonna get this done and this is what I'm supposed to do. Next! ... You could tell that she's just there for the paycheque.*

If you are around people experiencing homelessness enough in a service and support setting (or, in my case, as a researcher of those places), you will hear these sentiments a lot. It is sometimes in the form of a dichotomy between a service provider who cares and another who is perceived to be in the work for the paycheque, as highlighted in the second quote. Now, both/and would be more ideal than either/or in this case, with service providers both caring and receiving livable wages, but the perceptions are important. These quotes, which were from two participants in a study I led on what people with histories of homelessness want and notice when accessing health and social services, underscore that service delivery is fundamentally about relationships. This chapter provides an overview on how relationships shape and are shaped by homelessness experiences, with a focus on how service providers can foster meaningful and helpful working relationships with people experiencing and leaving homelessness.

Relationships and Homelessness

Social connection is recognized as a basic need, and human brains are hardwired to respond to the joys and pains that occur in social contexts (Seppala, Rossomando, and Doty, 2013). For example, a seminal neuroimaging study found that exclusion from a social activity activates the anterior cingulate cortex, an area of the brain that serves as a neural alarm system, in a similar way as physical pain (Eisenberger, Lieberman, and Williams, 2003). Research demonstrates that social connection has considerable health benefits in humans' lives (Holt-Lunstad, 2022), but the importance of relationships can be even greater during crises. It is perhaps unsurprising then that relationships are interwoven with and shape almost all aspects of homelessness, which is a period of profound instability and deprivation.

The effects of relationships begin even before homelessness. Adverse childhood experiences, many of which are relational in nature (e.g., parental and family separation, exposure to interpersonal violence, neglect), are independent risk factors for later homelessness and health problems (Liu et al., 2021). The majority of adults experiencing homelessness report four or more adverse childhood experiences, signaling heightened risk of health problems and early death, as well as attachment difficulties (Horácio, Bento, and Marques, 2023; Liu et al., 2021). Social network sizes have less of a role to play in pathways into homelessness (Nilsson, Nordentoft, and Hjorthøj, 2019); however, as Shinn and Khadduri (2020) caution, it is often not the lack of social resources that produces a risk of homelessness, but rather that individuals may exhaust the support that their social networks can provide (i.e., social capital), increasing the likelihood of their becoming homeless.

Episodes of homelessness greatly affect social networks and connections. People report weakened ties with friends and family after entering homelessness. Qualitative research on the pathways into family homelessness by Sylvestre et al. (2018) illustrated how changes in housing status could reveal the fair-weather friends in people's networks. As one participant of that study poignantly said, "When my skies are blue and sunny, I've got all the friends in the world, but if there's a cloud over my head, I'm dealing with it on my own" (p. 2278). Barriers at the service level can further exacerbate the negative consequences of homelessness on relationships and social connections. For example, many emergency shelters do not permit couples or families with adult children, which can force these family units to be split-up when accessing services. Similarly, shelter rules against animal companions can jeopardize another important type of relationship for some people experiencing homelessness (Kerman, Gran-Ruaz, and Lem, 2019b). These experiences and service barriers collectively contribute to a risk of social isolation, which has been shown to be a prevalent problem among people experiencing homelessness (Cummings et al., 2022; Lachaud et al., 2024), and a need for people to explore other ways of compensating for the social connection losses.

Over three decades ago, Grigsby et al. (1990) proposed a social process model of chronic homelessness. It theorized that homelessness disrupts social networks, yielding two different relational paths that lead to chronic homelessness: disaffiliation (continued loss of social support leading to isolation and health problems) or re-affiliation (establishment of connections to other people experiencing homelessness leading to a sense of belonging, but also street entrenchment). Although the theory has been largely unsupported with regard to the causes of chronic homelessness (structural factors, such as housing affordability and income inequality, have been found to be stronger predictors than social network-related ones; Shinn and Khadduri, 2020), it does highlight how people experiencing homelessness may attend to unmet needs for social connection. The disaffiliation path may be an intentional form of self-protection at a perilous time in people's lives. Maintaining a social distance from others has been described as a way of preventing victimization, avoiding substance use, and staying focused on the work needed to leave homelessness (Bender et al., 2014; Donley and Wright, 2012; Kerman and Sylvestre, 2020). This avoidance can also extend to health and social service providers due to past experiences of discrimination, which presents a risk of other needs going unmet (Canham et al., 2024). The re-affiliation path also offers self-protection and risks. Connections to peers in the context of homelessness protect against social isolation and provide a sense of belonging (Kerman et al., 2019a). Social relationships among people experiencing homelessness who use drugs can also be a protective factor against overdose fatalities when people do not use alone (Bardwell et al., 2018). However, re-affiliation presents victimization risks as well. Women, 2SLGBTQIA+ individuals, youth, older adults, and people with intellectual and developmental disabilities are at heightened risk of exploitation and abuse from peers and romantic partners experiencing homelessness (Kerman and Stergiopoulos, 2024). Thus, relationships in the context of homelessness can be double-edged swords, and it is imperative that the associated benefits and risks be recognized and considered in health and social service delivery practice, policy, and research.

Relationships as the Cornerstone of Service Delivery

People experiencing homelessness are one of the most serviced populations. As most people experiencing homelessness on any given night will stay in a shelter, individuals wake up and go to sleep in a service setting. During the day, they are likely to access food and other necessities via meal and drop-in programs. They may meet with case workers about housing, employment, income support applications, identification, and other fundamental needs. Given the high rates of mental and physical health conditions, use of healthcare services is also common. This makes the service provider a central figure in the lives of people experiencing homelessness, and these relationships can have tremendous impacts on both parties.

Much like psychotherapy, wherein common factors such as the working alliance are a key component of therapeutic outcomes (Wampold, 2015), the relationships between people experiencing homelessness and service providers are the cornerstone of service delivery across the four processes (survival, adaptation, integration, and precarity) of the Bridging the Transition Framework. Numerous studies have examined what people experiencing homelessness want when accessing health and social services. This research demonstrates that, at the core, people want to be seen, heard, and respected by service providers (Omerov et al., 2020). In practice, this looks like service providers who are welcoming, friendly, nonjudgmental, dependable, and responsive (Kerman et al., 2019a). People with histories of homelessness have described service providers with these qualities as contributing to reduced isolation because they have "at least one person in my corner" (Kerman and Sylvestre, 2020, p. 392). In addition to the emotional support benefits, continuity in service use is promoted when service providers are dependably available and perceived positively by people experiencing homelessness (Magwood et al., 2019). However, the opposite also occurs, with service providers who are perceived as judgmental and disrespectful being a risk factor for service discontinuation (Omerov et al., 2020; Thompson et al., 2006).

The life and service use histories of people experiencing homelessness also shape interactions with providers and warrant careful consideration in service delivery. Experiences of interpersonal trauma and abuse, both of which are prevalent among people experiencing homelessness, can hinder the development of trusting and safe relationships. It may take longer for people experiencing homelessness who have trauma histories to develop trust with service providers and may even mistrust them due to their authority roles (Briere and Scott, 2015). Similar challenges can arise from negative past service experiences. People experiencing homelessness who have encountered stigma and discrimination, felt abandonment, or merely had unmet needs within the health and social service systems may have understandable wariness toward providers. Accordingly, use of a patient, respectful, compassionate, and affirming approach in service delivery is critical to forming safe and trustworthy working relationships with service users who have histories of trauma and discrimination within health and social service systems (see Chapter 13 for more information on the use of a trauma-informed approach).

Relationships as an Essential Component of Work for Service Providers

The connection between people experiencing homelessness and service providers represents a dynamic relationship that affects both parties. Like service users, these relationships can have bidirectional effects on service providers. On the one hand, service users are a primary reason why providers report doing the work they do. As one service provider participant in a recent study I led said, "What keeps me going is the people that I work for. You know, especially when you see somebody getting better." Yet, the work is also challenging and, although many of the issues that make it this way are structural and systemic in nature, they can be felt acutely at the service delivery level. Providers, especially those in direct service roles, are often overworked and frequently encounter critical incidents, including fatalities, as well as other moral dilemmas in the workplace (Kerman et al., 2023; Lemieux-Cumberlege et al., 2024; Perez et al., 2024). They may also be insufficiently paid and have limited access to good fringe benefits. These experiences can be a threat to the mental health of service providers and, because of the relationship dynamic between service providers and people experiencing homelessness, the health of providers can ultimately affect service users. For example, a study from the United States of case managers working in a homeless service setting concluded that providers experiencing secondary traumatic stress could also encounter greater rapport development challenges with service users (Twis et al., 2022). The findings underscore the importance of supporting service providers with their own mental health needs in order for them to optimally support others at work.

Relationships are also a part of the antidote to workplace mental health difficulties. Greater perceived social support from colleagues has been found to be associated with lower posttraumatic stress symptoms and psychological distress among service providers to people experiencing homelessness

(Kerman et al., 2023). Emotional support from supervisors was also negatively correlated with distress (Kerman et al., 2023). Accordingly, agencies can support staff, with positive downstream effects for service users, by fostering cohesive team environments where providers can access mutual support from colleagues and regular supervision that is oriented to the emotional and practical needs of direct service providers.

Relationships during Transitions to Housing

Safe, affordable housing can provide a sense of ontological security (the feeling of well-being that is produced from constancy in people's social and material environments) that enables a secure base for identity development and self-actualization (Padgett, 2007). In the context of transitions to housing, this may include rebuilding relationships that predated homelessness, such as with family and friends, or developing new relationships within the community. Relationships with service providers during homelessness may or may not continue following transitions to housing. The same is also true of peer relationships that were developed during homelessness. Thus, transitioning into housing from homelessness is another critical and dynamic period for relationships.

Some people leaving homelessness require additional supports, either transitionally, such as during the survival to adaptation processes of the Bridging the Transition Framework, or on an ongoing basis inclusive of all four processes. Community mental health interventions of varying length and service intensity have been developed for these individuals. The most common of these interventions are permanent supportive housing and Housing First, which involve the provision of affordable housing or rent subsidies along with clinical supports in various models and structures. These interventions can affect the social connections and community integration of people leaving homelessness. Research has highlighted that Housing First is associated with more romantic partners and family members in social networks, as well as expanded social roles (Cummings et al., 2022; Nelson et al., 2015). However, people can also experience a loss of social support and barriers to community integration (Cummings et al., 2022; Marshall et al., 2020). Further, social isolation can be a key challenge among residents of permanent supportive housing and Housing First (Cummings et al., 2022). Hence, there is an important ongoing role for service providers working with individuals leaving homelessness to support their social connection and relational needs above what is provided by ontological security alone.

Relationships between service users and providers are an important component of transitions from homelessness. In the At Home/Chez Soi demonstration project, a randomized controlled trial of Housing First conducted in five Canadian cities, working alliance with intervention service providers had a significant positive effect on housing stability at six months (Sandu, Anyan, and Stergiopoulos, 2021). Working alliance was not a significant predictor, however, at the subsequent time points, underscoring the importance of these relationships during the initial transition out of homelessness, in particular. Similarly, in another demonstration project of a Housing First-oriented program in the United States, participants who had stronger working alliances with their case managers reported higher quality of life and perceived social support after three months than did those with lower alliances or no primary mental health provider (Tsai et al., 2013). However, these potential benefits can be overlooked in service providers' roles during this period. In a qualitative study by Marshall et al. (2022), one service provider participant reflected that too often the focus is only on housing sustainment, "We stick people in a house and say okay, you're housed. The problem is solved" (p. e6022). This sentiment was linked to other workforce-related issues described earlier in this chapter, most notably high caseloads and frequent crises. These issues can lead service providers to feel like they are relentlessly "putting out fires" in their work (Marshall et al., 2022, p. 6023). However, it is important that working relationships between service users and providers not be disconnected from the primary intervention objectives. Considering the aforementioned findings from the two demonstration projects, a focus on working relationships between providers and service users is an opportunity to strengthen housing and health outcomes associated with interventions, especially during transitions from homelessness.

Conclusion

Homelessness can have deleterious effects on people's relationships and social connections. Service providers are sometimes identified by people experiencing homelessness as the only source of support that they have (Cummings et al., 2022). Thus, relationships with service providers can be profoundly important and meaningful in the lives of people experiencing homelessness. When people feel seen, heard, and respected by service providers who are welcoming, friendly, nonjudgmental, dependable, and responsive, this creates a strong and stable support foundation during periods of homelessness instability and transitions. To that end, I present one last quote from the study where this chapter began. Describing the relational instability precipitated by homelessness, one participant reflected (Kerman and Sylvestre, 2020, p. 392):

> *The one thing through all of that – my friends bailed, everybody bailed – I had that case worker.*

References

Bardwell, G., Boyd, J., Kerr, T. and McNeil, R., (2018) Negotiating space & drug use in emergency shelters with peer witness injection programs within the context of an overdose crisis: A qualitative study. *Health & Place*, 53, pp. 86–93.

Bender, K., Thompson, S., Ferguson, K., Yoder, J. and DePrince, A. (2014) Risk detection and self-protection among homeless youth. *Journal of Research on Adolescence*, 25(2), pp. 352–65.
Briere, J.N. and Scott, C. (2015) *Principles of Trauma Therapy: A Guide to Symptoms, Evaluation, and Treatment* (2nd ed). Thousand Oaks: Sage.
Canham, S.L., Weldrick, R., Erisman, M., McNamara, A., Rose, J.N., Siantz, E., Casucci, T. and McFarland, M.M. (2024) A scoping review of the experiences and outcomes of stigma and discrimination towards persons experiencing homelessness. *Health & Social Care in the Community*, 2024, 2060619.
Cummings, C., Lei, Q., Hochberg, L., Hones, V. and Brown, M. (2022) Social support and networks among people experiencing chronic homelessness: A systematic review. *American Journal of Orthopsychiatry*, 92(3), pp. 349–63.
Donley, A.M. and Wright, J.D. (2012) Safer outside: A qualitative exploration of homeless people's resistance to homeless shelters. *Journal of Forensic Psychology Practice*, 12(4), pp. 288–306.
Eisenberger, N.I., Lieberman, M.D. and Williams, K.D. (2003) Does rejection hurt? An fMRI study of social exclusion. *Science*, 302(5643), pp. 290–292.
Grigsby, C., Baumann, D., Gregorich, S.E. and Roberts-Gray, C. (1990) Disaffiliation to entrenchment: A model for understanding homelessness. *Journal of Social Issues*, 46(4), pp. 141–46.
Holt-Lunstad, J. (2022) Social connection as a public health issue: The evidence and a systemic framework for prioritizing the "social" in social determinants of health. *Annual Review of Public Health*, 43, pp. 193–213.
Horácio, A.N., Bento, A. and Marques, J.G. (2023) Personality and attachment in the homeless: A systematic review. *International Journal of Social Psychiatry*, 69(6), pp. 1312–26.
Kerman, N., Ecker, J., Tiderington, E., Gaetz, S. and Kidd, S.A. (2023) Workplace trauma and chronic stressor exposure among direct service providers working with people experiencing homelessness. *Journal of Mental Health*, 28(2), pp. 424–433.
Kerman, N., Gran-Ruaz, S. and Lem, M. (2019b) Pet ownership and homelessness: A scoping review. *Journal of Social Distress and the Homeless*, 28(2), pp. 106–114.
Kerman, N., Gran-Ruaz, S., Lawrence, M. and Sylvestre, J. (2019a) Perceptions of service use among currently and formerly homeless adults with mental health problems. *Community Mental Health Journal*, 55, pp. 777–783.
Kerman, N. and Stergiopoulos, V. (2024) Addressing health needs in people with mental illness experiencing homelessness. *Nature Mental Health*, 2, pp. 354–366.
Kerman, N. and Sylvestre, J. (2020) Service use and recovery among currently and formerly homeless adults with mental illness. *International Journal of Social Psychiatry*, 66(4), pp. 389–396.
Lachaud, J., Yusuf, A.A., Maelzer, F., Perri, M., Gogosis, E., Ziegler, C., Mejia-Lancheros, C. and Hwang, S.W. (2024) Social isolation and loneliness among people living with experience of homelessness: A scoping review. *BMC Public Health*, 24, 2515.
Lemieux-Cumberlege, A.H., Griffiths, H., Pathe, E. and Burley, A. (2024) Posttraumatic stress disorder, secondary traumatic stress, and burnout in frontline workers in homelessness services: Risk and protective factors. *Journal of Social Distress and Homelessness*, 33(2), 329–340. https://doi.org/10.1080/10530789.2023.2191405
Liu, M., Luong, L., Lachaud, J., Edalati, H., Reeves, A. and Hwang, S. (2021) Adverse childhood experiences and related outcomes among adults experiencing homelessness: A systematic review and meta-analysis. *Lancet Public Health*, 6(11), E836–E847.
Magwood, O., Leki, V.Y., Kpade, V., Saad, A., Alkhateeb, Q., Gebremeskel, A., Rehman, A., Hannigan, T., Pinto, N., Sun, A.H., Kendall, C., Kozloff, N., Tweed, E.J., Ponka, D. and Pottie, K. (2019) Common trust and personal safety issues: A

systrematic review on the acceptability of health and social interventions for persons with lived experience of homelessness. *Plos One*, 14(12), e0226306.

Marshall, C.A., Boland, L., Westover, L.A., Marcellus, B., Weil, S. and Wickett, S. (2020) Effectiveness of interventions targeting community integration among individuals with lived experiences of homelessness: A systematic review. *Health and Social Care in the Community*, 28(6), pp. 1843–1862.

Marshall, C.A., Phillips, B., Holmes, J., Todd, E., Hill, R., Panter, G., Easton, C., Landry, T., Collins, S., Greening, T., O'Brien, A., Jastak, M., Ridge, R., Goldszmidt, R., Shanoff, C., Rudman, D.L., Carlsson, A., Aryobi, S., Perez, S. and Oudshoorn, A. (2022) 'We stick people in a house and say okay, you're housed. The problem is solved': A qualitative study of service provider and organisational leader perspectives on thriving following homelessness. *Health and Social Care in the Community*, 30(6), pp. e6018–e6029.

Nelson, G., Patterson, M., Kirst, M., Macnaughton, E., Isaak, C.A., Nolin, D., McAll, C., Stergiopoulos, V., Townley, G., MacLeod, T., Piat, M. and Goering, P.N. (2015) Life changes among homeless persons with mental illness: A longitudinal study of housing first and usual treatment. *Psychiatric Services*, 66(6), pp. 592–597.

Nilsson, S.F., Nordentoft, M. and Hjorthøj, C. (2019) Individual-level predictors for becoming homeless and exiting homelessness: A systematic review and meta-analysis. *Journal of Urban Health*, 96, pp. 741–750.

Omerov, P., Craftman, Å.G., Mattsson, E. and Klarare, A. (2020) Homeless persons' experiences of health- and social care: A systematic integrative review. *Health & Social Care in the Community*, 28(1), pp. 1–11.

Padgett, D.K. (2007) There's no place like (a) home: Ontological security among persons with serious mental illness in the United States. *Social Science & Medicine*, 64(9), pp. 1925–1936.

Perez, S., Kerman, N., Dej, E., Forchuk, C., George, C., Easton, C. and Marshall, C.A. (2024) When I can't help, I suffer: A scoping review of moral distress in service providers working with persons experiencing homelessness. *Journal of Mental Health*, advance online publication. DOI:10.1080/09638237.2024.2426986

Sandu, R.D., Anyan, F. and Stergiopoulos, V. (2021) Housing first, connection second: The impact of professional helping relationships on the trajectories of housing stability for people facing severe and multiple disadvantage. *BMC Public Health*, 21, p. 249.

Seppala, E., Rossomando, T. and Doty, J.R. (2013) Social connection and compassion: Important predictors of health and well-being. *Social Research: An International Quarterly*, 80(2), pp. 411–430.

Shinn, M. and Khadduri, J. (2020) *In the Midst of Plenty: Homelessness and What to do About it*. Hoboken: Wiley-Blackwell.

Sylvestre, J., Kerman, N., Polillo, A., Lee, C.M., Aubry, T. and Czechowski, K. (2018) A qualitative study of the pathways into and impacts of family homelessness. *Journal of Family Issues*, 39(8), pp. 2265–2285.

Thompson, S.J., McManus, H., Lantry, J., Windsor, L. and Flynn, P. (2006) Insights from the street: Perceptions of services and providers by homeless young adults. *Evaluation and Program Planning*, 29(1), pp. 34–43.

Tsai, J., Lapidos, A., Rosenheck, R.A. and Harpaz-Rotem, I. (2013) Longitudinal association of therapeutic alliance and clinical outcomes in supported housing for chronically homeless adults. *Community Mental Health Journal*, 49(4), pp. 438–443.

Twis, M., Petrovich, J., Cronley, C., Nordberg, A. and Woody, D. (2022) A mixed methods analysis of case manager stress at a homelessness services center. *Journal of Evidence-Based Social Work*, 19(1), pp. 19–41.

Wampold, B.E. (2015) How important are the common factors in psychotherapy? An update. *World Psychiatry*, 14(3), pp. 270–277.

5

THE "FOUR PROCESSES" OF LEAVING HOMELESSNESS

Carrie Anne Marshall

The functional and participation needs of individuals as they leave homelessness are known to evolve across the transition from unhoused to housed. The Bridging the Transition Framework describes Four Processes of leaving homelessness that are outlined in this chapter. These categories were developed from empirical research conducted to provide a foundation for the Bridging the Transition Framework. Initial categories were presented to a group of international practitioners and researchers with expertise in homelessness and refined further. This chapter describes the findings of the empirical research conducted to provide a foundation for this framework and contextualizes these findings in extant literature to characterize the experiences of individuals across the trajectory of unhoused to housing. Understanding the four processes of leaving homelessness will equip practitioners, researchers, and policymakers with a foundation for developing solutions for preventing homelessness through improving function and participation of individuals and families.

Component of the Bridging the Transition Framework Addressed in this Chapter

This chapter provides an overview of the "Four Processes of Leaving Homelessness" component of the Bridging the Transition Framework (see Figure 5.1). This part of the framework includes four components: (1) Survival, (2) Adaptation, (3) Integration, and (4) Precarity. These processes each represent experiences identified by individuals in previous research as they secure permanent housing and integrate into their communities following homelessness.

DOI: 10.4324/9781003541332-7

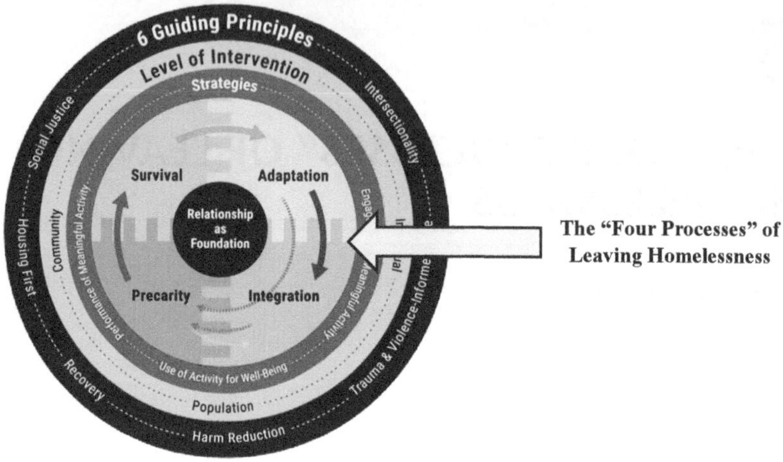

FIGURE 5.1 The "Four Processes" of Leaving Homelessness.

How this Chapter Guides Practice and Research in Homelessness Prevention

This chapter provides a foundation for practitioners, researchers, and policymakers as they contribute to solutions for improving the function and participation of individuals across the trajectory of unhoused to housing, with a goal of preventing ongoing homelessness. Practitioners will be provided with a summary of existing evidence on the transition to housing that will act as a foundation for inspiring strategies for supporting permanent transitions to housing. Researchers will be provided with evidence to inform directions for future research on the transition to housing from a functional and participation perspective in the interest of homelessness prevention. Finally, this chapter will provide policymakers with an understanding of the experience of transitioning to housing following homelessness from a functional and participation perspective as they develop policies and make decisions that affect the lives of individuals and families who are leaving homelessness.

Introduction

Existing literature exploring the transition to housing following homelessness indicates that individuals who secure housing frequently cycle through repeated episodes of homelessness in the process of becoming housed (Marshall et al., 2022b). The reasons for tenancy loss and ongoing difficulties with health and well-being among persons who experience homelessness are multiple and include individual, structural, and institutional factors (Aldridge, 2020; Warburton and Stahl, 2020; Pophaim and Peacock, 2021). These factors act as barriers that interfere with a person's ability to secure housing, sustain a tenancy, and to attain a basic degree of well-being during and following homelessness. Individual factors include challenges with mental illness and substance use disorders following homelessness that interfere with the ability to function effectively in daily life and participate fully in one’s community (Marshall et al., 2022d). Structural factors associated with tenancy loss and persistent challenges to well-being include ongoing poverty, increasing costs of living, and a lack of deeply affordable housing that combine to prevent individuals from adequately meeting their needs during and following homelessness (Shinn and Khadduri, 2020). Institutional factors include a lack of access to adequate housing and health supports during and following homelessness (Ramsay et al., 2019).

Perhaps the most widely known intervention for supporting transitions to housing following homelessness is Housing First, an intervention emphasizing the immediate provision of permanent supportive housing and psychosocial supports for sustaining a tenancy (Tsemberis, 2010). This intervention (explored in detail in Chapter 10) has consistently been demonstrated to be effective for helping individuals to secure a tenancy and sustain it for longer (Baxter et al., 2019). Housing First, however, has been poorly implemented outside of research initiatives that have demonstrated its effectiveness, thereby limiting its ability to support permanent tenancies in practice (Choy-Brown et al., 2021). While it is widely known to be effective for improving tenancy sustainment, Housing First has not been demonstrated to be effective for supporting a range of psychosocial outcomes following homelessness, including community integration, substance use, and indices of mental well-being (Marshall et al., 2020a; Woodhall-Melnik and Dunn, 2015), suggesting that there is a need for interventions that build on Housing First to more effectively address these outcomes. Approaches that meet the unique needs of individuals and families across the trajectory of unhoused to housing are needed. To inform these approaches, an appreciation of the priorities identified by persons with lived experience, service providers, and policy-makers during and following homelessness can provide a foundation for selecting interventions or informing the development of novel strategies.

The “Four Processes” of Leaving Homelessness

The Bridging the Transition Framework describes four processes of leaving homelessness that draw on existing interdisciplinary research and research conducted by the framework authors to provide a foundation for its development (Marshall et al., 2022c). This foundational research included 36 participants recruited from one moderate and one large urban centre in Ontario, Canada. In this research, qualitative interviews were conducted with individuals across the trajectory of unhoused to housing, including unhoused persons and persons housed for 1–3 months and 3–24 months following homelessness. Interviews focused on identifying the priorities of participants during homelessness, early in the transition to housing, and later in the transition to housing. Themes generated in the analysis of interviews described the experiences of individuals across the trajectory of unhoused to housing. These experiences were described as evolving as participants adapted to their new housing situations: (1) time use and participation in meaningful activity, (2) managing mental health and substance use, (3) emotional growth and change, (4) creating connection and community, and (5) managing new health concerns. These findings emphasized the need for attending to function and participation in different ways during and following homelessness.

The authors of the Bridging the Transition Framework used the findings of this research to develop four categories describing the various processes of leaving homelessness: (1) Survival (orange in Figure 5.1), (2) Adaptation (light green in Figure 5.1), (3) Integration (dark green in Figure 5.1), and (4) Precarity (red in Figure 5.1). Participants in the study that provided a foundation for the identification of these processes described that the length of time in which they experienced each was highly individual. This was emphasized further during the process of developing and refining the framework by seeking input from international practitioners and researchers (Marshall et al., 2023a). For this reason, the framework authors have not specified time frames that correspond to each process and encourage individuals who are using the framework to consider the individual factors involved in the timing of the four processes. The four processes and the findings of the research conducted to provide a foundation for the development of the Bridging the Transition Framework are discussed in the following sections.

The Survival Process

The Survival Process in the Bridging the Transition Framework describes a period during which a person is currently unhoused. By unhoused, the framework authors refer to circumstances in which a person is living in a shelter, in a location where they do not hold a tenancy (i.e. temporarily in a friend's home), directly on the street, in an encampment, or a combination of some or all of these living situations.

Priorities during the Survival Process

Time Use and Participation in Meaningful Activity

Consistent with previous research, individuals who were unhoused in the study providing a foundation for the framework discussed prioritizing survival activities during homelessness (Cunningham and Slade, 2019). Participants spent their time accessing basic resources from within the unhoused community and moving between organizations that supported them to meet their basic needs, a finding that has been demonstrated in a range of other studies exploring the time use of unhoused persons (Cunningham and Slade, 2019; Marshall et al., 2020b; Thomas et al., 2017; Illman et al., 2013). Although they expressed the desire for employment, their environmental circumstances frequently interfered with the ability to maintain work. Participants reported a lack of meaningful activity, resulting in boredom that imposed a negative influence on their mental well-being, a finding that aligns with a range of other studies on the time use of unhoused persons (O'Neill, 2014; Marshall et al., 2024a; Marshall et al., 2019). When discussing the lack of access to meaningful activity in this research, one participant summed up his experience of homelessness by describing that "you sit in the chair all day and feel like shit."

Managing Mental Health and Substance Use

Mental illness is known to be prevalent among individuals experiencing homelessness, with suicide representing a leading cause of mortality in this group (Hossain et al., 2020; Gutwinski et al., 2021). Mental well-being was a pressing concern for unhoused participants in the foundational study. Individuals who were unhoused recognized how substance use was a factor that sustained homelessness and expressed the desire to reduce their use or ultimately abstain. Not surprisingly, they experienced significant stress in their daily lives and required support to cope on a regular basis. Access to good quality mental health and substance use services was a challenge for participants, and they discussed the need to increase the availability of services during this time.

Emotional Growth and Change

In the study on which the framework was developed, participants who were unhoused expressed a high degree of self-judgement during homelessness. They reported feeling disappointed in themselves for allowing their homelessness to continue and expressed the desire for structure and routine in their lives.

Creating Connection and Community

In the study providing a foundation for the Bridging the Transition Framework, participants who were unhoused described living in challenging social environments that they struggled to navigate daily. Participants recognized the role of the social environments in which they were embedded and how these environments affected their well-being, and felt profoundly excluded. Many participants lacked family involvement in their lives, with one participant indicating: "I don't have family now. They're around, but they don't acknowledge me as that...family don't want nothin' to do with me." They tried to manage in this environment of exclusion by surrounding themselves with people who positively affected their mental health. This was challenging during homelessness given the many interpersonal conflicts that were reported to occur in shelters and on the street, a finding consistent with other existing literature (Marshall et al., 2020b; Marshall et al., 2023b; Gabrielian et al., 2018).

The Adaptation Process

During the Adaptation Process in the Bridging the Transition Framework, a person has recently left homelessness and has been living in transitional or permanent housing. At this time, the person is adapting to living in housing after leaving shelters, encampments, or the street. It is important to recognize that individuals leaving homelessness may have a range of experiences of homelessness, and that these experiences are likely to influence early adaptation to housing following this transition. For instance, some individuals may have experienced short-term homelessness before transitioning to housing again, whereas others may have experienced several episodes of homelessness over the course of years. Still, others may have been unhoused for several years prior to the transition to housing. These patterns of homelessness are likely to affect experiences of transitioning to housing after an episode of homelessness. For many individuals who are leaving homelessness, however, the transition to housing is not linear. In the research that provided a foundation for the Bridging the Transition Framework, participants described the early period of transition out of homelessness in the following way: "I'm in a transitory phase. Still getting used to not being homeless."

Priorities during the Adaptation Process

Time Use and Participation in Meaningful Activity

After leaving homelessness, participants in the study that provided a foundation for the framework discussed how their time use had changed from the need to engage in survival activities to no longer needing to perform these activities. As a result, they expressed frustration with being under-occupied. With little money, they were unable to occupy their time in meaningful ways and continued to struggle with high degrees of boredom, a finding consistent with existing literature on the transition to housing following homelessness (Marshall et al., 2024b). Simultaneously, they were trying to rediscover their own identities through activities that were personally meaningful, a journey that was sometimes satisfying and sometimes bewildering.

Managing Health Concerns

Homelessness is often described as an incredibly stressful experience. In our research conducted to provide a foundation for the Bridging the Transition Framework, participants who had been living unhoused described how they deprioritized physical health as they coped with stress and managed their survival needs. Once housed, participants noticed the impacts of physical health conditions in their lives that they had not noticed prior to securing housing and sought to access supports to manage these health problems more effectively. Accessing these services was a challenge, however, because they were described as frustratingly unavailable: "either you're on a waitlist, or it doesn't exist."

Creating Connection and Community

Participants who had recently left homelessness described becoming suddenly immersed in new social environments to which they needed to adjust. They found themselves involved in interpersonal conflicts that were difficult to resolve independently, and they recognized how this impacted on their mental well-being. Becoming immersed in new social environments and needing to manage interpersonal conflicts is an experience that has been reported in existing literature on the transition from homelessness (Marshall et al., 2023b). Yet, research also emphasizes the need for attaining belonging in one's community as an important component in promoting tenancy sustainment (Plett et al., 2023).

The Integration Process

During the Integration Process in the Bridging the Transition Framework, individuals who have left homelessness have been living in permanent housing and have overcome the initial period of this transition. Participants in the foundational study (Marshall et al., 2022c), and in other research (Marshall et al., 2023b), expressed that they continued to be in a period of adjustment to *being housed* following homelessness and described not being completely "settled" for months or years after securing housing: "I haven't been able to settle in there, and I've been there for almost a year." Individuals housed between 3 and 24 months in this foundational study expressed that they continued to work towards integrating into their communities during this time and struggled in finding a place for themselves within the social fabric of the community.

Priorities during the Integration Process

Time Use and Participation in Meaningful Activity

Participants reflected on the activities that they enjoyed in the past and expressed a desire to return to engaging in these activities. Many experienced boredom and a lack of meaningful time use, and described the need to alleviate this boredom by finding meaningful ways of spending their time. They recognized the importance of routine in their daily lives and strove to establish one with varying degrees of success. Although having limited financial resources was identified as a barrier to participating in activities that were meaningful, many participants were content with their time use and saw value in these activities. Participants discussed returning to school and work extensively, yet consistent with existing literature, also discussed how limitations imposed by health conditions were a barrier to engagement in these activities (Marshall et al., 2022a). Participants reported that they did not experience significant difficulties with independent living skills such as cleaning and self-care, and in fact talked about how important it was for them to return to being engaged in these activities after being housed. Participants described being proud of their ability to cook and take care of their apartments independently.

Managing Mental Health and Substance Use

Participants had a number of unmet mental health support needs later in the transition to housing following homelessness. They oscillated between hopefulness and hopelessness but found multiple ways of coping with psychological distress, including being in the outdoors, engaging in artwork, dog walking, improving their diet, and engaging in exercise. Participants had strong feelings about reducing or ending their substance use, but struggled to access services to support them with this overall objective (Marshall et al., 2023b; Marshall et al., 2018). Supports for participants who wanted to reduce their substance use were frustratingly unavailable, while they were able to access harm reduction services to maintain safety in the context of substance use in their communities.

Emotional Growth and Change

Participants in the research that provided a foundation for developing the Bridging the Transition Framework continued to struggle with adjusting to being housed later in the transition to housing following homelessness. They found themselves trying to manage as best they could with limited material resources. Several participants noted that food security was an issue after being housed for months following homelessness, while it hadn't been during homelessness. They recognized the need to sustain motivation to remain housed and continue to work towards identified goals in the face of these challenges. Participants described the value that they placed on self-compassion during this time. They used motivational strategies, including "giving themselves a push" and recalling past successes, to keep feeling positive about their housing and their futures. Participants described transformations that they were observing in themselves and expressed pride around their own independence. The stability provided by being housed helped participants to access and consistently utilize needed supports, which they recognized as critically important for maintaining their well-being.

Creating Connection and Community

Participants described a range of challenges that they faced in managing social relationships. They faced conflict with roommates and described experiences of feeling isolated from others, consistent with other studies exploring the transition to housing following homelessness (Marshall et al., 2018; Marshall et al., 2023b; Marshall et al., 2024b). Participants worked towards reconnecting and building relationships with family members with whom they had disconnected in the past, while limiting contact with individuals with whom they had experienced homelessness. In fact, they saw their housing as a foundation on which they could re-build family and community relationships. They discussed and celebrated new relationships with romantic partners and neighbours that they had cultivated since securing housing.

The Precarity Process

In the research conducted to provide a foundation for the Bridging the Transition Framework, participants who were at risk of tenancy loss were not specifically recruited. Although the authors did not interview participants who were at risk of homelessness, the importance of attending to the period that precedes housing loss is important to acknowledge in homelessness prevention efforts. The Precarity Process in the Bridging the Transition Framework draws on existing literature to emphasize the need for supporting individuals whose tenancies are at risk to prevent homelessness or a recurrence of homelessness. Not all individuals who have made the transition from homelessness experience housing precarity, yet it is important to recognize that this may occur. With the right kinds of supports, the loss of one's tenancy can be prevented. If supports are not available, the person may become or return to homelessness and will proceed through the processes of Survival, Adaptation, and Integration in the Bridging the Transition Framework.

Priorities during the Precarity Process

In the Bridging the Transition Framework, the primary priorities during the Precarity Process should be two-fold: (1) preventing homelessness and (2) providing emotional support to help the person who is at-risk of homelessness to cope with the enormously stressful experience of a possible tenancy loss. This period is one of crisis, and any strategy that prevents the loss of a tenancy needs to be emphasized. It is also important to note that the approach used needs to consider the causes of one's homelessness and use this information to respond effectively to the person's specific situation (Batterham, 2017). Still, loss of one's tenancy may still occur and should not be viewed as an individual failing of the person who has lost their housing, or the fault of a service provider who is providing support.

Conclusion

This chapter focused on describing the "Four Processes" component of the Bridging the Transition Framework. The four processes of leaving homelessness include Survival, Adaptation, Integration, and Precarity. During each of these processes, the support needs and priorities of individuals change along with the environments in which individuals are situated and the resources that are available to them. The priorities during each of the four processes were described and contextualized in the context of existing research, and research conducted to provide a foundation for the Bridging the Transition Framework. Practitioners, researchers, and policymakers may consider the ways in which functional and participation needs of individuals and families evolve across the process of leaving homelessness and use this information to inform their homelessness prevention efforts.

References

Aldridge, R. (2020) Homelessness: A barometer of social justice. *Lancet Public Health*, 5, e2–e3.

Batterham, D. (2017) Defining "At-risk of Homelessness": Re-connecting Causes, Mechanisms and Risk. *Housing, Theory and Society*, 36, 1–24.

Baxter, A. J., Tweed, E. J., Katikireddi, S. V. & Thomson, H. (2019) Effects of Housing First approaches on health and well-being of adults who are homeless or at risk of homelessness: Systematic review and meta-analysis of randomised controlled trials. *Journal of Epidemiology and Community Health*, 73, 379–387.

Choy-Brown, M., Tiderington, E., Tran Smith, B., Padgett, D. K. & Stefancic, A. (2021) Strategies for sustaining fidelity: A multi-state qualitative analysis in housing first programs. *Administration and Policy in Mental Health*, 48, 36–45.

Cunningham, M. J. & Slade, A. (2019) Exploring the lived experience of homelessness from an occupational perspective. *Scandinavian Journal of Occupational Therapy*, 26, 19–32.

Gabrielian, S., Young, A. S., Greenberg, J. M. & Bromley, E. (2018) Social support and housing transitions among homeless adults with serious mental illness and substance use disorders. *Psychiatric Rehabilitation Journal*, 41, 208–215.

Gutwinski, S., Schreiter, S., Deutscher, K. & Fazel, S. (2021) The prevalence of mental disorders among homeless people in high-income countries: An updated systematic review and meta-regression analysis. *PLOS Medicine*, 18, e1003750.

Hossain, M. M., Sultana, A., Tasnim, S., Fan, Q., Ma, P., Mckyer, E. L. J. & Purohit, N. (2020) Prevalence of mental disorders among people who are homeless: An umbrella review. *International Journal of Social Psychiatry*, 66, 528–541.

Illman, S. C., Spence, S., O'Campo, P. J. & Kirsh, B. H. (2013) Exploring the occupations of homeless adults living with mental illnesses in Toronto. *Canadian Journal of Occupational Therapy*, 80, 215–223.

Marshall, C., Cooke, A., Holmes, J., Bengall, J., Aryobi, S., Phillips, B., Lysaght, R. & Gewurtz, R. (2024a) "It's like your days are empty and yet there's life all around": A mixed methods, multi-site study exploring boredom during and following homelessness. *PLoS One*, *19*(5), 1–25.

Marshall, C. A., Boland, L., Westover, L. A., Goldszmidt, R., Bengall, J., Aryobi, S., Isard, R., Easton, C. & Gewurtz, R. (2022a) Effectiveness of employment-based interventions for persons experiencing homelessness: A systematic review. *Health & Social Care in the Community*, 30, 2142–2169.

Marshall, C. A., Boland, L., Westover, L. A., Marcellus, B., Weil, S. & Wickett, S. (2020a) Effectiveness of interventions targeting community integration among individuals with lived experiences of homelessness: A systematic review. *Health & Social Care in the Community*, 28, 1843–1862.

Marshall, C. A., Boland, L., Westover, L. A., Wickett, S., Roy, L., Mace, J., Gewurtz, R., Barbic, S. & Kirsh, B. (2020b) Occupational experiences of homelessness: A systematic review and meta-aggregation. *Scandinavian Journal of Occupational Therapy*, 27, 394–407.

Marshall, C. A., Cooke, A., Gewurtz, R., Barbic, S., Roy, L., Ross, C., Becker, A., Lysaght, R. & Kirsh, B. (2023a) Bridging the transition from homelessness: Developing an occupational therapy framework. *Scandinavian Journal of Occupational Therapy*, 30, 953–969.

Marshall, C. A., Cooke, A., Holmes, J., Bengall, J., Aryobi, S., Phillips, B., Lysaght, R. & Gewurtz, R. (2024b) "It's like your days are empty and yet there's life all around": A mixed methods, multi-site study exploring boredom during and following homelessness. *PlOS One*, 19, e0302900.

Marshall, C. A., Easton, C., Phillips, B., Boland, L., Isard, R., Holmes, J., Shanoff, C., Hawksley, K., Landry, T., Goldszmidt, R., Aryobi, S., Plett, P. & Oudshoorn, A. (2022b) Experiences of transitioning from homelessness: A systematic review and meta-aggregation of qualitative studies conducted in middle to high income countries. *Journal of Social Distress and Homelessness*, *33*(1), 28–49.

Marshall, C. A., Gewurtz, R., Ross, C., Becker, A., Cooke, A., Roy, L., Barbic, S., Lysaght, R. & Kirsh, B. (2022c) Beyond Securing a tenancy: Using the capabilities approach to identify the daily living needs of individuals during and following homelessness. *Journal of Social Distress and Homelessness*, 33, 81–95.

Marshall, C. A., Lysaght, R. & Krupa, T. (2018) Occupational transition in the process of becoming housed following chronic homelessness: *Canadian Journal of Occupational Therapy*, 85, 33–45.

Marshall, C. A., Phillips, B., Holmes, J., Todd, E., Hill, R., Panter, G., Easton, C., Landry, T., Collins, S., Greening, T., O'Brien, A., Jastak, M., Ridge, R., Goldszmidt, R., Shanoff, C., Laliberte Rudman, D., Carlsson, A., Aryobi, S., Perez, S. & Oudshoorn, A. (2022d) 'We stick people in a house and say okay, you're housed. The problem is solved': A qualitative study of service provider and organisational leader perspectives on thriving following homelessness. *Health & Social Care in the Community*, 30, e6018–e6029.

Marshall, C. A., Phillips, B., Holmes, J., Todd, E., Hill, R., Panter, G., Easton, C., Landry, T., Collins, S., Greening, T., O'Brien, A., Jastak, M., Ridge, R., Goldszmidt, R., Shanoff, C., Laliberte Rudman, D., Carlsson, A., Aryobi, S., Szlapinski, J., Carrillo-Beck, R., Pacheco, N., Perez, S. & Oudshoorn, A. (2023b) "I can't remember the last time I was comfortable about being home": Lived experience perspectives on thriving following homelessness. *International Journal of Qualitative Studies on Health and Well-being*, 18, 2176979.

Marshall, C. A., Roy, L., Becker, A., Nguyen, M., Barbic, S., Tjörnstrand, C., Gewurtz, R. & Wickett, S. (2019) Boredom and homelessness: A scoping review. *Journal of Occupational Science*, 27, 107–124.

O'Neill, B. (2014) Cast aside: Boredom, downward mobility, and homelessness in post-communist bucharest. *Cultural Anthropology*, 29, 8–31.

Plett, P., Oudshoorn, A., Gewurtz, R., Forchuk, C., Kfrerer, M., Perez, S., Easton, C. & Marshall, C. A. (2023) Experiences of belonging following homelessness: A systematic review and meta-aggregation. *Journal of Social Distress and Homelessness, 33*(2), 551–569.

Pophaim, J. P. & Peacock, R. (2021) Pathways into and out of homelessness: Towards a strategic approach to reducing homelessness. *Acta Criminologica: African Journal of Criminology & Victimology*, 34, 68–87.

Ramsay, N., Hossain, R., Moore, M., Milo, M. & Brown, A. (2019) Health care while homeless: Barriers, facilitators, and the lived experiences of homeless individuals accessing health care in a Canadian Regional Municipality. *Qualitative Health Research*, 29, 1839–1849.

Shinn, M. & Khadduri, J. (2020) *In the Midst of Plenty: Homelessness and What to Do about It*, John Wiley & Sons.

Thomas, Y., Gray, M. A. & McGinty, S. (2017) The occupational wellbeing of people experiencing homelessness. *Journal of Occupational Science*, 24, 181–192.

Tsemberis, S. (2010) *Housing First: The Pathways Model to End Homelessness for People with Mental Illness and Addiction Manual*. Hazeldon, Center City.

Warburton, K. & Stahl, S. M. (2020) Balancing the pendulum: Rethinking the role of institutionalization in the treatment of serious mental illness. *CNS Spectrums*, 25, 115–118.

Woodhall-Melnik, J. R. & Dunn, J. R. (2015) A systematic review of outcomes associated with participation in Housing First programs. *Housing Studies*, 31, 287–304.

6

INDIVIDUAL STRATEGIES FOR SUPPORTING FUNCTION AND PARTICIPATION IN DAILY LIFE

Leonie Boland

Individuals experiencing homelessness tend to have complex health needs that place significant challenges on their functional ability and ability to participate in daily life. This chapter outlines some of the challenges faced during and following homelessness to provide an understanding from an individual perspective. Guided by the Bridging to Transition framework, person-centred strategies to optimize the function and participation of individuals across the trajectory of homelessness are presented. Understanding function and supporting the development of strategies, habits or routines for individuals can facilitate optimal performance in meaningful activities, which have the potential to enhance well-being and create a sense of belonging following homelessness.

Component of the Bridging the Transition Framework Addressed in this Chapter

This chapter provides an overview of strategies that can be used to prevent homelessness by supporting function and participation in daily life with *individuals* during and following homelessness. By 'individual level', this part of the framework emphasizes support that can be provided across the trajectory of unhoused to housing that is focused on an individual person, as opposed to strategies for working with communities and populations (see Figure 6.1).

DOI: 10.4324/9781003541332-8

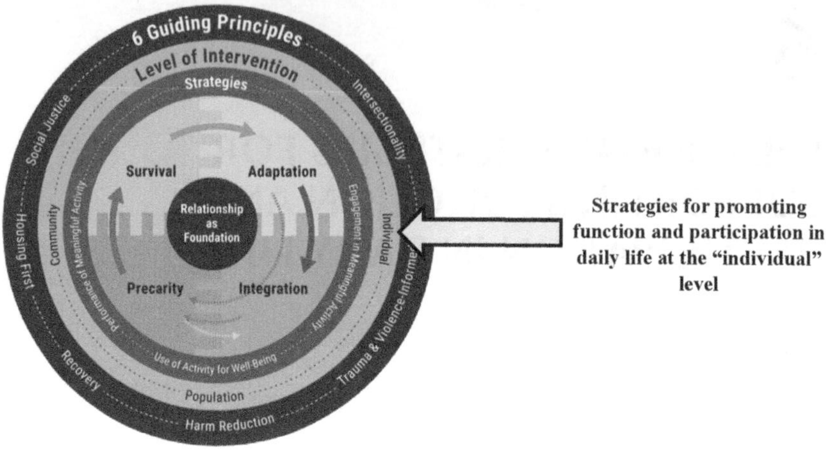

FIGURE 6.1 Individual-Level Strategies.

How this Chapter Guides Practice and Research in Homelessness Prevention

This chapter draws attention to the complexity of challenges faced by individuals within the homeless system, as well as those transitioning from homelessness into their own tenancies. It presents individual-level strategies for supporting function and participation in daily life across the trajectory of unhoused to housing to support homelessness prevention. Working with individuals is central to everyday practice within homelessness, and this chapter offers guidance to support meaningful activity participation. Guided by the Bridging to Transition framework, it explores person-centred strategies to optimize performance in daily activities by considering barriers and enablers to function. It offers practical strategies and approaches to increase engagement in meaningful activities for individuals caught in the cycle of homelessness.

The evidence base for these individual strategies in practice would benefit from development. Research could inform how best to measure meaningful activity participation outcomes in practice and help design studies, in partnership with individuals with lived experience and practitioners, to measure effectiveness.

Introduction

Homelessness is a complex and multifaceted social issue, experienced by a growing number of individuals internationally. Nearly nine of out ten adults experiencing homelessness have been exposed to at least one Adverse Childhood Experience (ACE)—early traumas that occur during childhood which are a strong risk factor for poor health and functioning—and over half have been exposed to four or more ACEs (Liu et al., 2021). The extreme health disparities faced by people using homelessness services have been well documented. They include a higher prevalence of acute and chronic mental and physical co-occurring conditions, higher rates of substance use disorders and a significantly shortened life expectancy (Fazel et al., 2014; Vallesi et al., 2021). For example, women experiencing homelessness are disproportionally affected by health issues (Aldridge et al., 2018) and have a higher prevalence of disability in comparison to women who are housed (Guillén et al., 2021). Compounding these complex health challenges and contributing to a higher risk of morbidity and premature mortality are structural barriers to accessing healthcare, e.g. availability, inflexible and poorly coordinated services (Siersbaek et al., 2021).

These complex factors can present significant challenges to a person's function and participation in daily life, which may precipitate and prolong homelessness. High rates of cognitive difficulties (Stone et al., 2019), traumatic brain injury (McMillan et al., 2015) and neurodiversity (Osborn & Young, 2024) have been found in studies of adults experiencing homelessness. These, in addition to childhood trauma, mental illness and alcohol and substance use, can affect an individuals' executive functioning. In everyday life, this contributes to individuals struggling to plan, problem solve and follow through on goals, which can be fundamental to using support services and moving on from homelessness.

Persons who experience homelessness are not a homogeneous group. Their pathways into and out of homelessness vary, are dynamic and non-linear. As outlined in the Bridging the Transition Framework, leaving homelessness has four distinct processes: survival, adaptation, integration and precarity. Each stage presents unique challenges to individuals, which are faced on a daily basis. In this chapter, some of these challenges are outlined before providing examples of strategies at an individual level to support function and participation across the trajectory of homelessness. It is informed by clinical experiences working for over fifteen years as an occupational therapist within homelessness services. Although the focus of this chapter is on strategies at an individual level, the role of social and structural systems in providing opportunities and influencing choices is acknowledged.

Reality of Daily Life during and following Homelessness

There is a significant body of literature illustrating how extremely difficult participating in everyday life can be for people within the homelessness system, as well as for those transitioning into their own tenancies. Studies describe the functional and participation experiences of people using homelessness services (Marshall et al., 2020a), experiences of refugees experiencing homelessness (Kaur et al., 2021), transgender people experiencing homelessness (McCann & Brown, 2021) and experiences of individuals transitioning from homelessness (Marshall et al., 2024a).

During the *survival* process, individuals are unhoused and may be sleeping rough, sofa surfing or in emergency shelters. This placement can be of assorted duration, provided without meaningful consideration of individual needs and have assorted staffing levels. In reality, adults may have to share rooms with a lack of personal space and have limited access to food preparation areas or food choices. Studies have clearly shown how time can be focused on survival occupations, including the use of services to meet basic needs (Cunningham & Slade, 2019), or depending on emergency services for health needs (Vohra et al., 2022). People can experience boredom, with its negative influence on well-being (Marshall et al., 2024b), and use substances for coping and structuring time (Marshall et al., 2020b). There can be a sense of feeling 'stuck' as individuals find themselves in the survival process for longer than expected (Boland, 2018).

When a person moves into independent or long-term supported accommodation, there is a process of *adaptation*. Although this is often the goal of housing services and what has been hoped for, it can take time to adjust. It is only the beginning of a process of rediscovering self (Marshall et al. 2024a). In reality, a tenancy can be a quiet and sometimes lonely place, in which new everyday routines need to be developed. Finding new or participating in existing meaningful activities can support the development of identity, belonging and connection, fundamental to *integration* (Boland et al., 2023). With a safe and secure tenancy providing the necessary foundation, the process of *integration* over time differs between individuals (Marshall et al., 2024a). Maintaining a focus on participation in daily meaningful activities, e.g. work, education, community services, provides a scaffold for individuals to build/re-build lives and thrive following homelessness.

As mentioned earlier, leaving homelessness is not a linear trajectory, and *precarity* is the risk of tenancy loss. It brings instability, increased anxiety, disruption to existing routines as well as the risk of returning to previous coping strategies that can put the ongoing tenancy at risk, e.g. substance use, avoiding meetings, concealing difficulties (Boland et al., 2023).

Individual Strategies for Supporting Participation

Central to all these processes is an individual, with their unique values, skills, strengths, challenges, health, trauma histories, interests, habits, hopes, sensory preferences, executive functioning, etc. All these aspects contribute to how a person functions in everyday life and participates on a daily basis, how they negotiate services and how they use opportunities and supports. Any approach to help people during or following homelessness must be person-centred, informed by the individual's unique strengths and difficulties and adapted for their specific context, e.g. survival, adaptation, etc. Given that leaving homelessness can be a complex process, individuals may have already struggled to transition from homelessness to being housed, and these past experiences may influence their current participation.

The Bridging the Transition framework outlines three strategies to support the process of leaving homelessness:

1 Support the person to increase engagement in meaningful activities
2 Support optimal performance in daily activities
3 Engage individuals in meaningful activities as a way of optimizing emotional, cognitive, physical and social well-being.

These strategies bring a functional and participation perspective—a focus on time use, meaningful activities, function, participation, engagement in 'doing' for well-being—largely overlooked in existing homelessness services. The following section will describe each one.

1 Support the person to increase engagement in meaningful activities

The disabling experience of homelessness and the reality of using services to meet basic needs mean that meaningful activity engagement can be a low priority. Individuals may have lost a sense of what they previously enjoyed or no longer have access to resources or places to carry out activities. Mental or physical health difficulties and substance use can present additional challenges. Engagement in activities that are subjectively meaningful to a person—based on their interests, values, past experiences, culture—cannot simply be prescribed.

Strategies to increase engagement to support participation include:

a Explore what is meaningful to the individual.
b Gauge what level of support and/or resources are necessary to facilitate engagement.
c Match the support to the person to increase engagement in meaningful activities.

a Explore what is meaningful to the individual.

This may be done through the completion of an Interest Checklist (University of Illinois, 2020) or Engagement in Meaningful Activities Survey (Eakman, 2012) but can also be gained from a conversation, listening to narratives, sourcing clues from passing comments or visuals, e.g. phone screensaver, tattoo. The process of identifying interests of meaning can take several sessions. It is enhanced by a trusting relationship and is informed by being clear about the link between engaging in doing and well-being. Remaining non-judgemental and curious about the meaning of non-health promoting activities is important in this process (Boland et al., 2020).

Balancing the skill and challenge level of a meaningful activity—the 'just-right' challenge—can enhance curiosity to try and provide an opportunity for the individual to demonstrate abilities and experience success. Engaging in an activity that provides a sense of control, complete concentration and distortion of time perception—a flow experience—can support well-being (Csikszentmihalyi, 1997). Also doing together can provide a chance to build rapport and groundwork for future work to support participation. Throughout all, maintaining a trauma-informed approach is critical (Wiewel & Hernandez, 2022). It is important to keep in mind that some individuals, due to socio-economic and socio-cultural factors, have had limited opportunities for engagement or have had their activity patterns and functional and participatory development disrupted long before becoming unhoused. Therefore, exploring what is meaningful may be challenging.

During and following homelessness, the process of exploring what is meaningful will remain similar. A home, however, provides the stability to reflect more deeply and allow for emotional and spiritual growth (Marshall et al., 2024a).

b Gauge what level of support and/or resources are necessary to facilitate engagement.

Through assessment and maintaining a strengths-based approach, a sense of the enablers and barriers to engagement can be identified. Barriers can include a lack of opportunity or resources, specific functional difficulties, e.g. physical, social, process and substance use. This can be explored in conversation, but a more complete understanding will be gained from observing the person carrying out activities or doing them together. Recognizing a person's readiness for change will also help inform the approach to facilitate engagement.

Despite a personal readiness for change, context is critical for achieving and maintaining change (Lord et al., 2021). Pragmatically, during the survival and adaptation processes, this may mean providing resources or being creative with limited supplies to facilitate engagement. Having a tenancy may allow more opportunities for doing, but personal factors always need to be considered.

c Match the support to the person to increase engagement in meaningful activities.

Remove as many external barriers to participation as possible, e.g., source services and resources if needed, offer choice on location and times, design individual or group-based activities and adapt the activity, e.g. reduce

TABLE 6.1 Strategies to Support Participation in the Gym

Example of strategies to support participation in the meaningful activity of going to the gym: • For the person who has the skills and confidence to attend but has limited resources—a reduced membership is negotiated with a public gym and they have an opportunity to buy necessities, e.g. lock, water bottle at a reduced rate from the service. • For the person who is unsure about committing but is interested, funding for one gym membership was sourced, which is shared between people on a monthly basis to help build the routine of going to gym. • For the person who has the skills but limited confidence, support is provided on a one-off visit to gain understanding of gym procedures, layout of changing rooms, etc. • For the person who benefits from regular support over a number of weeks to build confidence, support can be provided by a peer or assistant for an agreed number of weeks to build the habit of attending. • For the person who wants to go to the gym but requires 1:1 support, develop a one-hour weekly gym group, facilitated by a gym instructor and a health or social care provider.

complexity to encourage involvement initially. A full understanding of a person's strengths and challenges allows for the right level of support to facilitate participation. If a person is struggling to identify an area for change, motivational interviewing may be helpful (Miller & Rollnick, 2012), or a cognitive behavioural approach may help challenge unhelpful thoughts to allow participation (Donaghy et al., 2008). A more directive approach may be required initially for a person struggling with following directions, but this can become more facilitatory as engagement is increased or skills are developed. For others, a peer support relationship may be the 'just-right' match to increase engagement in meaningful activities (Marshall et al., 2020b).

This strategy needs regular review throughout all homelessness processes to ensure that support continues to align with the person's levels of needs and facilitates maintenance of participation.

Table 6.1 outlines different approaches to increase engagement in the meaningful activity of going to the gym.

Participation is enhanced by optimal performance in the activity, which is the second strategy of the Bridging to Transition framework.

2 ***Support optimal performance in daily activities.***

Understanding function and supporting the development of strategies, habits or routines can facilitate optimal performance in meaningful activities, which have the potential to rebuild a sense of identity and create a sense of belonging following homelessness (Marshall et al., 2024a). This is enabled by two key strategies:

a Collate a comprehensive person-centred assessment
b Support performance with strategies, habits and routines

a Collate a comprehensive person-centred assessment

Individuals can benefit from a person-centred comprehensive assessment to understand their skills, difficulties, habits and routines in the context of complex health and social care needs. This can include physical health factors, mental health, substance use and sensory preferences.

Health and social care professionals taking a functional and participation approach have a repertoire of assessment tools. Thoughtful consideration of their value, scheduling and limitations is important for their use during and following homelessness. Performance-based functional assessments can identify supports needed to transition into and maintain housing (Synovec et al., 2023). The assessment process can take time and may stretch over a number of sessions in various environments. Narrative interviewing builds trust and rapport. There is a risk that paperwork may put up barriers, but under the right circumstances it can be beneficial to help understand function. Keep a practical focus on doing and what is important and relevant to the person's current situation.

b Support performance with strategies, habits and routines

A comprehensive understanding of function provides the foundation for individualized skill and strategy development to support optimal performance. Skills for activities that people want to, or need to do, can be taught or practiced. Examples include pre-employment skills, education skills, maintaining a home, engaging in leisure and community resources, and organizational skills to access healthcare.

Together with skills, the use of strategies and routines supports performance in context. For example, functional cognition is the combination of a person's cognitive skills, with their use of strategies, habit and routines in the context of available resources (Synovec et al., 2023). Consider how to identify and develop routines that support participation, e.g. time of day to best get involved in a meaningful activity. A harm reduction approach will help individuals manage their use within the routines of their day by supporting engagement in meaningful activities.

Compensatory strategies can more easily be implemented within a person's own tenancy. They include environmental modifications (e.g. level access shower), environmental simplifications (e.g. keeping healthcare information together) and small devices (e.g. ear plugs in noisy rooms) to support optimal performance in daily activities to enhance well-being. Be mindful to match the strategy with the person's readiness for change, e.g. a self-management plan is helpful when the person has a sense of agency.

3 *Engage individuals in meaningful activities as a way of optimizing emotional, cognitive, physical and social well-being*

The experience of homelessness can contribute to boredom and the loss of recognizing the connection between doing and well-being. As described earlier, participation in meaningful activities has the potential to optimize well-being, build a sense of identity and create a sense of belonging and connection, all fundamental to preventing homelessness.

In the process of survival, well-being can be enhanced by doing personally meaningful activities. This practically means providing opportunities for engagement and being flexible, e.g. changing times or locations. Although the focus of engagement may be on the 'here and now', it provides a valuable opportunity to recognize strengths, identify hopes, build rapport and set the foundation for further plans.

A range of interventions have been developed internationally to support people to engage in meaningful activities, employment and integrate into their community. Systematic reviews synthesize the evidence on the effectiveness of interventions targeting community integration (Marshall et al., 2020b), meaningful activity participation (Marshall et al., 2024c), employment-based interventions (Marshall et al., 2022) and occupational therapy interventions (Marshall et al., 2021). These are varied in design and show mixed outcomes, but those demonstrating promise can be incorporated into service provision to support function and participation in daily life.

Conclusion

Engagement in activities that are subjectively meaningful to a person—based on their interests, values, past experiences—has the potential to rebuild a sense of identity and create a sense of belonging following homelessness. Practical strategies to support individuals to optimize their function and participation in meaningful activities are crucial to prevent homelessness. Strategies must be person-centred, informed by the person's unique strengths and difficulties, and adapted for their specific environmental context.

References

Aldridge, R. W., Story, A., Hwang, S. W., Nordentoft, M., Luchenski, S. A., Hartwell, G., … & Hayward, A. C. (2018). Morbidity and mortality in homeless individuals, prisoners, sex workers, and individuals with substance use disorders in high-income countries: A systematic review and meta-analysis. *The Lancet, 391*(10117), 241–250.

Boland, L. (2018). *Transitioning from homelessness into a sustained tenancy: What enables successful tenancy sustainment? (The Moving on Project)* (Doctoral dissertation, University of Plymouth).

Boland, L., Marshall, C. A., & Westover, L. A. (2020). Homelessness and occupation. In R. Twinley (Ed.), *Illuminating the Dark Side of Occupation* (pp. 57–64). Routledge.

Boland, L., Yarwood, R., & Bannigan, K. (2023). 'Making a home': An occupational perspective on sustaining tenancies following homelessness. *Housing Studies, 38*(7), 1239–1259.

Csikszentmihalyi, M. (1997). *Finding Flow: The Psychology of Engagement with Everyday Life*. Basic Books.

Cunningham, M. J., & Slade, A. (2019). Exploring the lived experience of homelessness from an occupational perspective. *Scandinavian Journal of Occupational Therapy, 26*(1), 19–32.

Donaghy, M., Nicol, M., & Davidson, K. M. (2008). *Cognitive Behavioural Interventions in Physiotherapy and Occupational Therapy*. Elsevier Health Sciences.

Eakman, A. M. (2012). Measurement characteristics of the engagement in meaningful activities survey in an age-diverse sample. *The American Journal of Occupational Therapy, 66*(2), e20–e29.

Fazel, S., Geddes, J. R., & Kushel, M. (2014). The health of homeless people in high-income countries: Descriptive epidemiology, health consequences, and clinical and policy recommendations. *The Lancet, 384*(9953), 1529–1540.

Guillén, A. I., Panadero, S., & Vázquez, J. J. (2021). Disability, health, and quality of life among homeless women: A follow-up study. *American Journal of Orthopsychiatry, 91*(4), 569.

Kaur, H., Saad, A., Magwood, O., Alkhateeb, Q., Mathew, C., Khalaf, G., & Pottie, K. (2021). Understanding the health and housing experiences of refugees and other migrant populations experiencing homelessness or vulnerable housing: A systematic review using GRADE-CERQual. *Canadian Medical Association Open Access Journal, 9*(2), E681–E692.

Liu, M., Luong, L., Lachaud, J., Edalati, H., Reeves, A., & Hwang, S. W. (2021). Adverse childhood experiences and related outcomes among adults experiencing homelessness: A systematic review and meta-analysis. *The Lancet Public Health, 6*(11), e836–e847.

Lord, A., Tickle, A., & Buckell, A. (2021). Change readiness in individuals experiencing homelessness and multiple complex needs. *Housing, Care and Support, 24*(1), 1–13.

Marshall, C. A., Boland, L., Westover, L. A., Goldszmidt, R., Bengall, J., Aryobi, S., … & Gewurtz, R. (2022). Effectiveness of employment-based interventions for persons experiencing homelessness: A systematic review. *Health & Social Care in the Community, 30*(6), 2142–2169.

Marshall, C. A., Boland, L., Westover, L. A., Isard, R., & Gutman, S. A. (2021). A systematic review of occupational therapy interventions in the transition from homelessness. *Scandinavian Journal of Occupational Therapy, 28*(3), 171–187.

Marshall, C. A., Boland, L., Westover, L. A., Marcellus, B., Weil, S., & Wickett, S. (2020b). Effectiveness of interventions targeting community integration among individuals with lived experiences of homelessness: A systematic review. *Health & Social Care in the Community*, *28*(6), 1843–1862.

Marshall, C. A., Boland, L., Westover, L. A., Wickett, S., Roy, L., Mace, J., … & Kirsh, B. (2020a). Occupational experiences of homelessness: A systematic review and meta-aggregation. *Scandinavian Journal of Occupational Therapy*, *27*(6), 394–407.

Marshall, C. A., Cooke, A., Holmes, J., Bengall, J., Aryobi, S., Phillips, B., … & Gewurtz, R. (2024b). "It's like your days are empty and yet there's life all around": A mixed methods, multi-site study exploring boredom during and following homelessness. *PLOS ONE*, *19*(5), e0302900.

Marshall, C. A., Easton, C., Javadizadeh, E., Holmes, J., Phillips, B., & Isard, R. (2024c). Effectiveness of interventions for meaningful activity participation in homelessness: A systematic review. *Canadian Journal of Occupational Therapy*, *91*(3), 256–271.

Marshall, C. A., Easton, C., Phillips, B., Boland, L., Isard, R., Holmes, J., … & Oudshoorn, A. (2024a). Experiences of transitioning from homelessness: A systematic review and meta-aggregation of qualitative studies conducted in middle to high income countries. *Journal of Social Distress and Homelessness*, *33*(1), 28–49.

McCann, E., & Brown, M. J. (2021). Homeless experiences and support needs of transgender people: A systematic review of the international evidence. *Journal of Nursing Management*, *29*(1), 85–94.

McMillan, T. M., Laurie, M., Oddy, M., Menzies, M., Stewart, E., & Wainman-Lefley, J. (2015). Head injury and mortality in the homeless. *Journal of Neurotrauma*, *32*(2), 116–119.

Miller, W. R., & Rollnick, S. (2012). *Motivational Interviewing: Helping People Change*. Guilford Press.

Osborn, E., & Young, R. (2024). Autistic and without a home: A systematic review and meta-ethnography of the presence and experiences of homelessness amongst autistic individuals. *Journal of Social Distress and Homelessness*, *33*(1), 10–27.

Siersbaek, R., Ford, J. A., Burke, S., Cheallaigh, C. N., & Thomas, S. (2021). Contexts and mechanisms that promote access to healthcare for populations experiencing homelessness: A realist review. *BMJ Open*, *11*(4), e043091.

Stone, B., Dowling, S., & Cameron, A. (2019). Cognitive impairment and homelessness: A scoping review. *Health & Social Care in the Community*, *27*(4), e125–e142.

Synovec, C., Boland, L., & Westover, L. (2023). Evaluation of functional cognition in people experiencing homelessness: A scoping review. *International Journal on Homelessness*, *3*(3), 302–338.

University of Illinois (2020). *Modified Interest Checklist*. https://moho-irm.uic.edu/productDetails.aspx?aid=38

Vallesi, S., Tuson, M., Davies, A., & Wood, L. (2021). Multimorbidity among people experiencing homelessness—insights from primary care data. *International Journal of Environmental Research and Public Health*, *18*(12), 6498.

Vohra, N., Paudyal, V., & Price, M. J. (2022). Homelessness and the use of emergency department as a source of healthcare: A systematic review. *International Journal of Emergency Medicine*, *15*(1), 32.

Wiewel, B., & Hernandez, L. (2022). Traumatic stress and homelessness: A review of the literature for practitioners. *Clinical Social Work Journal*, *50*(2), 218–230.

7

COMMUNITY-LEVEL STRATEGIES FOR SUPPORTING FUNCTION AND PARTICIPATION IN DAILY LIFE

Carrie Anne Marshall and Skye Barbic

Homelessness is shaped not only by the individual challenges that a person may experience during and following homelessness but also by forces that tend to vary from one community to another. Persons who experience homelessness face deep degrees of oppression and social exclusion which manifest differently in different communities, thereby necessitating the use of approaches that are uniquely attuned to the local context. Creating welcoming community spaces for persons who are leaving homelessness has the potential to contribute to homelessness prevention efforts by providing a foundation for function and participation in daily life, and ultimately, community integration.

Component of the Bridging the Transition Framework Addressed in this Chapter

This chapter provides an overview of strategies that can be used to prevent homelessness by supporting function and participation in daily life with *communities* during and following homelessness. By "community level", this part of the framework emphasizes support that can be provided across the trajectory of unhoused to housing that is designed and delivered in collaboration with communities instead of individuals and populations (see Figure 7.1).

How this Chapter Guides Practice and Research in Homelessness Prevention

In this chapter, we provide an introduction for practitioners, researchers, and policymakers on strategies for preventing homelessness using

DOI: 10.4324/9781003541332-9

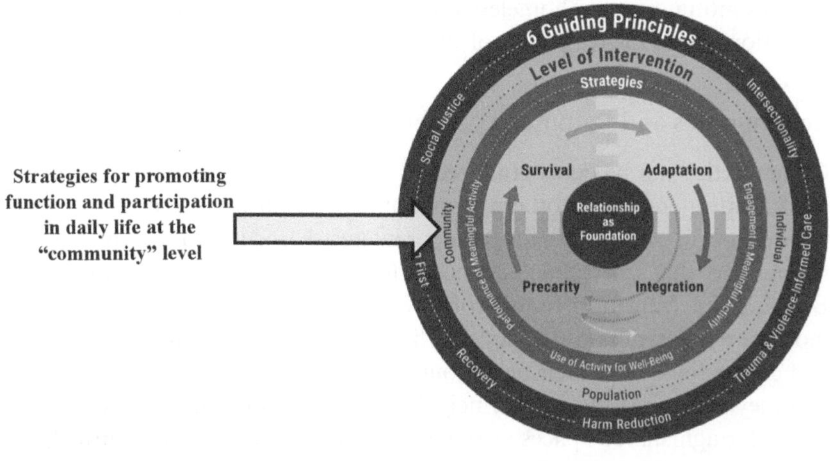

FIGURE 7.1 Community-Level Strategies.

community-level approaches that create the conditions for function and participation in daily life. Homelessness is not an individual or family problem but is often the consequence of problematic policies that have been implemented in a community or across a population, and for this reason, strategies for preventing homelessness need to be targeted at these levels. Further, the conditions in which many people with experiences of homelessness live are frequently determined by the community contexts in which they are situated – interpersonally and structurally. To create the conditions that can promote function and participation, and prevent ongoing homelessness, interventions that create inclusive communities are needed.

Introduction

The communities in which a person is embedded during and following homelessness can strongly influence their ability to function and participate in daily life. The availability of needed resources such as health and social care services, opportunities for social connection, access to basic needs such as affordable housing, food, and clothing, combined with local policies that directly affect the lives of unhoused, recently housed, and precariously housed individuals, is frequently determined within a single community. In contrast to population-level approaches in the Bridging the Transition Framework, which emphasizes the use of strategies relevant across multiple communities or municipalities, community-level strategies focus on single municipalities, neighbourhoods, or groups of people who come together around a common interest. In this chapter, we will describe a range of strategies that can be used for assessment and intervention with communities to increase their capacity for preventing ongoing homelessness through supporting function and participation across the trajectory of unhoused to housing.

Communities and Community-Level Approaches

Communities can be conceptualized as physical spaces in which people live, work, and interact with others. Communities can also be thought of as the various social, cultural, professional, or interest-based groups to which people belong and that can fulfil their needs for interpersonal connection. In the Bridging the Transition Framework, we recognize that people often occupy more than one community. They may have a neighbourhood in which they live and connections with their neighbours, but they may also have communities that they access outside of their neighbourhood. People often access communities through shared spaces, activities, online platforms, social networks, or common interests that connect them to others. While the communities that we are a part of vary across individuals, they are essential for our well-being (McNamara et al., 2021).

Often, people who experience homelessness face profound social exclusion due to the stigma of homelessness (Reilly et al., 2022), poverty (Inglis et al., 2022), and mental illness (Snow-Hill et al., 2024), and the inability to participate fully in their communities due to lack of financial resources to facilitate community engagement (Marshall et al., 2024a). The criminalization of homelessness (Herring, 2021) and the ongoing and repeated removal of homeless encampments despite a lack of available shelter beds and housing in many communities (Olson and Pauly, 2021) only deepen the feeling of social exclusion that many unhoused and previously unhoused people experience. The stigma of homelessness, mental illness, and substance use frequently layer over one another to contribute to deep degrees of oppression and exclusion during and following homelessness (Marshall et al., 2022, Marshall et al., 2023). During homelessness, individuals often find a sense of belonging in shelters, encampments, and the street but frequently struggle to attain these connections once they have been housed following homelessness (Marshall et al., 2024a, Plett et al., 2023). For many, this leads to feelings of wanting to leave their tenancies in search of the belonging that they once had access to while unhoused (Marshall et al., 2022, Marshall et al., 2023). Creating communities that include welcoming and inclusive spaces and social possibilities for individuals during and following homelessness is therefore an essential homelessness prevention and health promotion strategy.

Conducting Community-Level Assessments

To inform strategies implemented at the community level, approaches for identifying current strengths, challenges, and/or needs in the community can be useful. There are a range of approaches used to assess community strengths and needs for informing community-level solutions for homelessness prevention. The most common approaches include needs assessments, community asset mapping, and relationship-focused assessment approaches. Individuals who are conducting community assessments frequently use one or more of these approaches in the conduct of community-level assessments. It is important to note that assessing communities differs significantly from individual assessments of a person or family experiencing homelessness, which focus on their specific circumstances, challenges, and goals to provide personalized support. Overall, such assessments seek to uncover broader patterns to identify collective gaps and strengths that affect the entire community.

Needs Assessments

The most common assessment strategy used across communities is a "needs assessment". Needs assessments involve a range of data collection approaches where information is gathered using surveys, focus groups, community-level administrative data, and/or individual interviews to identify the needs of a particular community. In the gap between what the state of a community is for people who experience homelessness and what it "should be" based on this assessment reveals the "needs" of that community (Sleezer et al., 2014). By identifying community needs, such an approach tends to be focused and efficient, making it an attractive assessment strategy for working across a community.

Community Asset Mapping

Out of concerns that needs assessments unduly focus on the deficits of communities, Kretzmann and McKnight introduced the concept of identifying only community assets in the conduct of community assessments (1993). This approach, associated with "Asset-Based Community Development (ABCD)", begins with an assessment strategy, where social actors in a community come together to identify a common objective. This is followed by collaborating on the creation of a visual map of the assets in the community that could be mobilized to meet the identified objective (ABCD Institute, 2025). ABCD is built on a strengths-based philosophy positing that all communities have strengths, and that greater effectiveness at promoting change can occur by focusing on the assets in a community rather than its deficits (McKnight and Block, 2012). See Figure 7.2 for an example of a community asset map.

Relationship-Focused Community Assessment Approaches

Consistent with the Bridging the Transition Framework, community development scholars emphasize the importance of building and maintaining relationships with communities as a foundation for the conduct of successful and sustainable community development projects (McKnight and Block, 2012, Kretzmann and McKnight, 1993, McKnight, 1995). Learning about communities by engaging meaningfully with the members of that community can provide an important foundation for not only community-level intervention but also for assessing community needs and assets.

An important strategy for beginning the process of assessing communities is through the act of storytelling (Born, 2014). By sharing stories with one another about experiences of community, we can begin to feel emotionally and socially united, while also identifying community challenges that are meaningful to address collaboratively (Born, 2012, Born, 2014). In his book on the importance of community conversations as a foundation for community development, Paul Born identifies a range of relationship-based strategies that can build community while assessing its assets and needs (Born, 2012). Five of the ten approaches described by Born are summarized in Table 7.1.

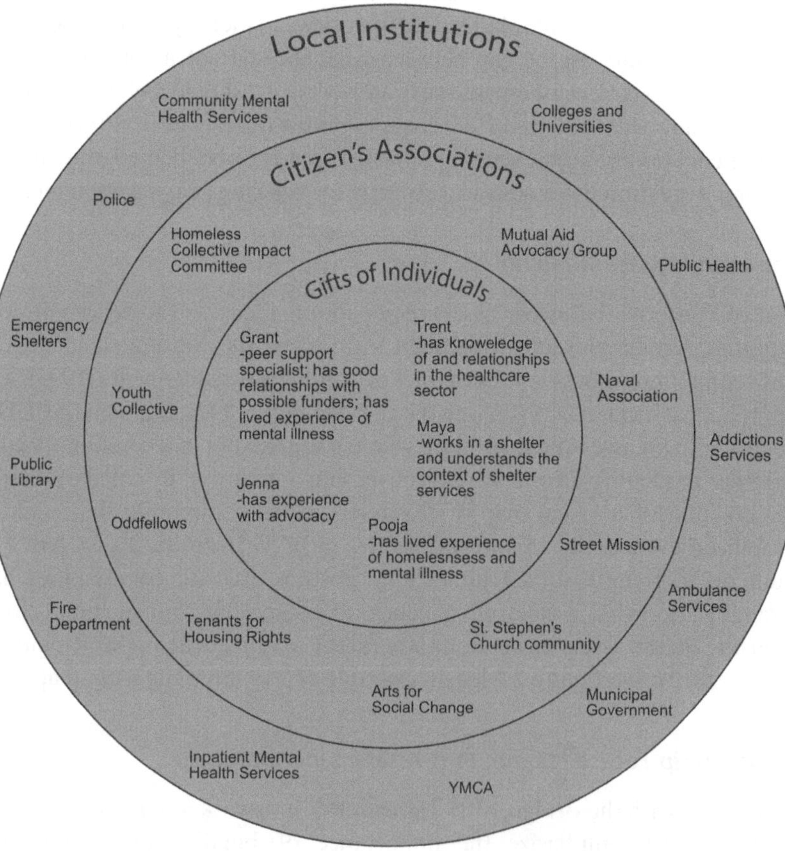

FIGURE 7.2 Community Asset Map.

TABLE 7.1 Key Relationship-Based Strategies for Understanding Community Needs and Assets

Strategy	*Description*
Conversation Café[1]	This approach involves posing questions to community members in a group setting and in an environment that is comfortable and hospitable. A conversation café is facilitated as follows: 1 Facilitators are placed at tables, the number of which corresponds to the number of questions that will be posed to participants, interest holders with knowledge of local issues. 2 Groups of 8–10 participants are then seated at a starting table where the facilitator poses a question regarding a social issue affecting participants' communities. The table facilitator encourages conversation among participants and records the conversation on large format paper. The conversation is allowed to proceed for a prescribed period of time (often 15–30 minutes). Participants at each table then shift to another table. 3 Once participants arrive at the next table, the facilitator begins by summarizing the discussion that occurred with the previous group(s) and then poses the new question to the new group. 4 This process continues until all participants have had an opportunity to visit each table. The number of questions that are posed is pre-determined, yet 2–3 questions are common. 5 Once participants have completed their discussions, facilitators at each of the tables summarize the conversations they heard across the groups. This is then presented back to the large group, who have an opportunity to provide additional context in a large group discussion. 6 A primary facilitator then engages the group in a collaborative discussion regarding how best to respond as a community to the findings of the conversation that unfolded.
Peer-to-Peer Conversations	Bringing together community members with decision-making capacity can be critical for identifying strategies for positive social change. In this structured conversation, a community leader is paired with another community leader (a peer) to discuss challenges that they are experiencing in manifesting planned initiatives. These two individuals discuss the issue that they are experiencing in front of a large group, sometimes with their chair turned away from the large group and one another to promote clearer thinking and comfort. The conversation is then facilitated by a group leader in the following manner: 1 ***Unpack (20 minutes)*:** During this part of the exercise, the person presenting the challenge discusses what they are experiencing. After this time has elapsed, the person who has just described the challenges they are experiencing asks a concrete question of their peers, who have been observing the conversation. 2 ***Question (20 minutes)*:** Peers in the large group are invited to ask clarifying questions of the participant. 3 ***Group discussion (30 minutes)*:** The peer group is invited to talk with one another about the question posed. The person who posed the question is discouraged from interrupting and is instead invited to listen. 4 ***Reflection (5–10 minutes)*:** The person who posed the question reflects on the process with the group.

(*Continued*)

TABLE 7.1 (Continued)

Strategy	*Description*
Top 100 Partners Exercise	In this exercise, participants in a community group identify influential community members with which to gather further information or partner on an initiative. The goal of this approach is to identify knowledge assets in the community that can be drawn upon during the assessment and implementation phases of community projects. The process unfolds in five steps: 1 ***Brainstorming a partner list*:** On a large paper or whiteboard, writing the names of people who may be influential regarding the initiative. 2 ***Rank the list by sector*:** The list of names is categorized by the group by sector. 3 ***Ranking the list by people*:** The names in the lists are ranked according to their level of influence and perceived willingness to partner. 4 ***Consider whom to approach first*:** Ranking the lists according to who to approach first, second, third, and so on. 5 ***Craft the "ask"*:** Decide as a group how you will contact each of the potential partners, and what information should be included in the invitation.
Food, Movies… and Conversations	This group of strategies emphasizes the use of food and movies to facilitate community conversations. As each of these approaches requires a pre-determined focus, we will list two strategies and illustrate each using the example of promoting food security for individuals during and following homelessness: 1 ***A progressive dinner*:** In this approach, the person(s) conducting the community assessment travels across a series of organizations where food is served, and conversations occur with each of these organizations over food. In the example of food insecurity following homelessness, the morning may consist of a conversation at a shelter where the person conducting the assessment eats food with shelter residents and staff while talking about community concerns. Following this, the person or group may go to a meal programme for lunch, followed by dinner at a permanent supportive housing community. During each of these meals, the person(s) conducting the assessment learns about the concerns of the community and assets that could be mobilized. 2 ***Movies*:** In this approach, a public viewing of a film is hosted by a community organization(s) for the purpose of inspiring conversation about a social issue in the community. To facilitate this approach, a movie is chosen that is provocative. The film is shown, usually in a comfortable environment with refreshments. Following the public viewing, a conversation about the social issue is facilitated with attendees. Using our example, the film could be a fiction or documentary film about the struggle to find nutritious food during and following homelessness. The facilitated conversation may then focus on how the issues depicted in the film correspond or deviate from the experiences of the community, and what assets could be mobilized to improve food security as a way of contributing to homelessness prevention efforts.

(*Continued*)

TABLE 7.1 (Continued)

Strategy	*Description*
Giving Voice to Photos[2,3]	This approach involves engaging community members in taking photographs of pressing social issues, followed by a public display of these photographs. Often, a conversation about the meaning of these photographs in relation to this social issue is facilitated during or following the public showing. This approach is used to: 1 Provide opportunities to describe the community's assets and challenges 2 Promote and elicit dialogue about community concerns 3 Engage policymakers so that they can bridge gaps between their perception of a community problem and the way that community members view the same problem. See Chapter 22 for an example of Photovoice used in revealing issues related to homelessness in the Global South

[1] Also known popularly as "World Café" (Brown and Isaacs, 2010).
[2] Born describes a range of strategies for using food and movies. We have provided only two examples here. We encourage readers to access Born's book for a more fulsome description of such strategies (Born, 2012).
[3] Also known popularly as "Photovoice" (Wang and Burris, 1997).

Community-Level Intervention Strategies

Once the community has identified, through an assessment process, the challenges that they would like to address, the contextual factors related to that challenge, and the assets that the community may have at their disposal, a range of strategies can be used for addressing these challenges. Jack Rothman, a social work scholar, has long identified three groups of strategies that can be used for community organizing (1974) that are still relevant today. These include locality development, social planning, and social action, which can be used as distinct approaches, and also in concert with one another (Rothman, 1974, Rothman, 1996).

Locality Development

Locality development is an approach to community organizing that is focused on bringing a range of community actors together who each have an interest in that community (Rothman, 1974). The philosophy underlying this approach is that members of a community each have an interest, knowledge, and assets to contribute to that community. Locality development strategies recognize that community resources can be organized in such a way that they create the conditions for mutual support and thriving for all involved. Such strategies aim to build the social and material capital of community members.

Examples of locality development related to homelessness prevention may include: creating resource sharing hubs where people with current or previous experiences of homelessness can access clothing and food to support their well-being; hosting a "living library" where people with experiences of homelessness share their personal stories directly with others in a structured, supportive format to create empathy and understanding between communities and persons with lived experiences of homelessness; building community gardens to improve food security and community connection for people who have been housed following homelessness; or developing local social businesses that provide opportunities for employment and social connection for individuals with histories of homelessness. For each of these examples, using a locality development approach means engaging persons with lived experiences of homelessness, service providers, advocates, and policymakers throughout the process of planning and implementation in order to gain support and resources for the success of such projects (Rothman, 1974).

Social Planning

Social planning is an approach that involves gathering and analysing data at a community level to inform needed changes in the community (Rothman, 1974). Instead of drawing on the expertise of persons with lived experiences of homelessness, service providers, and advocates, it instead draws on the expertise of researchers and policymakers who have expertise and access to data that may help to inform gaps and areas of saturation in community resources. This information is then used to inform policies, as well as the redirection and allocation of funding to programmes where gaps have been identified.

Examples of social planning related to homelessness prevention may be to: identify the amalgamated cost of supporting a person who is unhoused in emergency shelter, by-law enforcement, emergency room visits, ambulance costs, and criminal justice costs for a year in a given community, and comparing this with the cost of paying for permanent supportive housing to build an argument for funding more permanent supportive housing units; measuring indices of mental and social well-being among people with experiences of homelessness to inform the design of specialized mental health services; or interviewing people living with substance use disorders regarding their needs following homelessness to inform the re-design of permanent supportive housing services.

Social Action

When locality development and social planning fail to facilitate the conditions for preventing ongoing homelessness through the provision of housing, basic needs, and adequate services, there is often a need for placing political pressure on policymakers to act. Informed by a social justice philosophy, social action represents a series of strategies used to apply social force in order to communicate to decisionmakers the need for redistributing power and resources throughout a community (Rothman, 1974).

Examples of approaches that employ social action related to homelessness prevention include: writing an op-ed to a local paper highlighting ethical concerns associated with clearing encampments in a local community; presenting a city council delegation to provide information to city councillors regarding funding a permanent supportive housing complex; organizing a counter-protest against neighbours of a proposed permanent supportive housing community who are actively undermining attempts to establish this housing in their neighbourhood; and engaging the media in exposing the poor state of market housing available to people who are leaving homelessness.

Co-designing and Co-delivering Community-Level Approaches

Some of the community assessment and intervention approaches described in this chapter include the integration of persons with lived experience as an inherent component. Such approaches include: conversation or world cafés; food, movies, and conversations; photovoice; and locality development. All too often, however, we make decisions about persons with lived experiences of homelessness without asking them directly about their needs or including them in designing strategies that will affect their lives. Co-design is an approach that emphasizes a "nothing about us without us" mentality, where we meaningfully draw on the experiences of persons with lived experiences of homelessness, service providers, researchers, advocates, and policymakers to identify approaches based on knowledge gathered through a community assessment process (Donetto et al., 2015, Zamenopoulos and Alexiou, 2018). In a co-design approach, developmental and cultural needs must be considered to ensure that solutions are age-appropriate, contextually relevant, and respectful of a community's values, identities, and lived experiences.

Developing novel approaches in a community by drawing on the expertise of everyone whose lives will be affected by a policy change or practice innovation can promote trust in decisionmakers that they care about these perspectives and are willing to collaborate with individuals in the communities in which they work. A common pitfall in community-level work involving co-design is only inviting people who are perceived to be complacent, thereby "tokenizing" their involvement in the process. Instead, the best individuals to invite to projects involving co-design are people who have lived experience, experience in providing services, researchers, and policymakers who are collaborative and willing to challenge the status quo. When delivering these projects, leaders need to be prepared for disagreement and welcome opposing views and perspectives in a safe way in order to create solutions that are relevant for the communities in which they work.

One example of a co-design process focused on homelessness prevention was conducted by Marshall et al. (2024b). This project was a community-based participatory research study involving a community advisory board comprised of persons with lived experiences of homelessness, service providers, and organizational leaders in two mid-sized cities in Ontario, Canada (Hacker, 2013). The first part of the project involved a consultation with persons with lived experiences of homelessness, service providers, and organizational leaders regarding their perspectives on what individuals need to "thrive" following homelessness (Marshall et al., 2021a, Marshall et al., 2021b). This consultation revealed a gap in support following homelessness that could facilitate community integration. Information generated in this consultation was then used as a foundation for co-designing an intervention, called the Peer to Community (P2C) model, to support people leaving homelessness to integrate in their communities through meaningful activity engagement and relationship building. The model involves services facilitated by peer support specialists, social work, and occupational therapy (Marshall et al., 2024b). The community advisory board for this project co-designed the model itself, a fidelity measure, and educational modules for staff who would deliver the intervention in research evaluating this approach. The community advisory board then obtained funding to pilot the P2C model in one community, and the intervention was piloted between 2022 and 2024. Based on the findings of this pilot, the community advisory board will soon embark on making refinements to the P2C model. Throughout this entire process, persons with lived experience, service providers, and organizational leaders were meaningfully engaged – from designing research questions, conducting research interviews, presenting the findings of the consultation, to the public to co-designing all aspects of the intervention.

Conclusion

Community-level approaches move beyond focusing on individuals and families in homelessness prevention efforts and instead focus on understanding the contributions of communities to the perpetuation of ongoing homelessness. A range of approaches for assessing and intervening at the community level are available and can be used separately or in concert with one another. The language provided by the Bridging the Transition Framework may be useful for articulating how the community can be incorporated into strategies for improving the social contexts of people who are leaving homelessness. The profound social exclusion brought on by stigma and poverty means that working with communities to cultivate environments that are inclusive and supportive of people who are leaving homelessness is an essential component of any approach designed for homelessness prevention.

References

ABCD Institute (2025) *Asset-Based Community Development Institute*. Available at: https://abcdinstitute.org/ (Accessed: April 12, 2025).

Born, P. (2012) *Community conversations: Mobilizing the ideas, skills, and passion of community organizations, governments, businesses, and people*. Toronto: BPS Books.

Born, P. (2014) *Deepening community: Finding joy together in chaotic times*. San Francisco, CA: Berrett-Kohler.

Brown, J. & Isaacs, D. (2010) *The world café: Shaping our futures through conversations that matter*. San Francisco, CA: Berrett-Koehler.

Donetto, S., Pierri, P., Tsianakas, V. & Robert, G. (2015) 'Experience-based co-design and healthcare improvement: Realizing participatory design in the public sector', *The Design Journal*, 18(2), pp. 227–248.

Hacker, K. (2013) *Community based participatory research*. Los Angeles, CA: Sage.

Herring, C. (2021) 'Complaint-oriented "services": Shelters as tools for criminalizing homelessness', *The ANNALS of the American Academy of Political and Social Science*, 693, pp. 264–283.

Inglis, G., Jenkins, P., McHardy, F., Sosu, E. & Wilson, C. (2022) 'Poverty stigma, mental health, and well-being: A rapid review and synthesis of quantitative and qualitative research', *Journal of Community & Applied Social Psychology*, 33, pp. 783–806.

Kretzmann, J. & McKnight, J. (1993) *Building communities from the inside out: A path toward finding and mobilizing a community's assets*. Chicago: ACTA Publications.

Marshall, C. et al. (2021a) *"We need to genuinely listen to what people tell us they need": Identifying how to support individuals living with mental illness and/or substance use difficulties to thrive following homelessness in London, Ontario*. London, ON: Western University.

Marshall, C. et al. (2021b) *Beyond surviving: Identifying how to support individuals living with mental illness and/or substance use difficulties to thrive following homelessness in Kingston, Ontario*. London, ON: Social Justice in Mental Health Research Lab, Western University.

Marshall, C. et al. (2022) '"We stick people in a house and say okay, you're housed. The problem is solved": A qualitative study of service provider and organisational leader perspectives on thriving following homelessness', *Health & Social Care in the Community*, *30*(6), e6018–e6029.

Marshall, C.A. et al. (2023) '"I can't remember the last time I was comfortable about being home": lived experience perspectives on thriving following homelessness', *International Journal of Qualitative Studies on Health and Well-being*, 18, pp. 2176979.

Marshall, C.A., Cooke, A., Holmes, J., Bengall, J., Aryobi, S., Phillips, B., Lysaght, R. & Gewurtz, R. (2024a) '"It's like your days are empty and yet there's life all around": A mixed methods, multi-site study exploring boredom during and following homelessness', *PLOS ONE*, 19, e0302900.

Marshall, C.A. et al. (2024b) 'Co-designing the "Peer to Community (P2C) Model": An intervention for promoting community integration following homelessness', *International Journal on Homelessness*, pp. 1–23.

McKnight, J. (1995) *The careless society: Community and its counterfeits*. New York: Basic Books.

McKnight, J. & Block, P. (2012) *The abundant community: Awakening the power of families and neighborhoods*. San Francisco, CA: Berrett-Koehler Publishers.

McNamara, N. et al. (2021) 'Community identification, social support, and loneliness: The benefits of social identification for personal well-being', *British Journal of Social Psychology*, 60, pp. 1379–1402.

Olson, N. & Pauly, B. (2021) 'Homeless encampments: Connecting public health and human rights', *Canadian Journal of Public Health*, 112, pp. 988–991.

Plett, P. et al. (2023) 'Experiences of belonging following homelessness: A systematic review and meta-aggregation', *Journal of Social Distress and Homelessness*, 33, pp. 551–569.

Reilly, J., Ho, I. & Williamson, A. (2022) 'A systematic review of the effect of stigma on the health of people experiencing homelessness', *Health & Social Care in the Community*, 30, pp. 2128–2141.

Rothman, J. (1974) 'Three models of community organization practice', In *Strategies of community organization*, edited by F. Cox, J. Erlich, J. Rothman & J. Tropman, Itasca, IL: Peacock Publishing.

Rothman, J. (1996) 'The interweaving of community intervention approaches', *Journal of Community Practice*, 3, pp. 69–100.

Sleezer, C.M., Russ-Eft, D.F. & Gupta, K. (2014) *A practical guide to needs assessment*. John Wiley & Sons.

Snow-Hill, N.L., Reeb, R.N. & Bell, J.S. (2024) 'The stigma of homelessness as a function of mental illness comorbidity', *Stigma and Health*, online ahead of print.

Wang, C. & Burris, M.A. (1997) 'Photovoice: Concept, methodology, and use for participatory needs assessment', *Health Education & Behavior*, 24, pp. 369–387.

Zamenopoulos, T. & Alexiou, K. (2018) *Co-design as collaborative research*. Bristol: Bristol University/AHRC Connected Communities Programme.

8

POPULATION-LEVEL STRATEGIES FOR SUPPORTING FUNCTION AND PARTICIPATION IN DAILY LIFE

Tracy Smith-Carrier

Using human rights and the social determinants of health and mental health as lenses, this chapter explores how homelessness prevention strategies that bolster income security, promote housing stability, and improve mental health and well-being can be valuable in advancing housing access and retention at the population level. People with lived/living experience of hardship, health and social care practitioners, community partners, researchers, and advocates must work together to catalyse a social movement that has the potency to prompt transformative social change. To ensure housing, health, and well-being for all, the material conditions and environments in which people lead their lives must be altered and better reflect equity and social justice.

Component of the Bridging the Transition Framework Addressed in this Chapter

This chapter provides an overview of strategies that can be used to prevent homelessness in *populations* during and following homelessness. By "population-level," this part of the framework emphasizes research and practices that can be used across the trajectory of unhoused to housing that are designed to address the structural causes of homelessness rather than individual- or community-level approaches (see Figure 8.1).

DOI: 10.4324/9781003541332-10

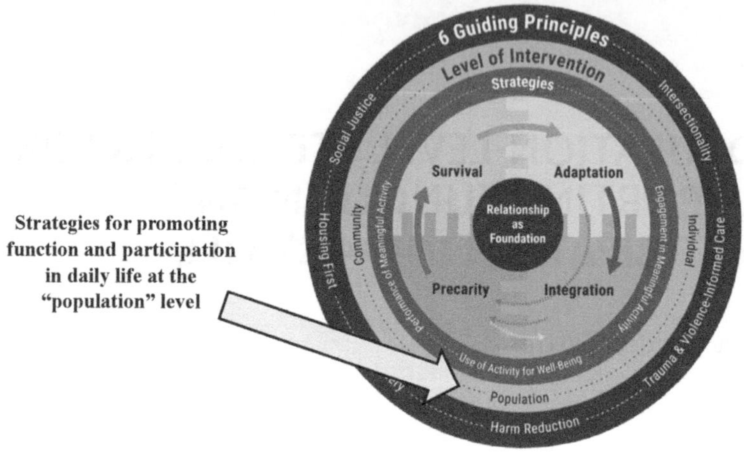

FIGURE 8.1 Population-Level Strategies.

How this Chapter Guides Practice, Research, and Policy in Homelessness Prevention

This chapter outlines valuable frameworks to anchor discussions about housing precarity and homelessness prevention, namely, human rights and the social determinants of health and mental health (SDoH and SDoMH). Researchers and health and social care practitioners are encouraged to recognize how income supports, housing and homelessness prevention strategies, and improved mental health and substance use services (built on harm reduction principles) can promote the SDoH and SDoMH, while also realizing the substantive human rights to housing, food, and an adequate standard of living. Recognizing the importance of these strategies at the population level, people with lived/living experience of hardship, non-profit leaders, researchers, practitioners, and advocates must band together to build a social movement that holds political actors accountable for their policy choices and rights infringements.

Introduction

This chapter explores homelessness prevention strategies aimed at improving income security, housing stability, and mental health and well-being at the population level. To anchor this discussion, we will first explore the lenses of substantive human rights, the SDoH and SDoMH, and consider how these can animate homelessness prevention strategies that promote and fulfil human rights, health equity, and social justice aims.

SDoH and SDoMH

Significant literature has amassed on the SDoH and their impacts on the health and well-being of populations broadly, and on equity-denied groups specifically (e.g., World Health Organization [WHO], 2008). The SDoH recognize that people's health is largely shaped by the material conditions and environments in which they lead their daily lives. They include: (a) income and income distribution, (b) education, (c) unemployment and job security, (d) employment and working conditions, (e) early childhood development, (f) food insecurity, (g) housing, (h) social exclusion, (i) social safety network, (j) health services, (k) Indigenous status, (l) gender, (m) race, and (n) disability (Mikkonen & Raphael, 2010). The WHO (n.d.) defines the SDoH as "the non-medical factors that influence health outcomes. They are the conditions in which people are born, grow, work, live, and age, and the wider set of forces and systems shaping the conditions of daily life" (para. 1). The WHO (2024) goes on to add "people's access to power, money and resources" (p. 1) as being central to contextualizing the SDoH.

Previous governmental and public health campaigns emphasized individual explanations of poverty and homelessness (i.e., "problems" inherent in the individual such as laziness, deficient work motivation, substance misuse, etc.) and fixated on shaping individual impulses and actions through behavioural modification techniques and nudges (Raphael, 2003). However, recent research shows that these social problems are largely structural and systemic in nature. Therefore, the perpetuation of poverty and homelessness is subject to, and contingent on, policy decisions made by state and sub-state actors (McCloskey, 2020). Of the many SDoH, income remains one of singular importance in influencing population health and well-being (Rachlis et al., 2013), and thus interventions aimed at ameliorating individuals' financial and social status should be of principal policy concern.

The SDoMH underscore how individual factors coalesce with structural, systemic, and environmental influences to intensify or reduce the risk and/or protective factors that promote mental illness or well-being (see Table 8.1). As differences in SDoMH largely develop from an unequal distribution of resources in society, they can therefore be redressed through social and economic policies that promote income and wealth redistribution (Alegría et al., 2018). While many of the constructs associated with the SDoMH align with those outlined in the SDoH literature, Handerer et al. (2022) find that they differ in relation to their etiological and epistemological orientations. The SDoH lean towards a focus on objective realities, whereas the SDoMH give greater attention to the perception of these realities.

TABLE 8.1 Social Determinants of Mental Health

Domains	*Proximal Factors*	*Distal Factors*
Demographic	Age, Gender, Ethnicity	Community Diversity, Population Density, Longevity, Survival
Economic	Income, Debt, Assets, Financial Strain, Relative Deprivation, Unemployment, Food Security	Economic Recessions, Economic Inequality, Macroeconomic Policy
Neighbourhood	Safety and Security, Housing Structure, Overcrowding, Recreation	Infrastructure, Neighbourhood Deprivation, Built Environment, Setting
Environmental Events	Trauma, Distress	Natural Disasters, Industrial Disasters, War or Conflict, Climate Change, Forced Migration
Social and Cultural	Individual Social Capital, Social Participation, Social Support, Education	Community Social Capital, Social Stability, Cultural

Adapted from Lund et al. (2018, p. 359); see also Smith-Carrier and Power (2025).

Human Rights

Although Canada has endorsed numerous human rights covenants and conventions since becoming one of the Founding Member States of the United Nations (Canada, 2024a) in 1945, social and economic rights (as well as cultural rights) have often been interpreted by political actors as having an aspirational texture. Consequently, UN Member States, including Canada, have often been quick to respect and protect such rights, but their policy actions to actively and robustly fulfil them have been sorely lacking. To do so, states would need to take direct measures, as they have committed to do, that apply the maximum of their available resources to progressively realize these rights. The courts have been reticent to mandate that state leaders comply with their rights obligations, given that these have been deemed to be policy matters, ones best addressed through actors afforded democratic legitimacy at the ballot box. At the same time, policymakers have, often by stealth, engaged various processes of neoliberalization that have reduced their involvement in health and social policy, and steadily decreased their budgetary expenditures (including income transfers and housing investments) to adequately fund them. Denied the accountability mechanisms that would hold state leaders responsible for their rights duties, social and economic rights, including the rights to housing, food, and an adequate standard of living, have been flagrantly violated or denied (Smith-Carrier & Manion, 2022).

While the right to housing has been identified in the National Housing Strategy Act (2019), it does not allow for individual claims to be enforced in court, and as such, it is not afforded the status of a constitutional right. The act does however provide some orientation to the practical implementation of the right to housing (Oren & Alterman, 2021) by legally enshrining the National Housing Strategy, forming the National Housing Council to advance housing policy, and creating the role of the independent, non-partisan Federal Housing Advocate to monitor and assess progress (Stadler & Collins, 2021). Regrettably, these measures have not necessitated that the federal government significantly step up its financial commitments to ensure dramatic increases in affordable and non-market housing stock in Canada.

When the National Housing Strategy was first announced in 2017, it included a $40 billion funding infusion and a commitment by the federal government to spend $75 billion over 10 years (Lee, 2022) to reduce chronic homelessness by 50%. Some, however, suggest that these numbers vastly exaggerate the financial expenditures actually allocated towards affordable housing over this time. Indeed, some argue that rather than applying federal resources to shore up the eroding non-market housing sector, the National Housing Strategy effectively enabled the ongoing financialization of Canada's housing market through the provision of low-interest loans to private developers seeking to build (more lucrative) market rental housing (Lee, 2022). Federal Budget 2024 did little to alleviate the worries of the non- or precariously housed, given the relentless preoccupation with increasing housing supply, providing little support to those being evicted, struggling to pay market rents, couch-surfing, or living rough on the streets (White & DiBellonia, 2024).

Income Supports for Homelessness Prevention

Policy innovations that provide people with greater income security can, alongside effective housing-related interventions, be valuable in preventing homelessness and promoting housing retention. Ample literature documents the benefits of a basic income guarantee (BIG) (e.g., Forget, 2018), also dubbed universal basic income (UBI), guaranteed annual income, citizen's wage, negative income tax, or unconditional cash transfers. Advocates in Canada generally employ the term BIG as it is associated with a specific form: a non-conditional benefit that is adequate (simply put, a liveable income), promotes dignity and autonomy, and is accessible to all who need it. It would thus act as an income replacement mechanism that is sensitive to individuals' income, i.e., decreasing the amount of the benefit as one's income increases to ensure greater equity (Basic Income Canada Network [BICN], 2023).

The *Consensus Statement on a Basic Income Guarantee* (BICN, 2023), crafted by BIG researchers and advocates across Canada, outlines the core elements (i.e., available to all residents and citizens aged 18–64; sufficient to cover basic needs and ensure no one falls into poverty; benefit amounts gradually reduced as other taxable income rises, paid to individuals on a regular schedule, etc.), design features (e.g., no behavioural conditionalities, developed in collaboration with the federal and provincial/territorial governments and Indigenous Peoples, etc.), possible interactions with other programmes (e.g., not as a replacement for other vital supports and services, etc.), and financing (e.g., promoting tax fairness and lowering income inequality) that the BIG movement is calling for. The BIG espoused here is income-tested and not a uniform (flat-rate) benefit available to everyone on the same terms (i.e., a universal demogrant model), as is commonly associated with the UBI model, which has garnered more rapt attention in the US. A BIG available to all, on the same terms, would likely yield a benefit of insignificant size, which for those with little to no forms of income (for reasons including parental leave, disability, etc.) would not be sufficient (Smith-Carrier, 2023).

Presently in Canada, we have forms of BIG that have proven to be advantageous in ameliorating poverty among specific groups. The suite of pension programmes, including Old Age Security (formerly a demogrant model before income clawbacks were introduced in 1989), a social insurance-oriented Canada/Quebec Pension Plan, and an income-tested Guaranteed Income Supplement, offers a clear policy success story in Canada (Béland & Marier, 2022) for BIG-like programmes (Emery et al., 2013). The income offered to older adults through pension programmes is meant to reduce poverty rates for this specific group, yet poverty, regrettably, continues to rise among older adults (Tabbara & Griffin, 2023) and all other demographic groups in Canada (Statistics Canada, 2024a).

Like the success of the BIG provided to older adults through Canada's pension programmes, significant changes were made in 2016 to improve Canada's child-tax benefits. At that time, the previous patchwork of tax-related benefits to families was transformed, jettisoning the Universal Child Care Benefit (a flat-rate benefit to parents of children under age 18), as well as the Canada Child Tax Benefit and National Child Benefit Supplement, in favour of one income-tested programme, the Canada Child Benefit (CCB). Providing a partial BIG to families, the CCB has been shown to be effective in reducing poverty for both single- and two-parent families alike (Baker et al., 2023). Partial BIG programmes (considered such because they are inadequate, are conditional, and/or not administered on a regular basis) have also been shown to be effective in reducing poverty. For example, the Canada Emergency Response Benefit, a temporary cash transfer to individuals, was beneficial in helping to financially stabilize the population during the Covid-19 pandemic (Statistics Canada, 2024b), despite some of its less-than-ideal design features (Burke, 2023).

A BIG, if provided at the population level at an adequate level, can eradicate poverty and address housing precarity by providing the wherewithal for people to more effectively manage their rent or mortgage payments. It would do so while also affording greater dignity (Hamilton & Mulvale, 2019) and less stigma (Calnitsky, 2016) to those receiving it, far more so than through existing social assistance programmes (Smith-Carrier, 2017). As food insecurity is invariably tied to income, offering an adequate BIG at the population level would also contribute to major reductions in hunger and food deprivation (Tarasuk, 2017).

Although a lacuna remains in the research on the efficacy of BIG programmes in meeting housing need specifically (Kerman, 2021), the literature is replete with studies documenting how BIG and its variants could be useful in promoting income security (Smith-Carrier & Green, 2017), a necessary condition for sustained housing tenure (Moore & Skaburskis, 2004). That said, simply providing more income to those who need it would not expressly address the speculation rife in the housing market, the intensifying soaring market rental and mortgage costs, or the dearth of non-market housing options in Canada. In addition to addressing income insufficiency, policies that remedy the other systemic causes of housing instability and homelessness are required.

De-Financialization and an Expansion of the Non-Market Housing Sector

A key concern reflected in many of Canada's housing strategies and initiatives has been about how to promote housing affordability, typically through, as noted, measures intended to increase housing supply. While some of these approaches have been valuable in creating more housing for Canadians, often of different type (e.g., congregate, individual unit, group homes, etc.) or form (e.g., apartments, townhouses, detached family homes, etc.) in the private market, increases in housing supply have not necessarily translated into greater affordability in the housing market overall. Indeed, the price of houses in Canada has skyrocketed in recent years (Mukherjee & Balu, 2024), much to the chagrin of housing developers who have witnessed a veritable boon in their construction sales (see RBC, 2024). Similarly, the private rental market, often beset by issues related to the lack of availability, has also seen its rental costs intensify (The Canadian Press, 2024), vastly outpacing the stagnating or declining wages of renters.

While housing in Canada is a policy domain involving multi-level governance (municipal, provincial/territorial, federal, and Indigenous), there appears to be few actions taken to dramatically curb the financialization of the housing sector over recent decades (Zhu et al., 2021). August (2022) documents this trend whereby housing has increasingly been seen more as a financial asset for investor profit and less as homes in which to live. Enabled by political actors, asset managers, private equity firms, real estate companies, and real estate investment trusts have dominated the market, acquiring housing for the purposes of profit generation and promoting the securitization of mortgages (allowing global investors to draw from packaged and traded securities offered through home loans). These same investors have also gained from the control and acquisition of short-term rental properties that have contributed to an increasingly tight and unaffordable rental market (August, 2022).

With home ownership becoming out of reach for many, activity in the rental market has skyrocketed, causing vacancies to decline. Consequently, in the absence of effective regulations, the housing market has steadily amplified wealth accumulation and inequalities, and housing instability and homelessness. Presently, 40% of Canadian households do not have sufficient income to afford today's average market rents (Burda & Chapple, 2024). As such, there is a need for policy interventions that not only redress the causes of housing unaffordability, but that also prioritize, enlarge, and maintain the non-market housing sector. Non-market housing takes myriad forms, including non-profit housing, co-op housing, government-owned housing, community land trusts, and Indigenous-led non-market housing. Canada's non-market housing is small relative to other high-income countries globally. In 2023, social housing represented a mere 3.5% of all housing stock in Canada: a rate significantly less than other OECD countries (e.g., the Netherlands at nearly 35%). Moreover, less than 5% of the units built through the National Housing Strategy to date can be considered affordable for those subjected to deep poverty. Thus, what is needed is a massive jump in non-market housing from 3.5% to 20% to adequately provide housing for those who cannot afford ever-rising private market rents (Canadian Human Rights Commission, 2023).

Investing in Mental Health and Substance Use Services

As housing encampments become larger, more common, and visible in Canada, some municipal leaders are now taking steps to acquire greater powers to dismantle them. Many seek to enlarge their discretionary authority to remove people denied housing by actively criminalizing, incarcerating, and/or displacing them (Draaisma, 2024). In lockstep with such manoeuvres, efforts underway by political actors have also sought to strip people of their rights and self-determination by forcing people into compulsory treatment and/or rehabilitation programmes (see Passafiume & Osman, 2024), which have been shown to have limited efficacy and are potentially laden with harms (Werb et al., 2016). Rather than advancing policies shown to promote housing stability, substance use recovery, and better mental health and well-being, policymakers in Canada appear to be shifting away from evidence-informed solutions.

Roughly one in five Canadians experience mental illness in any given year (CAMH, n.d.). Even before the Covid-19 pandemic brought about new disruptions in people's lives and heightened their levels of stress, isolation, fear, and grief, mental health and substance use disorders were the leading causes of disability in Canada. The development of mental health and substance use issues commonly begins during adolescence, and 70% of people living with a mental illness report experiencing symptoms before they reach the age of 18 (Canadian Institute for Health Information [CIHI], 2023). Thus, preventative and upstream interventions are needed that foster the conditions (i.e., environments responsive to the SDoH and SDoMH) and protective factors (e.g., perceived emotional support, positive networks, etc.) that promote wellness (Alegría et al., 2018), particularly among children and young people. Although mental health has been identified as a public health priority and "one of the most pronounced health inequities in Canada" (Canada, 2024b), mental health prevention and treatment services in Canada continue to be characterized by a lack of resources, lengthy wait times, and chronic underfunding (CIHI, 2023).

Possible solutions, grounded in empirical research, that government actors could pursue include bolstering Housing First programmes that ensure consumer choice in both housing and individualized supports; increasing access to mental health services (recognizing that such services receive a paltry 7% of all healthcare dollars in Canada; Bartram, 2017); and strengthening rehabilitation and recovery programmes applying a harm reduction model (O'Shaughnessy et al., 2024). The interventions and policies selected, however, must immediately redress urgent violations of the right to housing, and should be culturally and gender responsive and reflect a trauma-informed approach to care (Ranjbar et al., 2020).

Partnered Research Opportunities across Communities

While there are many individuals, public/private organizations, and civil society members working to advance more effective and humane approaches to tackling poverty and homelessness (e.g., Put Food Banks Out of Business campaign, etc.), it would be helpful for these commonly siloed efforts to be brought together. In so doing, a stronger and more formidable social movement could be forged that seeks to hold state and sub-state actors accountable for their rights duties, invoke measures to de-financialize and dismantle capital-led control of the housing market (Wijburg, 2021), and demand more progressive redistributive mechanisms (through, e.g., improved carbon, wealth, and corporate taxation; Smith-Carrier & Green 2017). These measures would not only help curb mass wealth accumulation and income inequality but would also engender the resources necessary to introduce a BIG (inclusive of the working-age population), ensure affordable private and non-market housing, and improve access to effective mental health and recovery supports.

Conclusion

Scholars and practitioners engaging in work on homelessness, poverty, mental health, and substance use treatment and recovery share common concerns about the systemic, structural, and environmental causes of social problems. Using the SDoH and SDoMH as anchors, researchers, health and social care professionals, community partners, advocates, and importantly, people with lived/living experience of hardship must work together to amplify knowledge mobilization efforts and build a strong social movement dedicated to transformative social change. It is only by remedying the material conditions and environments in which people lead their lives that we can redress the SDoH and SDoMH, ensuring health and wellness for us all.

References

Alegría, M., NeMoyer, A., Falgàs Bagué, I., Wang, Y., & Alvarez, K. (2018). Social determinants of mental health: Where we are and where we need to go. *Current Psychiatry Reports*, *20*(95), 1–13. https://doi.org/10.1007/s11920-018-0969-9

August, M. (2022, June). The Financialization of Housing in Canada. A Summary Report for the Office of the Federal Housing Advocate, Canadian Human Rights Commission. https://publications.gc.ca/collections/collection_2023/ccdp-chrc/HR34-7-2022-eng.pdf

Baker, M., Messacar, D., & Stabile, M. (2023). Effects of child tax benefits on poverty and labor supply: Evidence from the Canada Child Benefit and Universal Child Care Benefit. *Journal of Labor Economics*, *41*(4), 1129–1182. https://www.journals.uchicago.edu/doi/epdfplus/10.1086/721379

Bartram, M. (2017). Making the most of the federal investment of $5 billion for mental health. *Canadian Medical Association Journal*, *189*(44), E1360–E1363. https://doi.org/10.1503/cmaj.170738

BICN. (2023). Consensus statement on a basic income guarantee. https://basicincomecanada.org/wp-content/uploads/2023/03/Consensus-Statement-February-2023.docx.pdf

Béland, D., & Marier, P. (2022). How the guaranteed income supplement and old age security interact in Canada's pension system to tackle successfully poverty in old age. In *Policy success in Canada: Cases, Lessons, Challenges*, edited by E. A. Linquist, M. Howlett, G. Skogstad, & G. Tellier, & P. T. Hart, 206–224.

Burda, C., & Chapple, K. (2024, March). Housing supply mix strategy 4: Non-market housing. Supply mix research submitted to the Task Force for Housing https://schoolofcities.utoronto.ca/wp-content/uploads/2024/04/Housing-mix-strategy-4-Non-market-housing.pdf

Burke, A. (2023, March 15). Who won and lost with the Canada Emergency Response Benefit. *Policy Options*. https://policyoptions.irpp.org/magazines/march-2023/cerb-winners-losers/

Calnitsky, D. (2016). "More normal than welfare": The Mincome experiment, stigma, and community experience. *Canadian Review of Sociology/Revue canadienne de sociologie*, *53*(1), 26–71. https://doi.org/10.1111/cars.12091

CAMH. (n.d.). Mental illness and addiction: Facts and statistics. https://www.camh.ca/en/driving-change/the-crisis-is-real/mental-health-statistics

Canada. (2024a). Canada and the United Nations. https://www.international.gc.ca/world-monde/international_relations-relations_internationales/un-onu/index.aspx?lang=eng

Canada. (2024b). Inequalities in mental health, well-being and wellness in Canada. https://health-infobase.canada.ca/mental-health/inequalities/

Canadian Human Rights Commission. (2023, November). What We Heard Report: Nonmarket housing as a solution to the housing crisis National Right to Housing Day Virtual Panel, hosted by the Office of the Federal Housing Advocate. https://www.housingchrc.ca/sites/housing/files/2024-04/non-market-housing-as-a-solution-to-the-housing-crisis.pdf

CIHI. (2023, August 2). Canadians short on access to care for mental health and substance use. https://www.cihi.ca/en/taking-the-pulse-a-snapshot-of-canadian-health-care-2023/canadians-short-on-access-to-care-for

Draaisma, M. (2024, October 31). Ontario mayors ask Ford to use notwithstanding clause to clear homeless encampments. *CBC News*. https://www.cbc.ca/news/canada/toronto/ontario-big-city-mayors-notwithstanding-clause-encampments-1.7370210

Emery, J. H., Fleisch, V. C., & McIntyre, L. (2013). Legislated changes to federal pension income in Canada will adversely affect low income seniors' health. *Preventive Medicine*, *57*(6), 963–966. https://doi.org/10.1016/j.ypmed.2013.09.004

Forget, E. L. (2018). *Basic Income for Canadians: The Key to a Healthier, Happier, More Secure Life for All*. James Lorimer & Company.

Hamilton, L., & Mulvale, J. P. (2019). "Human again": The (unrealized) promise of basic income in Ontario. *Journal of Poverty*, *23*(7), 576–599. https://doi.org/10.1080/10875549.2019.1616242

Handerer, F., Kinderman, P., Shafti, M., & Tai, S. (2022). A scoping review and narrative synthesis comparing the constructs of social determinants of health and social determinants of mental health: Matryoshka or two independent constructs?*Frontiers in Psychiatry*, *13*, 848556. https://doi.org/10.3389/fpsyt.2022.848556

Kerman, N. (2021). The role of universal basic income in preventing and ending homelessness. *International Journal on Homelessness*, *1*(1), 3–13. https://doi.org/10.5206/ijoh.2021.1.13337

Lee, M. (2022, May 1). What happened to the National Housing Strategy? *Policynote*. https://www.policynote.ca/national-housing-strategy/

Lund, C., Brooke-Sumner, C., Baingana, F., Baron, E. C., Breuer, E., Chandra, P., Haushofer, J., Herrman, H., Jordans, M., Kieling, C., Medina-Mora, M. E., Morgan, E., Omigbodun, O., Tol, W., Patel, V., & Saxena, S. (2018). Social determinants of mental disorders and the Sustainable Development Goals: A systematic review of reviews. *The Lancet Psychiatry*, *5*(4), 357–369. https://doi.org/10.1016/S2215-0366(18)30060-9

McCloskey, S. (2020). Poverty is a political choice: A UN Rapporteur has delivered a withering critique of the international system. *Policy and Practice: A Development Education Review*, (31), 77–89. https://www.sloga-platform.org/wp-content/uploads/2021/03/Issue-31-Final-2.pdf#page=87

Mikkonen, J., & Raphael, D. (2010). *The Canadian Facts*. Toronto, ON: York University School of Health Policy and Management. https://www-preview.athabascau.ca/support-services/_documents/social_determinants_health_canadian_facts.pdf

Moore, E., & Skaburskis, A. (2004). Canada's increasing housing affordability burdens. *Housing Studies*, *19*(3), 395–413. https://doi.org/10.1080/0267303042000204296

Mukherjee, P., & Balu, N. (2024, July 17). Supply in Canada's property market surges as mortgage renewals loom. *CTV News*. https://www.ctvnews.ca/business/supply-in-canada-s-property-market-surges-as-mortgage-renewals-loom-1.6967278

Oren, M. & Alterman, R. (2021). The right to adequate housing around the globe: Analysis and evaluation of national constitutions. In *Rights and the City: Problems, Progress, and Practice*, edited by S. Agrawal, (pp. 1–27). University of Alberta Press.

O'Shaughnessy, B. R., Mayock, P., & Kakar, A. (2024). The recovery experiences of homeless service users with substance use disorder: A systematic review and qualitative meta-synthesis. *International Journal of Drug Policy*, *130*, 104528. https://doi.org/10.1016/j.drugpo.2024.104528

Passafiume, A., & Osman, L. (2024, October 11). Canada doesn't have enough beds to support involuntary addictions treatment, minister says. *CBC News*. https://www.cbc.ca/news/politics/canada-not-enough-beds-involuntary-addiction-care-1.7350485

Rachlis, M., Goel, R., Mackie, C., Pellizzari, R., & Simon, L. (2013). Policy and population approaches to poverty. *Ontario Medical Review*, *80*, 30–34. https://healthprovidersagainstpoverty.ca/wp-content/uploads/2015/07/part-5-policy-and-population.pdf

Ranjbar, N., Erb, M., Mohammad, O., & Moreno, F. A. (2020). Trauma-informed care and cultural humility in the mental health care of people from minoritized communities. *Focus*, *18*(1), 8–15. https://doi.org/10.1176/appi.focus.20190027

Raphael, D. (2003). Barriers to addressing the societal determinants of health: Public health units and poverty in Ontario, Canada. *Health Promotion International*, *18*(4), 397–405. https://doi.org/10.1093/heapro/dag411

RBC. (2024). Proof point: Rental housing construction picks up in Canada but will it be enough? https://thoughtleadership.rbc.com/proof-point-rental-housing-construction-is-finally-picking-up-in-canada-but-will-it-be-enough/

Smith-Carrier, T. (2017). Reproducing social conditions of poverty: A critical feminist analysis of social assistance participation in Ontario, Canada. *Journal of Women, Politics & Policy*, *38*(4), 498–521. https://doi.org/10.1080/1554477X.2016.1268874

Smith-Carrier, T. (2023). Advancing income security policy using universal design: The case of the Ontario Disability Support Programme in Ontario, Canada. In S. Robinson, & K. Fisher (Eds.), *Research Handbook on Disability Policy* (pp. 789–804). Edward Elgar Publishing.

Smith-Carrier, T., & Green, S. (2017). Another low road to basic income? Mapping a pragmatic model for adopting a basic income in Canada. *Basic Income Studies*, *12*(2), 1–25. https://doi.org/10.1515/bis-2016-0020

Smith-Carrier, T., & Manion, K. (2022). Bringing it all together: Leveraging social movements and the courts to advance substantive human rights and climate justice. *Human Rights Review*, *23*(4), 551–574. https://doi.org/10.1007/s12142-022-00674-0

Smith-Carrier, T., & Power, E. (2025). Structural violence and the social determinants of mental health: Exploring the experiences of participants on the Ontario Basic Income Pilot in Ontario, Canada. *Home and Social Care in the Community*, 1–18. https://doi.org/10.1155/hsc/7816069

Stadler, S. L., & Collins, D. (2021). Housing First programs from a right to housing perspective. *Education and Research Archive, University of Alberta Library*, 1–39. https://era.library.ualberta.ca/items/33c1b026-9af3-4d1e-95c2-7a22364004a3

Statistics Canada. (2024a). Dimensions of poverty hub. https://www.statcan.gc.ca/en/topics-start/poverty

Statistics Canada. (2024b, May 23). The role of the Canada Emergency Response Benefit in alleviating the impact of the COVID-19 pandemic on the employment income of racialized workers. https://www150.statcan.gc.ca/n1/daily-quotidien/240523/dq240523d-eng.htm

Tabbara, M-D., & Griffin, P. (2023, December 18). Canada does not know how many seniors live in poverty. *Policy Options*. https://policyoptions.irpp.org/magazines/december-2023/poverty-seniors-measurement/

Tarasuk, V. (2017). *Implications of a Basic Income Guarantee for Household Food Insecurity*. Thunder Bay: Northern Policy Institute. https://proof.utoronto.ca/resource/implications-of-a-basic-income-guarantee-for-household-food-insecurity/

The Canadian Press. (2024, January 31). Rent prices soared in 2023 as Canada saw lowest vacancy rate on record. *CBC News*. https://www.cbc.ca/news/business/rent-prices-rose-in-2023-1.7100571

Werb, D., Kamarulzaman, A., Meacham, M. C., Rafful, C., Fischer, B., Strathdee, S. A., & Wood, E. (2016). The effectiveness of compulsory drug treatment: A systematic review. *International Journal of Drug Policy*, *28*, 1–9. https://doi.org/10.1016/j.drugpo.2015.12.005

White, A., & DiBellonia, S. (2024, April 21). 2024 Federal Budget is full of actions, short on results for the most marginalized. *Maytree*. https://maytree.com/publications/2024-federal-budget-is-full-of-actions-short-on-results-for-the-most-marginalized/

WHO. (n.d.). Social determinants of health. https://www.who.int/health-topics/social-determinants-of-health#tab=tab_1

WHO. (2024, January 18). Operational framework for monitoring social determinants of health equity. https://www.who.int/publications/i/item/9789240088320

WHO. (2008). Closing the gap in a generation: Health equity through action on the social determinants of health. https://iris.who.int/bitstream/handle/10665/43943/9789241563703_eng.pdf

Wijburg, G. (2021). The de-financialization of housing: Towards a research agenda. *Housing Studies*, *36*(8), 1276–1293. https://doi.org/10.1080/02673037.2020.1762847

Zhu, Y., Yuan, Y., Gu, J., & Fu, Q. (2021). Neoliberalization and inequality: Disparities in access to affordable housing in urban Canada 1981–2016. *Housing Studies*, *38*(10), 1860–1887. https://doi.org/10.1080/02673037.2021.2004093

9

GUIDING PRINCIPLES OF THE BRIDGING THE TRANSITION FRAMEWORK

Social Justice

Ana Paula Serrata Malfitano and Ana Carolina da Silva Almeida Prado

From a socio-historical perspective, the current social mode of economic production is understood as a generator of inequities, directly impacting people's life possibilities. Due to the reconfiguration of the labor market, a significant portion of the population finds itself excluded from this social dimension. For many people, survival alternatives include living in shelters or on the streets. Homelessness is a complex, multifactorial, and socially produced phenomenon that cannot be understood in an individualized way. Professional work with this population requires interventions that bridge macro and micro-social spheres to fully understand the complexities of homelessness. Social justice emerges as a key element to guide policies aimed at redistributing resources and recognizing the unique needs of this population in addressing the inequities they experience.

Component of the Bridging the Transition Framework Addressed in this Chapter

This chapter describes social justice as a guiding principle in research and practice aimed at homelessness prevention. An overview of social justice theories and practices that can be used to support the daily life functioning, participation, and well-being of individuals across the trajectory of unhoused to housing is provided (see Figure 9.1).

DOI: 10.4324/9781003541332-11

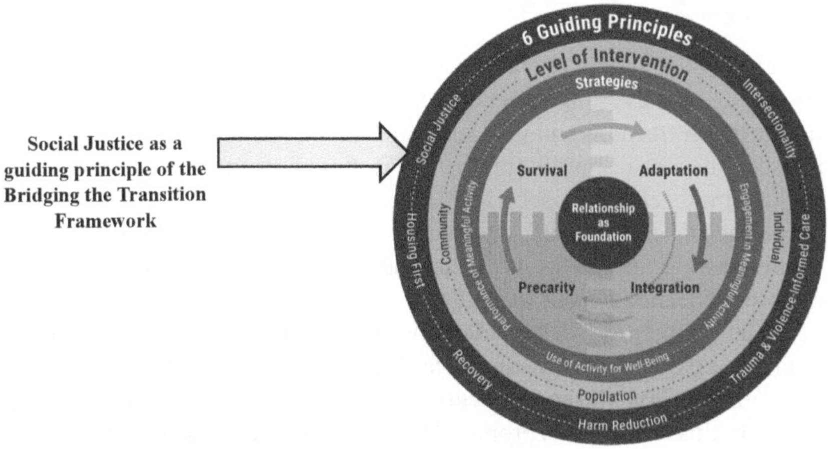

FIGURE 9.1 Social Justice as a Guiding Principle.

How this Chapter Guides Practice and Research in Homelessness Prevention

Currently, it is estimated that around 1.6 billion people worldwide, over 20 per cent of the world's population, do not have adequate and safe housing to live in, and it is estimated that 100 million people are homeless worldwide, following the last global survey attempted by the United Nations in 2005 (United Nations, 2020). There are differences in distributions of this phenomenon around the world, and the Global South has higher numbers of individuals living in conditions of poverty and consequently more people are homeless. To understand the worsening phenomenon of people experiencing homelessness, it is necessary to take a historically and socially contextualized perspective, because homelessness is an expression of the social relations within the current economic mode of production in a capitalist society. This foundation stems from the understanding that homelessness is often recognized as an individual issue but demands a collectivist approach, given that it is rooted in the structure of social organization at the macro level. As such, it is argued that professional work in various services dedicated to supporting the homeless population should be grounded in a macro and micro-social understanding of society to analyze this phenomenon in the complexity of its collective relationships.

Hence, prevention efforts targeting homelessness, interventions for those already living on the streets, and actions aimed at transitioning individuals to housing must fundamentally center on promoting social justice. This approach should be underpinned by policies focused on wealth redistribution and the recognition of differences, aiming to promote the participation of persons experiencing homelessness in society, thereby contributing to combating the inequities experienced daily by this population.

Introduction

Social justice is understood as the direction against oppressions lived in society, requiring the conjugation between individual and collective responsibilities, between freedom and justice (Freire, 1994), recognition of identity and redistribution of resources (Fraser, 1995). Based on an analysis grounded in the dynamic relationship between macro and micro-social elements that shape societal phenomena, this chapter offers an understanding of homelessness as a consequence of social inequity, a kind of oppression which requires collective actions to deal with.

Society is shaped by contradictions and inequalities, such that resources available are distributed unequally, leading to the accumulation of wealth for a few, and poverty and social exclusion for a significant portion of the population. In this context, it is proposed that professional work should be guided by actions against oppression, aimed at promoting social justice. To achieve this, Freire (2005) highlights the necessity of consciousness-raising through critical reflection and practices designed to challenge oppressive relationships experienced daily by people, which are considered "natural" or socially accepted. In the Freirean sense, the exercise of human reflection and action in the world, with the intention of transformation and social justice, is characterized as praxis (Freire, 2005). This process requires the conjunction between consciousness or recognition of the oppression and redistributions of resources acting to interrupt oppression (Freire, 1994, 2005; Fraser, 1995).

This conscious process requires a reading of the world, especially about the impacts of the current social mode of life production. It is understood that the capitalist mode of social production does not refer only to economic relations, but above all, to a specific set of established social relationships, involving political, cultural, and economic aspects, rooted in history. Within these elements, following the dialectical historical materialism approach, there is always a connection between the individual situation and the social structure, meaning that the appearance of phenomena and objects do not correspond with their essence. The domination of one human being over another constitutes the essence of the entire process, generating exclusion and inequality (Marx, 2013) manifested by social oppressions (Freire, 1994). In this social model of life production, labor is central even for people who are not in the labor market. It means that the contemporary reconfiguration of labor relations has led to a crisis that resulted in a significant number of individuals experiencing social exclusion, characterized by dual social vulnerability—lacking both employment and social support to sustain their lives. For Castel (2003), social exclusion and vulnerability consist of the interaction between the axes of social labor relationships and social support networks (Castel, 2003).

Here, the Marxian conception of labor is adopted, in which it is configured as an ontological dimension of human constitution; that is, the teleological capacity to meet a need. The organization of human activity is the core of this process. In essence, humanization occurs through labor; however, in the capitalist mode of social production, a process of dehumanization takes place, in which the individual is unable to recognize themselves in what they produce or not produce (Marx, 2013). There is an intensification of these social relations, in which a portion of the population is not incorporated into the productive process, either due to a lack of employment opportunities or because they do not possess the necessary capacity for such, remaining on the margins of social relations and not just labor relations. Since one of the central aspects of this economic system consists of the production of goods intended for sale and profit rather than meeting human needs, access to certain resources is determined by money rather than human necessity. As a result, different unequal processes are created because of individuals without available resources, such as people without safe and adequate housing, living in shelters or in the streets as a means of survival.

It is important to emphasize that homelessness can arise from multiple factors and often involves a combination of individual and collective characteristics in its manifestation. However, this chapter advocates for a collective understanding of this social phenomenon, grounded in the social inequity inherent to capitalism. We advocate for the importance of a professional role in society, imposing praxis against the processes of oppression, by focusing on understanding the individual and collective dimensions that encompass the phenomenon of homelessness. Further, the concept of social justice is presented, rooted in actions aimed at wealth redistribution and the recognition of difference, aiming to promote the status of participation in the social structure as a foundation for research and practice. Finally, examples of proposed actions are presented, focusing on the individuals' life context, aiming to support daily life, mediate processes of participation, recognition, and visibility of this group, and pursue initiatives guided by the principle of recognizing the worth of unhoused individuals, with access to historically constructed social goods. To achieve this, based on an understanding of the social relations to which these individuals are historically and contextually situated, it is essential to implement actions that address both macrostructural and microstructural aspects as integral elements of knowledge production and professional practice.

Social Justice as a Central Element to be Pursued in Working with Homeless People

The idea of social justice is present in different academic thought traditions, acquiring distinct meanings. Therefore, before beginning any discussion on the topic, it is essential to clarify from which perspective social justice will be addressed. In this chapter, the concept of social justice proposed by Fraser (2000, 2012) is used. The concept is based on three central principles: redistribution, recognition, and participatory parity.

The principle of redistribution focuses on the socioeconomic structure, targeting disadvantaged social classes or groups that demand economic restructuring. That is, a redistribution of wealth so that some level of social justice can be achieved for all. Injustices are, therefore, the result of problematic social and economic structures in society.

The second principle for achieving social justice is recognition, meaning that injustice is also understood as the product of a hierarchy of cultural values or a hierarchical revaluation. This paradigm focuses on cultural and identity-based injustices, in which the most exploited, oppressed, and inequitable groups are those with the least social prestige and esteem and whose injustices are deeply rooted in society (Fraser, 2000). Consequently, marginalized populations such as Indigenous people, immigrants from countries outside the Global North, Black people, among other groups, are considered socially disadvantaged and lack recognition of their equal status as citizens to achieve some level of social justice.

Finally, the third principle proposes participatory parity. According to Fraser (2000, 2012), participatory parity is necessary, and it can only be achieved through "reciprocal recognition" and "equality of status." In other words, there will be social justice if there are conditions for participation in society, which requires recognizing various socially invisible groups, as well as the redistribution of resources to ensure the necessary conditions for social justice to enable participation. Therefore, by ensuring the redistribution of wealth and recognizing differences, we have the elements for articulating a social system that fosters participatory parity, thus paving the way for the pursuit of social justice.

These principles are interconnected and should align redistribution and recognition policies, aiming to move closer to social justice. Both are dialectically related, enabling participation, therefore it is essential to consider them from their movement and a bidimensional perspective in the pursuit of justice. Through actions that promote social equality and recognize differences, subordinated groups can be addressed, which combine the demands of an exploited social class and marginalized cultural characteristics, emerging from economic spheres and false recognition, within dynamic relationships that mutually reinforce each other (Fraser, 2012).

As an example, we can consider the importance of this conception of justice in the lives of persons experiencing homelessness, aiming to overcome the context of marginalization they face in society. Since they are deprived of their basic rights, it is essential that, within the sphere of redistribution policies, actions should be implemented that promote their access to housing, work, income, food, health care, and other social goods. Furthermore, in light of the symbolic exclusion of unhoused individuals resulting from the stigma and prejudice they face, it is crucial to address discrimination related to race, geographic origin, substance use, lack of the desire to work, and other stigmas that are associated with homelessness.

Public policies focused on redistributing resources and recognizing individuals as citizens create the possibility for social participation, representation, and access to the basic dignity necessary for living. Discussing political actions aimed at persons experiencing homelessness, the role of professionals involves mediating social injustice.

The Crisis of the Labor Market Configuration and Life on the Streets: Notes from a Socio-historical Perspective

The theoretical foundation of this chapter is rooted in a socio-historical perspective that understands the direct impact of the current capitalist mode of economic production on people's life opportunities. In other words, the current state of social organization generates inequities experienced in individuals' daily lives, beyond the labor market, stemming from the structural inequality produced on a macrostructural level.

The fundamental premise of a socio-historical approach is that social phenomena are situated within historical time, thereby presenting specific challenges related to the production by human beings throughout history. This historical construction, within capitalism, is grounded in the world of labor as the regulator and organizer of social relationships. Therefore, to reflect on social phenomena, it is vital to understand the centrality of labor in individuals' daily lives. As Marx (2013) states, labor is a fundamental ontological category in the constitution of human beings. It refers to the capacity to anticipate, based on a need, a modification of nature; it is the possibility for humans to materialize their creative power in the products of this process. Essentially, it is through labor—namely, the transformation of nature to enable life—that we humanize ourselves.

However, in the current social mode of production, labor no longer corresponds to the fulfillment of human needs; its output is directed primarily toward profit, thus deviating from the principle of addressing human and social needs and focusing solely on generating wealth for a small group (Antunes, 2022). In this context, there is an intensification of labor exploitation, characterized by an expanded scale of domination. This process leads to dehumanization, as it becomes impossible to recognize oneself in what is produced. The result is a relationship of abstract domination, where the more it is reproduced, the more this domination is intensified (Antunes, 2022). Resistance to this process can come about through consciousness-raising about societal dynamics, intentional actions in response to knowledge of such dynamics, and praxis, to promote humanization and social justice (Freire, 1994).

As part of the metamorphosis of the central role of labor, contemporary society is experiencing a labor crisis. This crisis is characterized by the lack of universal access to work, an essential condition for participation in social dynamics. This situation arises from the reconfiguration of the social mode of production, marked by the degradation of working conditions and the elimination of certain jobs. These changes result in the individualization of social relationships, which Castel (2003) defines as a new social question; it means the labor crises associated with the individualism of personal relationships shape a new configuration of the social question.

According to Castel (2003), collective organization around this new social question occurs along two axes: integration (or lack thereof) into the labor market—which may be stable, precarious, or marked by total exclusion—and participation (or lack thereof) in social support networks. Social support networks, as defined by Castel (2003), provide resources for sustaining life. These networks can be formal, such as public policies, social benefits, and accessible social goods, or informal, such as initiatives from churches, unions, or autonomous groups. The interaction between the axes of labor and support networks defines various conditions: social integration, where individuals are fully incorporated into the labor market and have a strong social network; vulnerability, where they face precarious labor relationships and weakened social networks; social disaffiliation, characterized by exclusion from both the labor market and support networks; and assistance, where individuals are excluded from work but receive aid from formal (public) or informal assistance networks to ensure their survival.

Currently, there has been a significant increase in the number of people experiencing social disaffiliation, characterized as a mass of "superfluous" individuals—those on the margins of capitalist society (Castel, 2003). One group that exemplifies disaffiliation is people experiencing homelessness. Without access to basic necessities, such as conventional housing and food, streets and shelters often become their only means of survival. This group is particularly vulnerable to multiple forms of violence, facing numerous individual and collective challenges.

Considering the socio-historical understanding of inequalities, as experienced in contemporary times, the phenomenon of homelessness must be addressed dynamically and at multiple levels, as it is the interaction of these elements that contributes to this condition. Psychological distress, physical or mental disabilities, substance abuse, and the disconnection from both the labor market and social support networks are aspects that must be considered in an integrated manner when addressing the population of persons experiencing homelessness. In general, many persons experiencing homelessness face severe human degradation and social exclusion (Snow & Anderson, 1993).

What is observed in the individual lives of people who are unhoused reflects the contradictions historically produced within the macro social structure, which generates inequities and social oppression. For instance, situations experienced by individuals in similar conditions vary, as the processes of oppression are marked by stigmas and unequal access to opportunities, particularly affecting people living in poverty, women, Black individuals,

Latinos, and other groups. Therefore, the dialectic between the individual and the collective dimensions becomes an essential element for understanding social phenomena, such as life on the streets.

When different professionals work with these groups, the discussion should focus on building new forms of sociability, as the current economic structure has produced devastating effects on people's lives. Accordingly, when reflecting on the construction of new paths aimed at social transformation—that is, changing the structures that inherently create inequities—it is useful to draw on the concept of *aufheben*, as employed by Marx (2013). This concept is rooted in the dialectical movement of "elevating, preserving, and overcoming," where the progression of a specific phenomenon allows its contradictions to be recognized and transcended. In contemporary times, marked by increasing oppression, inequities, and exploitation under capitalism (Fraser, 2022), the concept of social justice emerges as a promising framework for driving transformative action.

The Role of Health and Social Care Practitioners and Researchers in the Pursuit of Social Justice

Despite a recognized theoretical debate about the social determination in life processes, the predominance of actions taken in society is often focused on the individual person, problematically taking individualized responses to problems that are collective (Conrad, 2007). Professional practices based on the idea of individualizing the problems experienced by individuals become insufficient to address the contexts of inequity they face, as in the case of persons experiencing homelessness, who present individual demands that reflect a collective inequality of the social organization itself.

Specifically, in working with persons experiencing homelessness, whether they are living on the streets or transitioning to housing, it is essential to combat ideologies that naturalize poverty, devalue people in these conditions, and create proposals and/or programs solely focused on the individual without acknowledging the social conditions that led to the problems they experience. Examples include how substance dependence and mental health problems are seen to be a problem of an individual person, and result in "teaching" motivation strategies or promoting decontextualized and individualized intervention approaches that fail to acknowledge the contribution of the social environment in which a person is embedded to the challenges that they experience. Commonly, the discourse of social justice is present in many of these narratives, creating a perverse confluence (Dagnino, 2007) that seldom addresses the social and collective dimension that leads many to live less dignified lives. The challenge lies in moving beyond discourse and, instead of considering the axes of subordination in isolation such as through individualizing explanations, it is essential to adopt a comprehensive understanding that reveals the contradictions between social inequity, the lack of recognition, and, consequently, their inability to acquire the ability to participate fully in society (Fraser, 1995).

To this end, professional practice must focus on people's life contexts, seeking ways to understand their social relationships, in a historical and situated way, aiming to find possibilities that allow actions for redistribution of resources, recognition of differences, and participation parity; that is, for social justice. The social context of people's lives must be addressed as an inherent element in all professional practices (Malfitano, 2021).

In the field of health and social care professions, where we are involved and conduct research on various professional actions with persons experiencing homelessness, among other groups in situations of social vulnerability, there has been a growing stance in several countries to establish alliances in the construction of knowledge and practices aimed at combating relationships of oppression, aiming to achieve social justice. Starting from a critical understanding of social injustice, whether local or global, it is recognized that these issues directly or indirectly affect the entire world. Thus, the aim is to promote a collective movement at the global level to combat the effects of capitalism, that is, social inequality and injustices (Leite Junior, Laliberte Rudman & Lopes, 2024).

In Brazil, since the 1970s, occupational therapists, among other professionals, have been dedicated to building knowledge and practices aimed at transforming the contexts of exclusion faced by populations in situations of vulnerability and social exclusion, for example, through social occupational therapy (Lopes & Malfitano, 2021). This involves the development of social approaches to be created and applied by professionals who base their practices on expanding the social participation possibilities of different social groups (Lopes; Malfitano, 2021). Its proposal arises from a critical perspective, grounded theoretically and methodologically, and providing tools to address the phenomenon of social injustice, such as in the case of homeless individuals to encompass the full complexity present in this way of life; that is: "The intervention with the homeless people presupposes action articulated through the policies and services available in the assistance network, including the macro-social questions, seeking action toward the people as well as the collectives of this population" (Malfitano, 2021, p. 52).

Considering the "Bridging the Transition to Housing" framework presented in this book, we believe it is necessary to perform a multifactorial analysis of elements that compose this framework. The work based on this framework is grounded in the principle of social justice, providing support during the transition from the streets or shelters to stable and secure housing, as well as the necessary assistance to ensure people can sustain themselves in this new context in a meaningful and satisfying way (Marshall; Gewurtz; Roy; Cooke, & Lysaght, 2023). As such, it is an important objective to work together with people in the search for constructing life projects that enable consciousness of their place in the world, expanding opportunities for social participation, and organizing actions aimed at lives worthy of being lived. To do this, it is necessary to propose policies and actions aimed at achieving social justice for people experiencing homelessness. One must consider the interdependent relationship between wealth redistribution and the recognition of differences, focusing on social participation. The pursuit of social justice, grounded in social participation, should aim to create new and better life opportunities, where different ways of living are made available.

From a critical, collective, and solidarity-based construction of knowledge, the aim is to combat power relationships that seek to oppress and exploit historically marginalized populations. In this way, a movement is proposed to think and build collectively, creating structures of social solidarity in pursuit of the constructing political and social emancipation, against the grain of the neoliberal way of life, in which relationships are increasingly individualized and fragmented, blaming people for their social condition (Leite Junior, Laliberte Rudman & Lopes, 2024).

Conclusion

The worsening of social issues, driven by unemployment, reduced access to basic rights, such as housing, food, and healthcare, and the increasing number of people experiencing homelessness, is a social product of capitalism resulting in inequalities. This scenario demands professional approaches that are both theoretically and practically grounded in a non-fragmented understanding of society, recognizing this reality in its entirety, to guide their practice against oppression through the enactment of social justice. Working with people experiencing homelessness must involve an understanding of the reality that encompasses both the macro and micro-social contexts in which people are situated, recognizing that this phenomenon is multifactorial. It means professionals should consider efforts aimed at coordinating a support network that facilitates access to employment, healthcare, leisure, and education activities, through specific programs that work together according to everyone's needs and particularities. This approach would integrate these dimensions, providing tailored support and ensuring that individuals receive comprehensive care. All actions are always connected to a political-professional role, which is directed toward social mobilization for the construction of social policies that truly address needs of this population. Therefore, the focus should be on work grounded in social justice, where redistribution of resources and recognition of differences are essential for expanding access to rights and social participation for all people, including people experiencing homelessness as part of society.

References

Antunes, R. (2022). *Farewell to Work? Essays on the World of Work's Metamorphoses and Centrality*. Haymarket Books.

Castel, R. (2003). *From Manual Workers to Wage Laborers: Transformation of the Social Question* (R. Boyd trans). Routledge.

Conrad, P. (2007). *The Medicalization of Society: On the Transformation of Human Conditions into Treatable Disorders*. Johns Hopkins University Press.

Dagnino, E. (2007). Citizenship: A perverse confluence. *Development in Practice*, *17*(4–5), 549–556. https://doi.org/10.1080/09614520701469534

Fraser, N. (1995). From redistribution to recognition? Dilemmas of justice in a 'post-socialist' age. *New Left Review*, *212*, 68–93. https://newleftreview.org/issues/i212/articles/nancy-fraser-from-redistribution-to-recognition-dilemmas-of-justice-in-a-post-socialist-age

Fraser, N. (2000). Redistribution, recognition and participation: towards an integrated concept of justice. In *UNESCO. World Culture Report, 2000: Cultural Diversity, Conflict and Pluralism*. https://unesdoc.unesco.org/ark:/48223/pf0000121058

Fraser, N. (2012). Social justice in the age of identity politics: redistribution, recognition, and participation. In (1999). *Culture And Economy After the Cultural Turn*, edited by L. Ray, & A. Sayer. SAGE Publications Ltd, https://doi.org/10.4135/9781446218112. Online 2012

Fraser, N. (2022). *Cannibal Capitalism: How Our System Is Devouring Democracy, Care, and the Planet and What We Can Do About It*. Verso.

Freire, P. (1994). *Pedagogy of Hope: Reliving Pedagogy of the Oppressed*. New York: The Continuum Publishing Company (Original work published 1992).

Freire, P. (2005). *Pedagogy of the Oppressed* (30th anniversary ed.). Continuum.

Leite Junior, J. D., Laliberte Rudman, D., & Lopes, R. E. (2024). Alliances between social occupational therapy and critical occupational science: propositions to mobilize social justice. *Journal of Occupational Science*, *32*(1), 54–70. https://doi.org/10.1080/14427591.2024.2374308

Lopes, R. E.; Malfitano, A. P. S. (2021). *Social Occupational Therapy: Theoretical and Practical Designs*. Elsevier.

Lopes, R. E. (2021). Citizenship, rights, and social occupational therapy. In *Social Occupational Therapy: Theoretical and Practical Designs*, edited by R. E. Lopes & A. P. S. Malfitano (Orgs.). (pp. 1–10). Elsevier.

Malfitano, A. P. S. (2021). Social context and social action: generalizations and specificities in occupational therapy. In *Social Occupational Therapy: Theoretical and Practical Designs*, edited by R. E. Lopes & A. P. S. Malfitano (Orgs.). (pp. 48–56). Elsevier.

Marshall, C. A., Gewurtz, S. B., Roy, L., Cooke, A., & Lysaght, R. (2023). *Bridging the Transition to Housing: A Social Justice Framework to Guide the Practice of Occupational Therapists and Other Professionals with Experiences of Homelessness* (2nd ed), London, ON: Western University. https://doi.org/10.13140/rg.2.2.24013.41443

Marx, K. (2013). *Capital: A Critique of Political Economy Part I the Process of Capitalist Production*. (Original work published 1867). Cosimo Classics.

Snow, D. A. & Anderson, L. (1993). *Down on their Luck: A Study of Homeless Street People*. KDPPR.

United Nations. (2020). *First-ever United Nations Resolution on Homelessness*. Available at: www.un.org/development/desa/dspd/2020/03resolution-homelessness/. Access on Fev 24th 2025.

10

GUIDING PRINCIPLES OF THE BRIDGING THE TRANSITION FRAMEWORK

Housing First

Julia Woodhall-Melnik

Housing First is an evidence-based philosophy that guides programmes and service provision for individuals who experience chronic homelessness. Its main premise is that all individuals are housing ready and housing readiness does not need to be achieved. However, fidelity to key programme principles is fundamental to providing Housing First. This chapter describes the principles of Housing First and how their application to supporting the participation of individuals across the trajectory of unhoused to housing. An overview of each of Tsemberis' five principles of Housing First is provided and alongside evidence that demonstrates their importance to individuals who are on the trajectory of unhoused to housing. Evidence on Housing First indicates that it has several limitations, and these are discussed alongside practices to overcome these barriers.

Component of the Bridging the Transition Framework Addressed in this Chapter

This chapter describes Housing First as a guiding principle in research and practice to respond to and prevent homelessness. An overview of Housing First, its principles and their connection to the Bridging the Transition Framework (see Figure 10.1), and challenges associated with its implementation are provided. Recommendations for service providers on how to implement Housing First in light of challenges are provided.

DOI: 10.4324/9781003541332-12

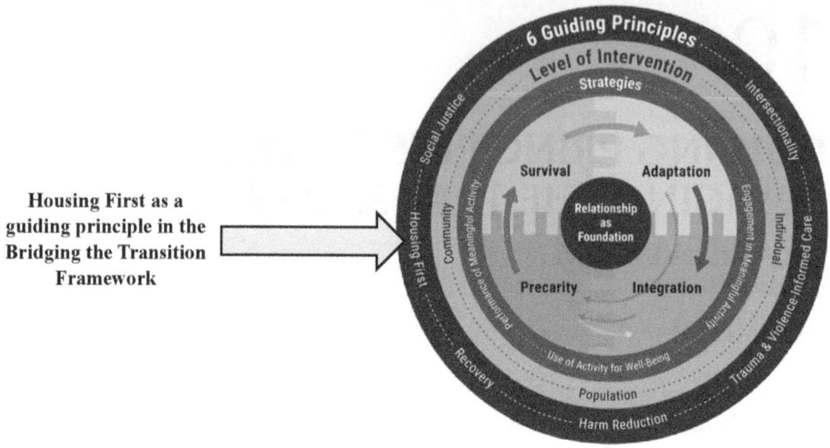

FIGURE 10.1 Housing First as a Guiding Principle.

How this Chapter Guides Practice, Research, and Policy in Homelessness Prevention

Drawing on the extensive research that exists on Housing First, this chapter demonstrates the importance of adherence to the principles of Housing First for service providers who engage in homelessness response and prevention. It discusses the continued importance of measuring fidelity to these principles and notes that future research should focus on the role of Housing First in recovery from substance use and/or psychiatric diagnoses. Further, it provides common challenges that are experienced by practitioners who employ Housing First. In light of increasingly constrained rental markets with expensive rents and low vacancy rates, challenges to housing individuals using Housing First will likely persist. Recommendations for overcoming these challenges are provided.

Introduction

Housing First emerged as both a philosophical approach and programme model in the late 1990s through Sam Tsemberis' design of the principles of Housing First and their application in the Pathways to Housing programme in New York City. Pathways to Housing specifically offered rapid access to housing for individuals who lived with psychiatric disabilities and experienced street-based homelessness. This programme was evaluated over five years and Tsemberis and Eisenberg (2000) found that 88% of Pathways to Housing participants maintained their housing, compared to 47% of participants in New York's residential treatment programme. This initial work demonstrated the efficacy of Housing First as a philosophy and programme model that contributed to higher rates of housing stability. Subsequent research finds that Housing First is not only associated with increased stability but also decreased expenses (Latimer et al., 2019). Housing First, in philosophy, aligns well with the understanding that housing is a human right (Stadler & Collins, 2023). In other words, Housing First can be more effective, cheaper, and more ethical than traditional responses to homelessness.

As a philosophy, Housing First understands stable, permanent housing as a precursor to growth in other areas of life. This draws on Abraham Maslow's hierarchy of needs. This well-known theory postulates that basic physiological needs (e.g. food, water, clothing, and shelter) must be met before other needs for safety and security, love and belonging, self-esteem and self-actualization can be addressed (Maslow & Lewis, 1987). In following this theoretical assumption, the philosophy of Housing First proposes that one must have access to shelter before they can work on other life goals. Hence, unlike previous programme philosophies and models, such as treatment first approaches which require that individuals demonstrate housing readiness through sobriety and treatment of mental health concerns, Housing First prioritizes access to stable and permanent housing as a precursor to improved quality of life.

This chapter describes the principles of Housing First and their application to supporting the participation of individuals across the trajectory of unhoused to housing. To do so, it provides an overview of each of Tsemberis' (2010) five principles of Housing First and discusses their importance to individuals who are on the trajectory of unhoused to housing. This chapter concludes with a discussion of the barriers to successful implementation of Housing First—of which every practitioner should be aware—and ways to overcome these barriers.

The Principles of Housing First

As noted above, Housing First is a philosophy which guides the work of Housing First programmes. It dictates the need for rapid access to stable and permanent housing for individuals who experience homelessness before other individual needs are addressed (Woodhall-Melnik & Dunn, 2016). However, there are other elements that are fundamental to the success of Housing First. Tsemberis (2010) identifies the five core principles of Housing First as: (1) immediate access to permanent housing with no requirement to demonstrate housing readiness, (2) self-determination and choice, (3) recovery orientation, (4) client-driven supports that are individualized, and (5) social and community integration.

The principles of Housing First differentiate the philosophy and associated programmes from other programmes that also use housing as the first and primary intervention for individuals who experience homelessness. For example, rapid rehousing programmes are becoming increasingly popular in North America. Where Housing First programmes prioritize access to permanent housing, rapid rehousing instead provides flexible, but time-limited, access to assistance that is meant to immediately remove individuals and households from homelessness and reduce the harm of spending any time unhoused (Byrne et al., 2023). Herein, the first core principle of Housing First does not apply in that rapid rehousing is meant to be temporary.

Although Housing First programmes need to respond to homelessness within diverse local contexts while simultaneously being responsive to the needs, priorities, and motivations of programme participants (Greenwood et al., 2013), fidelity to the core principles of housing first is associated with improved outcomes for individuals who experience homelessness. For example, higher fidelity to the principles of Housing First is associated with increased housing stability, community functioning, and quality of life (Goering et al., 2016). The Pathways Housing First Fidelity Scale (Stefancic et al., 2013) is commonly used to assess the adherence of Housing First programmes to the principles of Housing First.

The present author attended a talk hosted at McMaster University by prominent Boston-based paediatrician and researcher Dr Megan Sandel. Afterward, Housing First was informally discussed at length, and Dr Sandel made an excellent argument on Housing First and fidelity. She noted that a doctor would not prescribe a patient half a course of antibiotics and expect to successfully cure strep throat. Fidelity to the principles of Housing First should be viewed the same way as administering a course of medication. Doctors would not provide half a course of antibiotics and expect it to work, so why would a Housing First programme that does not adhere to the core principles of fidelity expect to provide an effective response to homelessness? This metaphor, although quite pathologizing, calls upon practitioners to rigorously employ the principles of Housing First within programming. Further, it also calls upon researchers to work alongside community organizations to assist with fidelity assessments and to ensure that these assessments are accessible to organizations that often experience hardships from high caseloads and practitioner burnout (Lemieux-Cumberlege & Taylor, 2019).

Housing First is the second guiding principle of the Bridging the Transition Framework; however, the other five principles of this framework overlap considerably with the core principles of Housing First. The alignment between the principles of the Bridging the Transition Framework and Housing First demonstrates cohesive synergy and suggests that Housing First—as a mechanism for homelessness response and prevention—is well suited to practitioners' and researchers' comprehensive and effective engagement with the framework. The following sub-sections outline the five original principles of Housing First, as presented by Tsemberis (2010).

Principle #1: Provide Immediate Access to Permanent Housing with No Readiness Requirements

Housing First is considered a housing-based intervention to respond to and prevent homelessness. Although it may seem common sense to fix a lack of housing with the provision of housing, traditional approaches fail to provide this immediate access to housing and instead favour treatment first. Treatment first approaches require that individuals demonstrate housing readiness through sobriety from substances and/or treatment for psychiatric diagnoses before they receive permanent housing (Tsemberis, 2010). However, treatment first violates the principle of social justice, as the human right to housing is not met. Housing First remedies this as permanent housing is provided before anything else.

Although varied measures of residential stability are used (e.g. maintained residence in first housing unit, days spent stably housed, proportion of days stably housed over a period, etc.), research finds that Housing First produces more residential stability than traditional service-based approaches to housing individuals who experience homelessness (Pearson et al., 2009). The more time that an individual spends homeless, the greater risk they experience of poor health, social and economic outcomes (Fazel et al., 2014). Hence, in addition to meeting the human right to housing, providing immediate access to permanent housing with no readiness requirements serves a harm reduction function.

Principle #2: Prioritize Consumer Choice and Self-Determination

Self-determination is a core concept within the fields of psychology, social work, and disability studies (Kirzner & Miserandino, 2023; Wehmeyer & Shogren, 2016), which refers to one's ability to make intentional choices based on their preferences. Individual choice and self-determination are easier to exercise if one has what Wehmeyer and Shogren (2016) refer to as positive action-control beliefs. Individuals who possess these beliefs trust that they have the ability, means, and capability to achieve their goals. In a study of a street-based intervention, which serves as a precursor to the Pathways to Housing programme, Tsemberis (2013) finds that individuals who experience homelessness and psychiatric diagnoses desire housing. Housing First programmes provide the means and capacity for permanent and stable housing for those who want to be housed and are not. This involves offering clients choice in housing through scattered site housing models.

Client choice and self-determination in housing are instrumental to Housing First. This involves choice in housing itself and in how one lives in their housing. In their study of a Housing First programme for men who experience chronic homelessness in Hamilton, Ontario, Woodhall-Melnik et al. (2017) find that permanent and affordable housing is important to individuals with histories of long-term homelessness; however, they also find that housing that provides independence and control is important. Individuals' choice of how to live in their home provides a sense of stability and a desire to be at home and maintain place. Seemingly small comforts like a television set for entertainment can enhance well-being for individuals with histories of homelessness. Piat et al. (2020) find that choice in life activities (e.g. what to cook, when to eat, establishing cleaning routines, etc.) can help to build a sense of home. The ability to exercise choice and self-determination in place is important, as many individuals with histories of homelessness are previously exposed to trauma and violence at home, which are precursors to homelessness and produce negative attachments to home and place (Woodhall-Melnik et al., 2018). Practitioners, such as those implementing the Bridging the Transition Framework, who use trauma- and violence-informed care approaches, should focus on ensuring choice in neighbourhoods and home environments, whenever possible, to allow for housing that meets the needs and desires of their clients.

Principle #3: Operate with a Recovery Orientation

Both the Bridging the Transition Framework and Housing First employ the principle of operating with a recovery orientation. Service providers who work in teams that prioritize a recovery orientation give clients the benefit of the doubt, celebrate small wins, withhold judgement, and focus on the positive (Barrenger et al., 2015). Barrenger et al. (2015) find that using positive, non-pathologizing language creates more positive discussions between service providers and their clients' landlords, which can improve housing stability in light of minor setbacks. Further, perceived stigma and humiliation are antithetical to recovery for individuals who use substances and/or have psychiatric diagnoses (Reilly et al., 2022; Wright, 2012).

Housing First is best practice for housing persons experiencing chronic homelessness, as it promotes housing stability; however, research on substance use and psychiatric symptomology is mixed. For example, Tinland et al. (2020) find no evidence of improved recovery in their assessment of France's Housing First programme. They suggest that a longer study period may be needed to demonstrate significant recovery outcomes. Despite this, research does show an improvement in both community functioning and quality of life in Housing First participants in Canada (Aubry et al., 2015).

Principle #4: Ensure Supports Are Individualized and Client Driven

Housing First involves the disconnection of housing from supports and services (Tsemberis, 2010). In other words, housing is not dependent on, and is separate from, the use of services. In this vein, supports are intended to be individualized and client driven. Individuals with histories of homelessness work with Intensive Case Management (ICM) or Assertive Community Treatment (ACT) teams to identify personal goals and work towards them.

ICM for Housing First employs case managers to work with clients. Case managers meet with their clients on a regular basis in the community and in their homes and develop a trusting relationship that is focused on client-defined recovery and self-selected goals (Employment and Social Development Canada, 2018). ACT teams are less frequently used in Canada and are designed to provide more intensive supports to individuals with complex needs. These teams are multi-disciplinary (e.g. primary health practitioners, social workers, psychiatrists, addictions specialists, etc.) and are designed to provide wrap-around supports (Nelson & Aubry, 2018). Practitioners who provide individualized and client-driven supports acknowledge the diversity of needs within homeless populations and acknowledge that recovery means different things for different people. They allow client choice in goals, services, and supports that are not connected to the ability to receive or keep housing.

Individualized and client-driven approaches to support and service provision allow for movement away from traditional staircase approaches, wherein clients complete predetermined tasks and goals (Oudshoorn et al., 2023). In practice, clients who have a choice of services form stronger relationships with service providers and are more capable of expressing their needs (Piat et al., 2020). Strong relationships with service providers are associated with improvements in community integration and quality of life for individuals enrolled in Housing First programmes (Stergiopoulos et al., 2014).

Principle #5: Prioritize Social and Community Integration

Social and community participation are fundamental to the maintenance of stable housing. O'Campo et al. (2022) test a theory of change for Housing First at 24 months of engagement with Housing First and find that health and social status at study enrolment and subsequent health status and social connectedness impact recovery and quality of life. They note that it is important to link clients with health and social services, support participants' choices to engage with community members and family, and provide resources to improve and maintain good health. This study demonstrates the importance of case management and support workers to recovery and well-being.

Strong case management can enhance recovery for individuals housed with Housing First, and practitioners using the Bridging the Transition Framework should consider the importance of engaging clients, when interested, with a variety of social and community-based supports.

Social isolation and loneliness are identified as barriers to stable housing, health, and well-being. Individuals who are housed through Housing First are more likely to experience loneliness and social isolation than those who receive usual services (Ferreiro et al., 2021). For example, individuals who are lonely after being housed may choose to continue contact with unsupportive networks and may bring individuals from these networks home, which can threaten housing stability (Stergiopoulos et al., 2014). Service providers should work with clients to identify relationships that clients would like to (re)build and assist with building community connections.

Challenges with Implementing Housing First

Although Housing First is one of the primary mechanisms for responding to and preventing homelessness in North America, practitioners experience significant difficulties with its implementation. In Canada, like many other nations, there is a significant shortage of affordable rental housing, which makes it extremely challenging for service providers to locate immediate housing options for clients and limits the choice that clients can exercise in housing type and locations (Anderson-Baron & Collins, 2019). Stadler and Collins (2023) argue that Housing First, in principle, views housing as a human right; however, housing shortages prevent the actualization of this right. Jurisdictions across Canada have long and growing waitlists for access to subsidized housing. All levels of government must prioritize investment in, and the rapid development of, publicly owned subsidized housing units (e.g. public or social housing), non-profit run housing, and cooperative housing units. Programmes that engage with private sector landlords to house clients are in a better position to rapidly respond to housing need than those that are reliant on social and community housing with long waitlists (Oudshoorn et al., 2023); however, as vacancy rates remain low, finding private market housing still presents challenges. To remedy this, some communities use Rapid Rehousing programmes to immediately respond to housing need. Rapid Rehousing is not designed to provide permanent, ideal housing situations; however, these models can provide short-term relief of housing need while permanent solutions that follow Housing First models are sought.

In addition to housing shortages, Housing First experiences other challenges to implementation. Clients with complex needs may refuse or have inconsistent engagement with services. Oudshoorn et al. (2023) find that service providers identify challenges with balancing the need to assertively engage clients and simultaneously allow for consumer choice. They also note that the placement of services can limit client choice in housing, especially in jurisdictions with limited public transportation. Further, power differences between clients and providers and providers and funders limit clients' abilities to exercise true choice (Oudshoorn et al., 2023). Pressure and stress experienced by providers can negatively impact relationships. In light of these constraints, Oudshoorn et al. (2023) suggest that Housing First providers ensure that the programmes do not establish processes that are antithetical to the core principles of Housing First, are clear and upfront about what housing is or is not available, work with clients even if they decline available housing, conduct honest fidelity assessments, and prioritize consumer choice above all other principles.

Conclusion

Housing First is an integral part of the Bridging the Transition Framework and aligns well with its core principles. The philosophy engages with a housing-driven approach to homelessness response and prevention. Despite its limitations, practitioners should focus on prioritizing a Housing First approach to service provision and assess programme fidelity to the core principles of Housing First. Practitioners should remove readiness requirements for housing, provide client choice in both housing and supports, operate with a recovery orientation, and foster social connections and community integration.

References

Anderson-Baron, J. T., & Collins, D. (2019). 'Take whatever you can get': Practicing Housing First in Alberta. *Housing Studies*, *34*(8), 1286–1306.

Aubry, T., Nelson, G., & Tsemberis, S. (2015). Housing first for people with severe mental illness who are homeless: A review of the research and findings from the at home—Chez Soi demonstration project. *The Canadian Journal of Psychiatry*, *60*(11), 467–474.

Barrenger, S. L., Stanhope, V., & Atterbury, K. (2015). Discursive processes creating team culture and recovery orientation among housing first providers. *American Journal of Psychiatric Rehabilitation*, *18*(3), 247–264.

Byrne, T., Huang, M., Nelson, R. E., & Tsai, J. (2023). Rapid rehousing for persons experiencing homelessness: A systematic review of the evidence. *Housing Studies*, *38*(4), 615–641.

Employment & Social Development Canada (2018). *Toolkit for Intensive Case Management in Canada: A Resource for Those Using a Case Management Program for the Housing First Model*. Government of Canada: Ottawa, ON.

Fazel, S., Geddes, J. R., & Kushel, M. (2014). The health of homeless people in high-income countries: Descriptive epidemiology, health consequences, and clinical and policy recommendations. *The Lancet*, *384*(9953), 1529–1540.

Ferreiro, I. C., Abad, J. M. H., & Cuadra, M. A. R. (2021). Loneliness in homeless participants of a housing first program: Outcomes of a randomized controlled trial. *Journal of Psychosocial Nursing and Mental Health Services*, *59*(3), 44–51.

Goering, P., Veldhuizen, S., Nelson, G. B., Stefancic, A., Tsemberis, S., Adair, C. E., ... & Streiner, D. L. (2016). Further validation of the pathways housing first fidelity scale. *Psychiatric Services*, *67*(1), 111–114.

Greenwood, R. M., Stefancic, A., Tsemberis, S., & Busch-Geertsema, V. (2013). Implementations of Housing First in Europe: Successes and challenges in maintaining model fidelity. *American Journal of Psychiatric Rehabilitation*, *16*(4), 290–312.

Kirzner, R. S., & Miserandino, M. (2023). Self-determination theory and social work values. *Research on Social Work Practice*, *33*(6), 656–665.

Latimer, E. A., Rabouin, D., Cao, Z., Ly, A., Powell, G., Adair, C. E., ... & At Home/Chez Soi Investigators. (2019). Cost-effectiveness of Housing First intervention with intensive case management compared with treatment as usual for homeless adults with mental illness: Secondary analysis of a randomized clinical trial. *JAMA Network Open*, *2*(8), e199782.

Lemieux-Cumberlege, A., & Taylor, E. P. (2019). An exploratory study on the factors affecting the mental health and well-being of frontline workers in homeless services. *Health & Social Care in the Community*, *27*(4), e367–e378.

Maslow, A., & Lewis, K. J. (1987). Maslow's hierarchy of needs. *Salenger Incorporated*, *14*(17), 987–990.

Nelson, G., & Aubry, T. (2018). *Assertive Community Treatment (ACT) and Housing First in Canada*. Toronto: EENet, Ontario Housing First Regional Network Community of Interest.

O'Campo, P., Stergiopoulos, V., Davis, O., Lachaud, J., Nisenbaum, R., Dunn, J. R., ... & Tsemberis, S. (2022). Health and social outcomes in the Housing First model: Testing the theory of change. *EClinicalMedicine*, *47*, 1–12.

Oudshoorn, A., Smith-Carrier, T., Hall, J., Forchuk, C., Befus, D., Caxaj, S., ... & Parsons, C. (2023). Understanding the principle of consumer choice in delivering housing first. *Housing Studies*, *38*(5), 841–859.

Pearson, C., Montgomery, A. E., & Locke, G. (2009). Housing stability among homeless individuals with serious mental illness participating in housing first programs. *Journal of Community Psychology*, *37*(3), 404–417.

Piat, M., Seida, K., & Padgett, D. (2020). Choice and personal recovery for people with serious mental illness living in supported housing. *Journal of Mental Health*, *29*(3), 306–313. https://doi.org/10.1080/09638237.2019.1581338

Reilly, J., Ho, I., & Williamson, A. (2022). A systematic review of the effect of stigma on the health of people experiencing homelessness. *Health & Social Care in the Community*, *30*(6), 2128–2141.

Stadler, S. L., & Collins, D. (2023). Assessing Housing First programs from a right to housing perspective. *Housing Studies*, *38*(9), 1719–1739.

Stefancic, A., Tsemberis, S., Messeri, P., Drake, R., & Goering, P. (2013). The Pathways Housing First fidelity scale for individuals with psychiatric disabilities. *American Journal of Psychiatric Rehabilitation*, *16*(4), 240–261.

Stergiopoulos, V., Gozdzik, A., O'Campo, P., Holtby, A. R., Jeyaratnam, J., & Tsemberis, S. (2014). Housing First: Exploring participants' early support needs. *BMC Health Services Research*, *14*, 1–15.

Tinland, A., Loubière, S., Boucekine, M., Boyer, L., Fond, G., Girard, V., & Auquier, P. (2020). Effectiveness of a housing support team intervention with a recovery-oriented approach on hospital and emergency department use by homeless people with severe mental illness: A randomised controlled trial. *Epidemiology and Psychiatric Sciences*, *29*, e169.

Tsemberis, S. (2010). Housing First: Ending homelessness, promoting recovery and reducing costs. *How to House the Homeless*, 37–56.

Tsemberis, S. (2013). Housing first: Implementation, dissemination, and program fidelity. *American Journal of Psychiatric Rehabilitation*, *16*(4), 235–239.

Tsemberis, S., & Eisenberg, R. F. (2000). Pathways to housing: Supported housing for street-dwelling homeless individuals with psychiatric disabilities. *Psychiatric Services*, *51*(4), 487–493.

Wehmeyer, M. L., & Shogren, K. A. (2016). Self-determination and choice. In N. N. Singh (Ed.), *Handbook of Evidence-Based Practices in Intellectual and Developmental Disabilities*, 561–584. Springer.

Woodhall-Melnik, J. R., & Dunn, J. R. (2016). A systematic review of outcomes associated with participation in Housing First programs. *Housing Studies*, *31*(3), 287–304.

Woodhall-Melnik, J., Dunn, J. R., Svenson, S., Hamilton-Wright, S., Patterson, C., Waterfield, D., … & Matheson, F. I. (2017). Finding a place to start: Exploring meanings of housing stability in Hamilton's male housing first participants. *Housing, Theory and Society*, *34*(3), 359–375.

Woodhall-Melnik, J., Dunn, J. R., Svenson, S., Patterson, C., & Matheson, F. I. (2018). Men's experiences of early life trauma and pathways into long-term homelessness. *Child Abuse & Neglect*, *80*, 216–225.

Wright, A. G. (2012). Social defeat in recovery-oriented supported housing: Moral experience, stigma, and ideological resistance. *Culture, Medicine, and Psychiatry*, *36*, 660–678.

11

GUIDING PRINCIPLES OF THE BRIDGING THE TRANSITION FRAMEWORK

Recovery

Skye Barbic

This chapter explores the concept of recovery in the context of homelessness, emphasizing the importance of understanding recovery at individual, community, and population levels. Individual recovery focuses on personal healing from mental illness (substance use disorders), while community-level recovery creates supportive environments that foster inclusion, social connections, and access to resources. Population-level recovery addresses the systemic factors that contribute to homelessness, such as housing instability, poverty, and discrimination, and works toward creating structural changes that promote long-term recovery for entire populations. By integrating these three levels of recovery, the chapter highlights how a comprehensive approach can address both immediate needs and the root causes of homelessness. Key strategies discussed include providing stable housing, accessible and integrated healthcare and social services, peer support, and community engagement, as well as the need for cross-sector collaboration. Ultimately, understanding recovery at all levels is essential for fostering lasting, meaningful recovery for individuals and communities affected by homelessness.

Component of the Bridging the Transition Framework Addressed in this Chapter

This chapter describes the recovery model as a guiding principle in research and practice aimed at homelessness prevention. An overview of the recovery model, and how it can be used in research and practice to support the daily

DOI: 10.4324/9781003541332-13

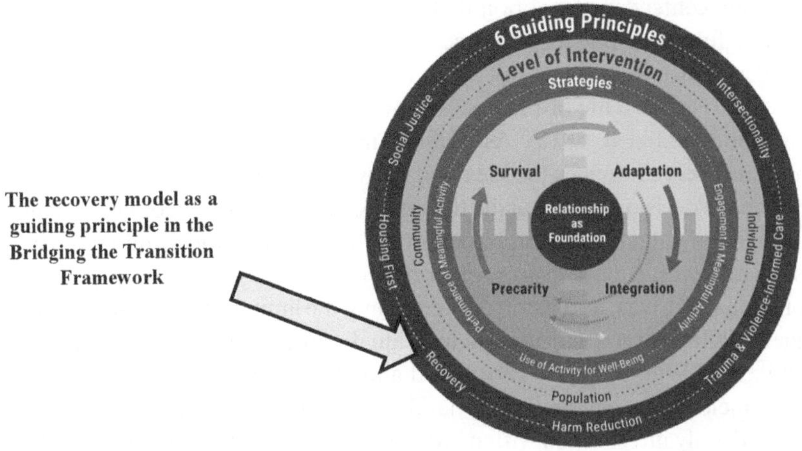

FIGURE 11.1 Recovery as a Guiding Principle.

life functioning, participation, and well-being of individuals across the trajectory of unhoused to housing, is discussed in this chapter (see Figure 11.1).

How this Chapter Guides Practice and Research in Homelessness Prevention

Understanding recovery as a process of living a full and meaningful life despite mental illness (Drake and Whitley, 2014) is crucial for both practice and research in homelessness. By redefining recovery as the pursuit of purpose and dignity, not just the absence of symptoms, this approach shifts the focus from managing mental illness to fostering well-being and social inclusion. The *Bridging the Transition from Homelessness* framework emphasizes stable housing as a foundation for recovery, integrating mental health care, social support, and personal growth. It promotes trauma-informed, harm reduction practices that address the complex needs of individuals facing both homelessness and mental illness. For researchers and practitioners alike, it highlights the importance of studying and implementing holistic, integrated support systems that lead to sustainable recovery and community integration.

Introduction

Recovery, particularly in the context of mental illness, is often misunderstood as merely the absence of symptoms or a return to a previous state of functioning (Davidson et al., 2007). However, a more comprehensive and evidence-based definition centers on the notion that recovery is the process of living a full and meaningful life despite the presence of mental illness (Deegan, 1997, Drake and Whitley, 2014). Recovery is not about returning to what was, but rather moving forward to create a life of purpose, dignity, and connection (Leamy et al., 2016, Slade and Longden, 2015). As outlined in the *Bridging the Transition framework*, recovery embraces the idea that individuals can regain control over their lives, make decisions, and pursue their goals, even with the ongoing challenge of managing mental health conditions, other health conditions, and the precarity associated with a past history of homelessness. Recovery is deeply personal, contextually driven, and involves overcoming the limitations imposed by mental illness while also recognizing the individual's inherent strengths and resilience (Drake and Whitley, 2014, Thornicroft and Slade, 2014).

Homelessness, on the other hand, is a complex and multifaceted issue that is deeply intertwined with mental health and the recovery process. Many individuals experiencing homelessness face mental health and/or substance use challenges, and conversely, mental illness can exacerbate or contribute to the conditions that lead to homelessness (Kidd et al., 2019). Mental illness can disrupt a person's ability to maintain stable housing, access services, and build or maintain social connections (Jones et al., 2022, Jones et al., 2015, Vila-Rodriguez et al., 2013). The isolation, trauma, and instability of homelessness often worsen the symptoms of mental illness, creating a cycle that is incredibly difficult to break.

Recovery is possible, even in the face of homelessness, and everyone has the right to a life of dignity, hope, and meaning. It requires access to mental health care, stable housing, social support, and opportunities for engagement. While the journey may be complex, with the right resources and community commitment, individuals can build new futures. The *Bridging the Transition framework* emphasizes integration as the ultimate goal, urging communities to create stronger, more inclusive support systems.

Recovery and Homelessness: A Personal, Community, and Population-Level Approach

Homelessness is a complex, global issue marked by instability, social exclusion, and often poor mental and physical health. It is closely linked to mental illness and substance use, with each reinforcing the other. In this context, recovery offers a vital pathway toward stability, purpose, and social inclusion. Recovery from mental illness, as defined by the *Substance Abuse and Mental Health Services Administration* and others (Drake and Whitley, 2014, Davidson, 2016), is a process of living a full and meaningful life, *in and despite* the mental illness. This understanding of recovery is not about curing or eliminating symptoms but about empowering individuals to live lives that have personal meaning and purpose, supported by hope, autonomy, and community. When applied to individuals experiencing homelessness, recovery takes on a unique set of challenges and opportunities.

The *Bridging the Transition framework* is useful for understanding how individuals who have experienced homelessness can be supported through the recovery process. This framework emphasizes the importance of not just providing housing but ensuring that individuals are *integrated* into society, provided with opportunities for social participation, and supported in their mental and physical health needs. It offers a pathway through which individuals can move from a state of homelessness to one of recovery, stability, and meaningful engagement. The following sections use the framework to understand recovery from the individual, community, and population perspectives.

Understanding **Individual** *Recovery in the Context of Homelessness*

Individual recovery, in the context of mental illness, is defined by more than just symptom reduction. It is about reclaiming control over one's life, pursuing a sense of purpose, and engaging meaningfully with society. Recovery is often described as deeply individual; what recovery looks like for one person may be entirely different for another, depending on their values, needs, and aspirations (Davidson, 2016). Although there are many different definitions of recovery, the key elements that constitute recovery include hope, personal responsibility, self-advocacy, meaningful roles, and social connection. These are defined more clearly in Table 11.1.

Recovery is especially difficult for people experiencing homelessness due to the trauma, instability, and lack of access to care. Homelessness worsens existing mental health and substance use issues, while also increasing the risk of developing conditions like depression, anxiety, and serious psychiatric disorders (Castillo et al., 2019). The stress and deprivation of life without stable housing make recovery nearly impossible without basic supports. Thus, for those experiencing both mental illness and homelessness, recovery requires more than just treatment. It requires access to stable housing, social support, and resources that foster healing, growth, and integration into society.

TABLE 11.1 Common key elements that constitute recovery

- **Hope**: Belief that recovery is possible, regardless of the severity of the mental illness or substance use disorder.
- **Personal responsibility**: Taking charge of one's life and making decisions that support well-being.
- **Self-advocacy**: Empowering individuals to speak up for their needs and goals.
- **Meaningful roles**: Engaging in work, community, and relationships that are valued by the individual.
- **Social connection**: Developing relationships and being part of a community that supports well-being.

Understanding Community Recovery in the Context of Homelessness

The *Bridging the Transition framework* offers a valuable approach to supporting individuals as they move from homelessness to stability and recovery. It emphasizes that recovery is not just an individual journey but a collective one, requiring strong community involvement. Recovery-oriented communities recognize the need for safe, affordable housing, inclusive and compassionate environments, integrated health services, peer support, and opportunities for education and employment. Recovery-oriented communities are built on the belief that everyone has the potential to integrate, grow, and thrive, regardless of their past struggles. The framework highlights how addressing these areas can foster integration, stability, and long-term recovery.

Creating Safe, Stable, and Affordable Housing

One of the most essential components for people in recovery, especially those who have experienced homelessness or housing instability, is access to stable housing. A safe and permanent place to live provides the foundation for individuals to begin their recovery journey. Without stable housing, individuals are often unable to focus on their mental health or recovery goals, as their immediate survival needs take priority. Communities need to ensure there are affordable and accessible housing options for individuals in recovery, especially for those with mental health or substance use disorders. Housing-first models (Tinland et al., 2020, Kozloff et al., 2016), which prioritize providing stable housing before requiring individuals to engage in treatment, have proven to be effective in supporting recovery and preventing relapse.

Building a Culture of Community Compassion and Inclusivity

For nearly half a century, extensive literature has highlighted how recovery is often an isolating experience, particularly for individuals who may have faced stigma due to their mental illness (Tanner, 1946, Eissler, 1947, McCusker et al., 1982). The *Bridging the Transition framework* outlines how communities can actively work to reduce stigma by fostering an inclusive and compassionate culture. This includes educating the public about mental health and recovery, promoting empathy, and dismantling stereotypes about people with lived experiences of mental illness or addiction. A compassionate community provides people in recovery with a sense of belonging and acceptance. Social inclusion is critical to recovery because isolation can exacerbate feelings of shame, hopelessness, and disconnection. Communities that embrace people in recovery create an environment where individuals feel valued and supported, which in turn can enhance their self-esteem and motivation to continue their recovery journey.

Increasing Access to Integrated Health and Mental Health Services

As noted above, recovery is often a complex and ongoing process that requires access to a range of services, including mental health care, substance use treatment, physical health care, and social services. Communities need to ensure that there are accessible, affordable, and effective services for individuals in recovery. Strong emerging evidence suggests that these services should be integrated and culturally relevant, addressing not only the symptoms of mental illness or addiction but also the social, emotional, developmental, and practical needs of individuals (Barbic et al., 2024, Henderson et al., 2018). In addition, integrated health and social systems must be flexible and responsive to the needs of people in recovery, including managing co-occurring physical health and cognitive issues and ensuring that individuals are able to maintain their well-being as they work on their recovery and transition from homelessness (Barbic et al., 2024, Henderson et al., 2023, McGorry et al., 2022).

Social Support and Peer Networks

Extensive literature supports that peer support is an integral part of recovery (Ow et al., 2022, Foerster et al., 2021). Communities should foster opportunities for people in recovery to connect with others who have had similar experiences (including homelessness), as peer support has been shown to be an effective mechanism for recovery and transitioning from homelessness or states of precarious housing. Peer support groups and recovery communities offer individuals a space to share their experiences, receive encouragement, and learn from others who understand their struggles. Community programs, such as support groups, club-houses, recovery-oriented events, and mentorship opportunities, can be instrumental in helping individuals feel less alone and more connected to others. These networks can provide emotional support, practical advice, and a sense of accountability that can encourage sustained recovery. Furthermore, peer support helps challenge the isolation that often accompanies the recovery process, creating a positive feedback loop where individuals feel empowered and encouraged (Peate, 2020).

Supported Employment and Education in Recovery

For individuals and communities in recovery, finding and offering meaningful work or engaging in educational opportunities can be pivotal to building self-worth, financial independence, and a sense of purpose. As noted throughout the *Bridging the Transition from Homelessness*, communities need to create pathways to employment and education for people in recovery, recognizing that stable work and ongoing learning are essential aspects of a person's recovery journey. Communities can support people in recovery by offering job training programs, workforce development initiatives, and educational opportunities that are tailored to individuals with a history of mental illness, substance use, and/or homelessness (Poremski and Hwang, 2016, Poremski et al., 2015). Additionally, creating inclusive workplaces that offer accommodations for mental health and recovery needs can help ensure that people in recovery have fair access to employment opportunities and are able to thrive in their roles (Knapp et al., 2013, Latimer et al., 2011).

Prioritizing How to Address the Root Causes of Recovery Barriers in Communities

Finally, for this work to be sustainable, communities need to recognize and address the underlying social determinants that can make recovery more difficult for individuals, such as poverty, unemployment, discrimination, and a lack of access to resources (Rafla-Yuan et al., 2022, Turpel-Lafond, 2020). For people in recovery, overcoming these barriers can be critical to their success. Communities can offer programs that target these root causes, such as financial literacy classes, housing support, legal aid, and anti-discrimination initiatives. By addressing the broader social issues that contribute to mental health and substance use challenges and homelessness, communities create a more supportive environment where individuals in recovery can thrive. Moreover, communities can offer support to those who face systemic barriers due to race, gender, or socioeconomic status, ensuring that recovery is inclusive and equitable for all members of society.

In summary, this section highlights that supporting people in recovery requires a holistic approach that encompasses a wide range of services, social connections, and opportunities for growth. Communities have the power to create environments that nurture recovery by offering safe housing, reducing stigma, providing comprehensive health services, supporting peer networks, and promoting social inclusion. Ultimately, understanding what communities need to do to support people in recovery means recognizing that recovery is not an individual effort but a collective one. By working together, communities can help individuals find hope and build lives that are meaningful, stable, and connected to others.

Understanding Population-Level Recovery in the Context of Homelessness

Perhaps the most unique contribution of the *Bridging the Transition from Homelessness framework* is the need to consider population-level recovery in the context of homelessness as involving and recognizing recovery as a multifaceted and collective process that transcends the individual and community and addresses the *systemic and societal factors* that contribute to both homelessness and intersecting mental health and substance use struggles. As noted by Llewellyn-Beardsley and colleagues, "Nothing's changed, baby" (Llewellyn-Beardsley et al., 2023). While individual recovery focuses on the personal journey of healing and rebuilding life after mental illness or substance use, and community-recovery focuses on increasing access to the things a person needs to recovery, population-level recovery emphasizes large-scale efforts aimed at creating an environment where individuals, particularly those who have experienced homelessness, can access the resources, support, and opportunities needed to recover and thrive. There have long been calls in research and practice for sustainable funding and policy to support population-level approaches to supporting recovery of all people, including those who experience homelessness (Davidson et al., 2007, Davidson et al., 2007, Kidd et al., 2014b, McKenzie, 2013).

This approach goes beyond addressing the immediate needs of people experiencing homelessness and focuses on creating an inclusive, supportive environment that promotes recovery for entire populations. It involves understanding how systems of care, housing policies, and community-level interventions can collectively contribute to the recovery of individuals while fostering broader societal change (Jones et al., 2021, Kerman and Sylvestre, 2020).

Structural Barriers

Population-level recovery requires an understanding of the broader structural barriers that contribute to homelessness, such as poverty, housing instability, inequality, and lack of access to healthcare and social services. These systemic issues are key determinants of whether or not individuals can achieve lasting recovery. Recovery in this context means addressing the root causes of homelessness and mental illness and substance use, not just treating symptoms once they appear. *The Bridging the Transition from Homelessness framework emphasizes the steps to exit homelessness but also takes a careful perspective on prevention and early intervention to prevent homelessness*. For example, a lack of affordable housing for all is a significant barrier to recovery for those experiencing homelessness. Without secure housing, people are unable to focus on mental health or substance use recovery, which ultimately hinders their chances of successful reintegration into society. Additionally, individuals from marginalized groups (such as racial minorities, 2SLGBTQIA+ populations, and those with disabilities) often face higher rates of homelessness due to systemic discrimination, further complicating their process of recovery. Therefore, tackling these systemic issues through policy reform, affordable housing development, anti-discrimination initiatives, and equitable access to resources is essential for population-level recovery (Kidd and Davidson, 2009, Kidd et al., 2014a).

Prevention and Early Intervention

A key part of population-level recovery is the focus on prevention and early intervention. Rather than waiting for individuals to experience homelessness or crisis, communities and systems of care should prioritize efforts to prevent homelessness from occurring in the first place, especially for populations at risk (e.g., people leaving institutional settings, those with mental illness or substance use issues, youth aging out of foster care). Preventative measures may include early intervention such as mental health and harm reduction services, eviction prevention programs, access to affordable healthcare and integrated social services, and community-based outreach, including peer support (Samji et al., 2021). By identifying and addressing risk factors early, communities can help individuals avoid the trauma of homelessness and better support their long-term recovery. A population-level approach should ensure that interventions are proactively addressing the needs of equity-deserving groups before they fall into homelessness and crisis.

Collaboration Across Sectors and Prioritizing Community-driven Solutions

Population-level recovery is most successful when collaboration occurs across various sectors, including housing, mental health, healthcare, law enforcement, employment, and social services. These sectors must work together to provide coordinated and holistic support for individuals recovering from homelessness and mental illness. Unfortunately many funding structures place agencies in silos and often make them compete for funding, therefore diluting the motivation to collaborate. From a policy perspective, healthcare providers, social service agencies, housing organizations, and legal aid services must be supported and funded to coordinate efforts to help individuals navigate the complex systems of care, data collection, and reporting. By sharing information, collecting robust data, and ensuring that individuals and communities in recovery receive the appropriate services at the right time, these sectors can create a more effective safety net and streamline the recovery process for people who have experienced homelessness or who are at risk of homelessness. Population-level recovery must also incorporate the voices and experiences of people who have lived through homelessness and recovery (Kulik et al., 2011, Llewellyn-Beardsley et al., 2023).

In summary, population-level recovery from homelessness requires a holistic, systemic approach that addresses both individual needs and the structural factors driving homelessness and mental health challenges. It involves building inclusive, resilient communities through prevention, early intervention, comprehensive services, and cross-sector collaboration. With sustained resources and collective effort, communities can create conditions that support long-term recovery, promote social inclusion, and make recovery accessible for all.

Conclusion

Understanding recovery at the individual, community, and population levels is key to developing a sustainable response to homelessness. Individual recovery focuses on personal healing, community recovery builds supportive environments, and population-level recovery addresses systemic issues. Together, these levels offer a holistic approach that meets immediate needs, tackles root causes, and promotes inclusion and resilience. Frameworks like *Bridging the Transition from Homelessness* help integrate these efforts into a more effective and compassionate system of support.

References

Barbic, S., Mallia, E., Wuerth, K., Ow, N., Marchand, K., Ben-David, S., Ewert, A., Turnbull, H., Gao, C., Ding, X., Dhillon, A., Hastings, K., Langton, J., Tee, K. & Mathias, S. (2024) 'Implementing Foundry: A cohort study describing the regional and virtual expansion of a youth integrated service in British Columbia, Canada', *Early Intervention in Psychiatry*, 18, pp. 877–887.

Castillo, E.G., Ijadi-Maghsoodi, R., Shadravan, S., Moore, E., Mensah, M.O., 3rd, Docherty, M., Aguilera Nunez, M.G., Barcelo, N., Goodsmith, N., Halpin, L.E., Morton, I., Mango, J., Montero, A.E., Rahmanian Koushkaki, S., Bromley, E., Chung, B., Jones, F., Gabrielian, S., Gelberg, L., Greenberg, J.M., Kalofonos, I., Kataoka, S.H., Miranda, J., Pincus, H.A., Zima, B.T. & Wells, K.B. (2019) 'Community interventions to promote mental health and social equity', *Current Psychiatry Reports*, 21, p. 35.

Davidson, L. (2016) 'The recovery movement: Implications for mental health care and enabling people to participate fully in life', *Health Affairs (Millwood)*, 35, pp. 1091–1097.

Davidson, L., Tondora, J., O'Connell, M.J., Kirk, T., Jr., Rockholz, P. & Evans, A.C. (2007) 'Creating a recovery-oriented system of behavioral health care: Moving from concept to reality', *Psychiatric Rehabilitation Journal*, 31, pp. 23–31.

Deegan, P.E. (1997) 'Recovery and empowerment for people with psychiatric disabilities', *Social Work in Health Care*, 25, pp. 11–24.

Drake, R.E. & Whitley, R. (2014) 'Recovery and severe mental illness: Description and analysis', *Canadian Journal of Psychiatry*, 59, pp. 236–42.

Eissler, K.R. (1947) 'Objective (behavioristic) criteria of recovery from neuropsychiatric disorders', *Journal of Nervous and Mental Disease*, 106, pp. 550–64.

Foerster, V., Tallon, C., Turuba, R., Amarasekera, A., Brockmann, V., Darnay, K., Helfrich, W., Henderson, J., Mathias, S. & Barbic, S. (2021) *Peer support for young people and substance use*. Foundry.

Henderson, J.L., Chiodo, D., Varatharasan, N., Andari, S., Luce, J. & Wolfe, J. (2023) 'Youth Wellness Hubs Ontario: Development and initial implementation of integrated youth services in Ontario, Canada', *Early Intervention in Psychiatry*, 17, pp. 107–114.

Henderson, J.L., Hawke, L.D. & Relihan, J. (2018) 'Youth engagement in the YouthCan IMPACT trial', *CMAJ*, 190, pp. S10–S12.

Jones, A.A., Cho, L.L., Kim, D.D., Barbic, S.P., Leonova, O., Byford, A., Buchanan, T., Vila-Rodriguez, F., Procyshyn, R.M., Lang, D.J., Vertinsky, A.T., MacEwan, G.W., Rauscher, A., Panenka, W.J., Thornton, A.E., Barr, A.M., Field, T.S. & Honer, W.G. (2022) 'Pain, opioid use, depressive symptoms, and mortality in adults living in precarious housing or homelessness: A longitudinal prospective study', *Pain*.

Jones, A.A., Vila-Rodriguez, F., Leonova, O., Langheimer, V., Lang, D.J., Barr, A.M., Procyshyn, R.M., Smith, G.N., Schultz, K., Buchanan, T., Krausz, M., Montaner, J.S., MacEwan, G.W., Rauscher, A., Panenka, W.J., Thornton, A.E. & Honer, W.G. (2015) 'Mortality from treatable illnesses in marginally housed adults: A prospective cohort study', *BMJ Open*, 5, p. e008876.

Jones, N., Atterbury, K., Byrne, L., Carras, M., Brown, M. & Phalen, P. (2021) 'Lived experience, research leadership, and the transformation of mental health services: Building a researcher pipeline', *Psychiatric Services*, 72, pp. 591–593.

Kerman, N. & Sylvestre, J. (2020) 'Service use and recovery among currently and formerly homeless adults with mental illness', *International Journal of Social Psychiatry*, 66, pp. 389–396.

Kidd, S.A. & Davidson, L. (2009) 'Homeless youth: The need to link research and policy', In *Finding home: Policy options for addressing homelessness in Canada*, edited by Hulchanski, J., Campsie, P., Chau, S., Hwang, S.C. & Paradis, E., Toronto: University of Toronto.

Kidd, S.A., McKenzie, K.J. & Virdee, G. (2014a) 'Mental health reform at a systems level: Widening the lens on recovery-oriented care', *Canadian Journal of Psychiatry - Revue Canadienne de Psychiatrie*, 59, pp. 243–249.

Kidd, S.A., McKenzie, K.J. & Virdee, G. (2014b) 'Mental health reform at a systems level: Widening the lens on recovery-oriented care', *Canadian Journal of Psychiatry*, 59, pp. 243–249.

Kidd, S.A., Thistle, J., Beaulieu, T., O'Grady, B. & Gaetz, S. (2019) 'A national study of Indigenous youth homelessness in Canada', *Public Health*, 176, pp. 163–171.

Knapp, M., Patel, A., Curran, C., Latimer, E., Catty, J., Becker, T., Drake, R.E., Fioritti, A., Kilian, R., Lauber, C., Rossler, W., Tomov, T., Van Busschbach, J., Comas-Herrera, A., White, S., Wiersma, D. & Burns, T. (2013) 'Supported employment: Cost-effectiveness across six European sites', *World Psychiatry*, 12, pp. 60–68.

Kozloff, N., Stergiopoulos, V., Adair, C.E., Cheung, A.H., Misir, V., Townley, G., Bourque, J., Krausz, M. & Goering, P. (2016) 'The unique needs of homeless youths with mental illness: Baseline findings from a Housing First trial', *Psychiatric Services*, appips201500461.

Kulik, D.M., Gaetz, S., Crowe, C. & Ford-Jones, E.L. (2011) 'Homeless youth's overwhelming health burden: A review of the literature', *Paediatrics & Child Health*, 16, p. e43–e47.

Latimer, E.A., Bond, G.R. & Drake, R.E. (2011) 'Economic approaches to improving access to evidence-based and recovery-oriented services for people with severe mental illness', *Canadian Journal of Psychiatry*, 56, pp. 523–529.

Leamy, M., Clarke, E., Le Boutillier, C., Bird, V., Choudhury, R., MacPherson, R., Pesola, F., Sabas, K., Williams, J., Williams, P. & Slade, M. (2016) 'Recovery practice in community mental health teams: National survey', *British Journal of Psychiatry*, 209, pp. 340–346.

Llewellyn-Beardsley, J., Rennick-Egglestone, S., Callard, F., Pollock, K., Slade, M. & Edgley, A. (2023) '"Nothing's changed, baby": How the mental health narratives of people with multiple and complex needs disrupt the recovery framework', *SSM Mental Health*, 3, p. 100221.

McCusker, E.A., Rudick, R.A., Honch, G.W. & Griggs, R.C. (1982) 'Recovery from the "locked-in" syndrome', *Archives of Neurology*, 39, pp. 145–147.

McGorry, P.D., Mei, C., Chanen, A., Hodges, C., Alvarez-Jimenez, M. & Killackey, E. (2022) 'Designing and scaling up integrated youth mental health care', *World Psychiatry*, 21, pp. 61–76.

McKenzie, K. (2013) 'How do social factors cause psychotic illnesses?', *Canadian Journal of Psychiatry - Revue Canadienne de Psychiatrie*, 58, pp. 41–43.

Ow, N., Leon, A., Thom, B., Herwynen, J., Mathias, S.M. & Barbic, S. (2022) '"I felt supported by the peers in my group": Analyzing experiences of youths with mental health challenges of a supported employment program in Canada', *Journal of Occupational Rehabilitation*, 1, pp. 1–11.

Peate, I. (2020) 'Self-isolation and the homeless population', *British Journal of Nursing*, 29, p. 387.

Poremski, D. & Hwang, S.W. (2016) 'Willingness of Housing First participants to consider supported-employment services', *Psychiatric Services*, 67(6), pp. 667–670. doi: 10.1176/appi.ps.201500140

Poremski, D., Rabouin, D. & Latimer, E. (2015) 'A randomised controlled trial of evidence-based supported employment for people who have recently been homeless and have a mental illness', *Administration and Policy in Mental Health*, pp. 1–11.

Rafla-Yuan, E., Moore, S., Carvente-Martinez, H., Yang, P., Balasuriya, L., Jackson, K., McMickens, C. & Robles-Ramamurthy, B. (2022) 'Striving for equity in community mental health: Opportunities and challenges for integrating care for BIPOC youth', *Child and Adolescent Psychiatric Clinics of North America*, 31, pp. 295–312.

Samji, H., Dove, N., Ames, M., Barbic, S., Sones, M. & Leadbeater, B. (2021) 'Impacts of the COVID-19 pandemic on the health and well-being of young adults in British Columbia', Unpublished report.

Slade, M. & Longden, E. (2015) 'Empirical evidence about recovery and mental health', *BMC Psychiatry*, 15, p. 285.

Tanner, J.M. (1946) 'Treatment and recovery of a case of anxiety state', *Nursing Mirror & Midwives Journal*, 82, p. 441.

Thornicroft, G. & Slade, M. (2014) 'New trends in assessing the outcomes of mental health interventions', *World Psychiatry*, 13, pp. 118–124.

Tinland, A., Loubière, S., Boucekine, M., Boyer, L., Fond, G., Girard, V. & Auquier, P. (2020) 'Effectiveness of a housing support team intervention with a recovery-oriented approach on hospital and emergency department use by homeless people with severe mental illness: A randomised controlled trial', *Epidemiology and Psychiatric Sciences*, 29, p. e169.

Turpel-Lafond, M.E. (2020) *In plain sight: Addressing Indigenous-specific racism and discrimination in B.C. Health Care*. Government of British Columbia. https://engage.gov.bc.ca/app/uploads/sites/613/2020/11/In-Plain-Sight-Full-Report.pdf

Vila-Rodriguez, F., Panenka, W.J., Lang, D.J., Thornton, A.E., Vertinsky, T., Wong, H., Barr, A.M., Procyshyn, R.M., Sidhu, J.J., Smith, G.N., Buchanan, T., Krajden, M., Krausz, M., Montaner, J.S., MacEwan, G.W. & Honer, W.G. (2013) 'The hotel study: Multimorbidity in a community sample living in marginal housing', *American Journal of Psychiatry*, 170, pp. 1413–1422.

12

GUIDING PRINCIPLES OF THE BRIDGING THE TRANSITION FRAMEWORK

Harm Reduction

Abe Oudshoorn

Harm reduction is a conceptual approach to addressing substance use health, itself made up of several principles. It is a pragmatic approach that recognizes individuals as experts in their own recovery, that using substances comes with harms, and that there are ways to mitigate these harms inclusive of but not only through abstinence. While grounded in theory, harm reduction is actualized as a variety of programs that support individuals to optimize their wellness in the context of potentially continued substance use. In this chapter, the principles of harm reduction are presented in the context of the Bridging the Transition Framework, along with examples of harm reduction programs, and the particularities of supporting substance use health in the transition from homeless to housed.

Component of the Bridging the Transition Framework Addressed in this Chapter

As harm reduction is a guiding principle of the Bridging the Transition Framework (see Figure 12.1), this overview of harm reduction will support researchers, service providers, policymakers, and lived experts in providing quality transitions to housing in the context of substance use (see Figure 12.1).

DOI: 10.4324/9781003541332-14

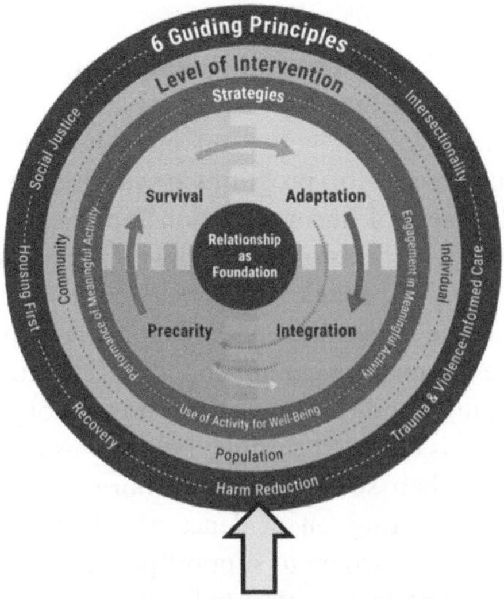

Harm reduction as a guiding principle in the Bridging the Transition Framework

FIGURE 12.1 Harm Reduction as a Guiding Principle.

How this Chapter Guides Practice and Research in Homelessness Prevention

Building on decades of evidence supporting Housing First models, research demonstrates that swift access to housing, coupled with comprehensive wraparound services, results in the most favorable health and social outcomes for individuals exiting homelessness (Aubry, Nelson & Tsemberis, 2015). For exits from homelessness to be rapid and efficient, there needs to be no pre-requirements or pre-conditions on the individual. This includes no requirement for sobriety or no requirement to have started on one's personal recovery journey (as outlined in Chapter 11). Otherwise, those most likely to experience chronic homelessness would be systematically screened out of re-housing services. Instead, housing is the context in which people can start to create new goals for their health and well-being. This chapter explains how harm reduction serves as a key practice in the transition to housing, acting as a tool for secondary homelessness prevention. By addressing substance use in practical ways, harm reduction helps prevent individuals from cycling back into homelessness. By meeting people where they are at and reducing harms related to substance use, those working in the sector can help to enhance the likelihood of long-term housing stability.

Introduction

While harm reduction is a theory and guiding principle in the Bridging the Transition Framework, in that it provides explanations for how delivering services in certain ways leads to better outcomes, it is frequently conceptualized as a program or series of programs to support people who use substances. The development of harm reduction approaches, interventions, and programs represents evolutions of best and wise practices in health services. This includes co-design approaches that include the lived and living experience of people who use substances, researchers, service providers, and decision-makers. While this chapter cannot encompass the full scope of evidence on these care modalities and their evolution, it is important to acknowledge that the knowledge has emerged through continuous iterations of practical interventions, rather than solely through laboratory research or abstract theory. Ultimately, reflecting on evidence-based practices such as harm reduction should allow providers to support people across a variety of contexts and individual experiences, essentially 'meeting them where they are'. In a historical context of substance use healthcare that at times has been paternalistic and punitive (Bruzelius et al., 2024), harm reduction offers an alternative situatedness where collaboration is central (Claborn et al., 2023) (Table 12.1).

Harm reduction is a pragmatic approach to the use of substances. Herein, the term 'substances' is used broadly, recognizing that this can be legal substances, such as alcohol, or criminalized substances, such as crystal methamphetamine. That said, the focus here is narrowed to substances rather than other aspects of addiction, such as gambling disorders, for which harm reduction principles might also be of use but which are not primarily covered within the research evidence on harm reduction. The pragmatism of harm reduction stems from its foundation in years of both practical service delivery and research evidence (Marlatt & Witkiewitz, 2010; Ritter & Cameron, 2006). The term is used intentionally to highlight that there are alternative approaches to substance use disorders, often rooted in personal beliefs, philosophies, or political views. While these approaches may seem effective to those who share similar belief systems, they may be less effective in achieving long-term positive substance use health outcomes (Musalek, 2013). The fundamental definition of harm reduction is, not surprisingly, to reduce harms particular to substance use. Therefore, while all treatments have a common goal of the health of the individual, harm reduction is distinguished from other more dated treatment modalities, such as forced abstinence, by recognizing that some individuals may continue to use substances and they can still improve their health throughout use (Vakharia, 2024). Indeed, harm reduction remains neutral on the idea of abstinence. If the individual has

TABLE 12.1 Conceptualizing Harm Reduction

As a theory	People who use drugs have inherent value and their rights and choices must be respected and protected. The negative consequences of drugs can be reduced without requiring abstinence.
As practices	Working collaboratively with people who use drugs to find ways to reduce the harms of substance use regardless of their interest in abstinence, but also allowing for abstinence if that is the goal.
As programs	Including but not limited to: safe supply, supervised consumption, needle exchange or distribution, provision of clean drug using equipment, naloxone distribution, opioid agonist therapy, withdrawal symptom management
Principles of Harm Reduction	1 Drug use is an inherent human activity and the harms related to this use can be reduced; 2 Some ways of using drugs are safer than others; 3 Well-being of people who use drugs and communities is more important than abstinence; 4 Supports around drug use should not be coercive; 5 People who use drugs should be a part of the leadership of programs addressing drug use; 6 Social inequities and inequality impact the ability of individuals to reduce the harms of substance use; 7 Drug use does come with risks and harms.

Adapted from National Harm Reduction Coalition (2024)

abstinence as their goal, harm reduction programs and providers can support them in this goal, but they can also support them in many other ways if this is not the current or a perceivable future goal. This is congruent with the fundamental principle in harm reduction that the individual sets their goals related to substance use health and well-being. However, this approach is not without awareness of the potential harms associated with all substances, including financial, social, health, and psychological impacts. The question underpinning the modality is how best the individual wants to address these harms while also recognizing the real harms substance use can have on the individual, those around them, and the broader community.

Harm Reduction for Substance Use Health

Combining the principles of pragmatism, recovery-orientation (Chapter 11), and client/patient/person-centeredness, it can be considered how someone who uses a substance might be protected from some of the harms while acknowledging these approaches do not eliminate all harms. For example, providing clean injection equipment to people who inject drugs may reduce the likelihood of acquiring or transmitting an infectious disease. However, this equipment itself does not reduce the risk of overdose/drug poisoning. One harm is reduced, but not all harms are reduced. That said, the actual provision of the equipment is an important point of connection between the individual and a health service provider. Through this health service, relationships might be built that create a supportive space to ask questions about other forms of reducing harms that may be of interest (see Chapter 4 for discussion on the importance of relationship).

'Judgment-free service' is a principle that is fundamental in aligning harm reduction with best evidence around motivational theories of recovery (Engel et al., 2021). Recognizing that people will only be successful in their personal goals related to substance use if the goals are indeed their own and if their goals are accepted (Groshkova, 2010), then harm reduction can be seen as congruent with substance use disorder treatment generally and should not be perceived as an alternative to treatment, but rather a set of tools to support positive treatment outcomes and experiences. Many decades of evidence indicate that *non-person-centered* approaches such as periods of forced abstinence, for example, lead to exceptionally high rates of relapse once the barrier to use has been removed (Larney, Mathers & Dolan, 2007; Tyndall, 2020). A pertinent example of this is people who are incarcerated. While recognizing that substances are often maintained or obtained while in jail, those who are incarcerated and stop using substances because of their incarceration are still highly likely to return to using substances upon release from jail (Western & Simes, 2019).

Another core principle of harm reduction is that 'people who use substances are experts in their own lives and have the right to set their own goals' (Hawk et al., 2017). This is not to negate the expertise of people such as health or social service professionals, but rather to recognize that expertise takes a variety of forms and one of these forms is lived and living experience. Therefore, service delivery of harm reduction modalities should include people with lived and living experiences of substance use disorders in the planning, co-design, and implementation of these services. Thus, it is not surprising that peer support models or peer service delivery are frequently found within harm reduction services (Parkes et al., 2019). There is coherence in these ideas of seeing the individual as an expert in their own health and their own goals that coincides nicely with seeing lived expertise as valuable for service delivery. To reiterate however, for the purposes of countering criticisms of harm reduction as being naïve to the harms of substance use, harm reduction as a philosophy acknowledges that substances can and do create harm. Therefore, the inclusion of lived and living expertise is not to the purpose of negating scientific realities of biology and chemistry, or the realities of social science and human science research, but rather to acknowledge that different sources of expertise and wisdom can absolutely go hand-in-hand. Accepting that substances create harms also allows us to consider that there are less harmful ways to use substances. Centering the expertise of lived experience empowers us to recognize that these individuals are key to identifying and implementing safer approaches that are person and community centered.

An example of harm reduction helps to clarify these foundational theoretical principles. Consider a modality that has garnered significant media and political attention: 'safe supply'. The idea of safe supply is to medically prescribe a substance that matches the substance use needs of an individual who lives with a substance use disorder (Ivsins et al., 2020). The concept is to prescribe drugs to people who are 'addicted' to drugs (the term 'addiction' is used herein for clarity purposes and is not generally used within health and social services due to its stigmatizing nature).

If we consider the example of an individual who may live with a substance use disorder that involves injection drug use and who is living on the streets in an urban city in Canada, we recognize that if unsupported, this carries a high risk of morbidity and increased likelihood of mortality (Mathers et al., 2013). The rates of overdose/drug poisoning for street-level injection drug use are as high as ever in Canada (Government of Canada, 2024). This has particularly escalated at this moment in time due to very high use of fentanyl, although newer forms of synthetic opioids are continuously entering the illicit drug supply. Fentanyl, which started mostly as an additive to other substances, is now increasingly used as a primary substance (Armenian, 2018). The widespread availability of fentanyl, coupled with the lack of consistent dosage or purity in illicitly manufactured substances, means that individuals injecting street-purchased drugs often have no knowledge of what is in their supply. This uncertainty increases the risk of unintentional overdose, or more accurately, drug poisoning. The less that the individual knows about their substance (i.e., such as its source, how it should look, and how other people have responded to use of this particular batch), the more deadly the situation may be when using. At the street level, individuals often rely on local knowledge, such as identifying trusted dealers who can provide a more consistent product with a reliable dosage. This has a slight protective effect as most people who deal drugs do not want to permanently harm the people to whom they sell their product. Therefore, they too are trying to seek a consistent supply of strong but predictable drugs. In this, we can actually see some of the principles of harm reduction in practice. A safer supply of drugs is one that is as explicitly understood as possible, so that people can use a controlled and safe amount, an amount they understand their body can tolerate. In the unregulated environments of the street or in the context of homelessness, this is often not done well or consistently (Browne, Gold, & Martin, 2021). Not surprisingly, many countries across the world are facing a catastrophic crisis of drug poisonings that are devastating individuals, communities, and populations (Government of Canada, 2024). Addressing this issue for people who are homeless is crucial because they are particularly vulnerable to substance use-related harms and overdose, often lacking access to stable housing, healthcare, and harm reduction resources.

Safe supply takes the pragmatic harm reduction principles and integrates them into health and social care services, including supporting a person to exit homelessness. If a physician is working with a person who injects drugs and that person is not ready to stop or switch to agonist treatments like Methadone or Suboxone, the physician can best support them by focusing on reducing the risk of drug poisoning. This is achieved by prescribing the individual with a known substance, at a known dose, that is going to be consistent for the individual. This is called safe supply. 'Safe', in this context, is a particular use of the term that does not indicate that injection drug use is free of harm, but indicates that substances that are manufactured in a controlled manner are always going to be safer to consume than substances which have been bought off the street. Safe supply is delivered intentionally and in a controlled manner as the health provider (often a physician or nurse practitioner) works within a therapeutic provider-patient relationship to understand the individual, to understand their other health risks or risks related to side effects, and titrates the safe supply prescription cautiously. The health provider will start treatment at a dose that balances how accustomed a person may already be to narcotic medication, without risking an over-supply. This complex balance demonstrates why safe supply is delivered within the context of a therapeutic relationship between a health provider and a patient. For people who are homeless or exiting homelessness, this process is complicated because they may face inconsistent access to healthcare, lack stable living conditions, and have challenges building a consistent therapeutic relationship with a service provider. These factors can make it difficult to achieve the delicate balance between providing adequate medication and avoiding overdose, as well as meeting their broader health goals and managing risks in a safe, individualized manner.

This presentation of safe supply stands in contrast to ways in which it has been misrepresented by its opponents as simply distributing large quantities of narcotics to anyone who asks. However, rather than mass quantities, the prescribed dose is intended to be matched to the patient and their particular needs to the purpose of completely reducing use of an unregulated supply. Use is often monitored (Ivsins et al., 2020), for example via urine drug screens, and if the person is supplementing with a street supply because their cravings are not adequately addressed, the dosage may be increased. If the patient is alternatively diverting the safe supply (i.e., selling), a portion or all of their prescription to others, the prescription will usually be reduced or cancelled (McNeil et al., 2022). Again, harm reduction acknowledges the harms that come with substance use. This includes harms of diversion of prescribed drugs to the streets, or harm related to how the prescribed drugs might be consumed, such as via injection. The response in safe supply is not to ignore these harms nor punish the person using substances, but rather to work collaboratively within the confidentiality of the provider-patient relationship to meet shared goals of substance use health.

In a final side note related to safe supply and diversion of prescribed opioids to the street, this may not be an ideal situation and has knock-on effects related to social harms such as crime. However, again from a pragmatic lens, someone choosing to use a pill that is untainted and in a known dose, diverted from a safe supply prescription, is going to be safer than using a street-manufactured synthetic opioid containing some unknown quantity of fentanyl. So while diversion is not wanted and efforts are taken to reduce diversion, even diverted prescribed medications can presumably reduce some of the harms of drug poisoning as a safer alternative when replacing street drugs. This is particularly relevant to people who are homeless because they often have limited access to regulated healthcare and face higher exposure to the risks of using illicit substances.

Harm Reduction to Bridge the Transition from Homelessness to Housing

As noted previously in this chapter, harm reduction takes many forms (Table 12.2), including but beyond substance use, and safe supply is simply one illustration how to reduce harms. Next, we will examine the unique considerations involved in delivering harm reduction services to individuals transitioning from homelessness to stable housing. Recognizing that some proportion of people exiting homelessness live with a substance use disorder and considering that becoming housed does not mean stopping using substances, harm reduction is a core modality of service provision in the sector. This means that staff, peer workers, and volunteers who are supporting people transitioning from homelessness should understand and recognize that while housing is the foundational intervention, there are other specific interventions related to substance use that can support this housing transition and long-term success.

Given the diversity of harm reduction approaches noted in Table 12.2, there are many ways that housing support workers can address substance

TABLE 12.2 Harm Reduction Modalities

Provision of clean injection equipment
Provision of clean smoking equipment
Needle exchange
Safe supply
Opioid agonist or antagonist, or receptor antagonist treatments (replacement therapies)
Nicotine gums or patches Condoms
Replacement of cigarette smoking with vaping
Transition from opioid use to THC use
Supervised drug consumption sites/overdose prevention sites
Drug testing
Community distribution and training on Naloxone

use. These modalities provide alternatives to more punitive approaches that instead allow for an ongoing supportive relationship based on the honest acknowledgment of substance use. If people are being invited into low-barrier housing with no pre-conditions, this needs to be held up via not then punishing substance use in the form of evictions. Conversely, however, supporting people who live with a substance use disorder in housing does not mean simply ignoring, avoiding, or downplaying the impacts of substance use. Quite the opposite, in that the transition from homelessness to housed is actually a high-risk period related to drug poisonings and overdose deaths (Fleming et al., 2024). Research suggests that this is because people who have been living in more congregate settings have been protected from overdoses via staff and other residents but may lose some of this natural protection when they are in a private apartment and may be using alone (Fleming et al., 2024). This is particularly dangerous because they may not be noticed for hours-to-days on end and therefore a potentially reversible poisoning may lead to death. This was illustrated during the COVID-19 pandemic where initially moving people from congregate shelters to motel rooms led to an increase in overdoses, and staff had to then adopt ways to collaboratively work with people to provide more protective support. Although it can be challenging in a housing setting where individuals have a right to privacy, and where openness and honesty are central to the support relationship, most residents are generally receptive to agreed-upon methods for housing staff to check in and ensure their safety.

As noted in the Bridging the Transition Framework, harm reduction is not only at the individual level, but also important considerations are needed at the community and population levels. To deliver harm reduction services within supported or supportive housing means that organizational policies must be in place to enact these practices. Organizations (and sometimes regions or jurisdictions) can best support staff and programs by making sure that policies acknowledge that some people use substances, some people continue to use substances once housed, and some people may start using substances while housed who had not done so before. It is unhealthy for both staff and residents when staff, recognizing the practicality of harm reduction, implement such approaches without the support of administration and policy. Many health and social service providers who worked in the early 2000s will recall the days of giving out clean needles to people without support of their organizations or legislation and in doing so put themselves at risk of being criminalized around carrying and distribution of 'drug paraphernalia'. The opposite of this situation is organizations who are explicit about the type of services they are able to provide, how they are provided, and the role staff play in providing these services to target populations.

An interesting example of policy addressing reality is how organizations deal with the fact that some people will purchase their substances from illicit providers. Conceivably, people who are selling drugs may be entering an apartment building to make such sales. Unaddressed, this has several potential negative impacts both for the individual themselves and for other residents of the building or in the community. Complaints and eviction requests often arise from uninvited visitors being brought into a building. Instead of punishing the resident, proactive approaches can acknowledge that people will likely purchase illicit drugs and focus on how agreements can minimize the potential harms associated with this reality. Where trust may exist between the housing provider and residents, it may be easier to have an honest conversation about best practices to support the individual and the community. Boundaries, rules, and agreements are all part of harm reduction practices. The key is co-developing them mutually. No one is well served by either pretending that people don't buy illicit drugs, or by just evicting anyone who is letting guests in the building who are causing trouble. Hence the pragmatism of harm reduction.

Other harm reduction strategies in a housing environment designed to transition people out of homelessness could include safer or supervised consumption spaces. Designing such a program would require careful planning to ensure it doesn't negatively affect other tenants, but it would provide a safer environment for substance use compared to individuals using drugs unsupervised in their own apartments. It could also include training on and provision of medications to reverse overdoses, such as Naloxone. Finally, peer support programs to discuss the use of substances and safer ways to use substances are common harm reduction approaches and can be delivered within housing environments.

As noted in the Bridging the Transition Framework, homelessness and homeless precarity may complicate harm reduction solutions such as safe supply and supervised consumption sites because individuals experiencing homelessness often lack stable housing, which makes it challenging to implement consistent, controlled harm reduction strategies like supervised consumption spaces. People may not have access to the resources, support, or privacy needed for such programs to be effective. Additionally, the transient nature of homelessness may mean that residents may be more difficult to engage in long-term rehabilitation or peer support programs. The instability of their living situations may also hinder the coordination needed to ensure safety, reduce harm, and foster long-term trust between residents and staff in these harm reduction initiatives.

Conclusion

Harm reduction is built upon the wisdoms of research, lived and lived experience of substance use, and service delivery experience. For transitions to housing to work for all people, recognition is important that for some this means ongoing substance use challenges. While abstinence may be an outcome with the least direct harms, it is often not the immediate or long-term reality for everyone as recovery journeys depend on the individual and their communities. Therefore, housing providers need to be familiar with harm reduction modalities, and decision-makers need to co-design and implement policies in place to support these modalities. Ultimately, all people are 'houseable', and reducing the harms of substance use is one necessary means to achieve this.

References

Armenian, P., Vo, K. T., Barr-Walker, J., & Lynch, K. L. (2018). Fentanyl, fentanyl analogs and novel synthetic opioids: A comprehensive review. *Neuropharmacology, 134*, 121–132.

Aubry, T., Nelson, G., & Tsemberis, S. (2015). Housing first for people with severe mental illness who are homeless: A review of the research and findings from the at home—chez soi demonstration project. *The Canadian Journal of Psychiatry, 60*(11), 467–474.

Browne, T., Gold, M. S., & Martin, D. M. (2021). The rapidly changing composition of the global street drug supply and its effects on high-risk groups for COVID-19. *Current Psychopharmacology, 10*(2), 138–154.

Bruzelius, E., Underhill, K., Askari, M. S., Kajeepeta, S., Bates, L., Prins, S. J., Jarlenski, M. & Martins, S. S. (2024). Punitive legal responses to prenatal drug use in the United States: A survey of state policies and systematic review of their public health impacts. *International Journal of Drug Policy, 126*, 104380.

Claborn, K., Samora, J., McCormick, K., Whittfield, Q., Courtois, F., Lozada, K., Sledge, D., Burwell, A., Chavez, S., Bailey, J., Bailey, C., Dalton Pederson, C., Zagorski, C., Conway, F.N., Holleran Steiker, L., Chance, J. & Potter, J. (2023). "We do it ourselves": Strengths and opportunities for improving the practice of harm reduction. *Harm Reduction Journal, 20*(1), 70.

Engel, L. B., Bright, S. J., Barratt, M. J., & Allen, M. M. (2021). Positive drug stories: Possibilities for agency and positive subjectivity for harm reduction. *Addiction Research & Theory, 29*(5), 363–371.

Fleming, T., Boyd, J., Gagnon, M., Kerr, T., & McNeil, R. (2024). Using drugs alone in single room occupancy housing: Understanding environmental drivers of overdose risk. *International Journal of Drug Policy*, *128*, 104444.

Government of Canada (2024). Opioid- and stimulant-related harms in Canada. Retrieved September 27, 2024 from https://health-infobase.canada.ca/substance-related-harms/opioids-stimulants/

Groshkova, T. (2010). Motivation in substance misuse treatment. *Addiction Research & Theory*, *18*(5), 494–510.

Hawk, M., Coulter, R. W., Egan, J. E., Fisk, S., Reuel Friedman, M., Tula, M., & Kinsky, S. (2017). Harm reduction principles for healthcare settings. *Harm Reduction Journal*, *14*, 1–9.

Ivsins, A., Boyd, J., Beletsky, L., & McNeil, R. (2020). Tackling the overdose crisis: The role of safe supply. *International Journal of Drug Policy*, *80*, 102769.

Larney, S., Mathers, B., & Dolan, K. A. (2007). *Illicit Drug Treatment in Prison: Detoxification, Drug-free Units, Therapeutic Communities, and Opioid Substitution Treatment*. National Drug and Alcohol Research Centre, University of New South Wales.

Marlatt, G. A., & Witkiewitz, K. (2010). Update on harm-reduction policy and intervention research. *Annual Review of Clinical Psychology*, *6*(1), 591–606.

Mathers, B. M., Degenhardt, L., Bucello, C., Lemon, J., Wiessing, L., & Hickman, M. (2013). Mortality among people who inject drugs: A systematic review and meta-analysis. *Bulletin of the World Health Organization*, *91*, 102–123.

McNeil, R., Fleming, T., Mayer, S., Barker, A., Mansoor, M., Betsos, A., Austin, T., Parusel, S., Ivsins, A. & Boyd, J. (2022). Implementation of safe supply alternatives during intersecting COVID-19 and overdose health emergencies in British Columbia, Canada, 2021. *American Journal of Public Health*, *112*(S2), S151–S158.

Musalek, M. (2013). Reduction of harmful consumption versus total abstinence in addiction treatment. *Neuropsychiatry*, *3*(6), 635.

National Harm Reduction Coalition (2024). Principles of Harm Reduction. Retrieved July 17, 2025 from https://harmreduction.org/about-us/principles-of-harm-reduction/

Parkes, T., Matheson, C., Carver, H., Budd, J., Liddell, D., Wallace, J., Pauly, B., Fotopoulou, M., Burley, A., Anderson, I., MacLennan, G. & Foster, R. (2019). Supporting Harm Reduction through Peer Support (SHARPS): Testing the feasibility and acceptability of a peer-delivered, relational intervention for people with problem substance use who are homeless, to improve health outcomes, quality of life and social functioning and reduce harms: Study protocol. *Pilot and Feasibility Studies*, *5*, 1–15.

Ritter, A., & Cameron, J. (2006). A review of the efficacy and effectiveness of harm reduction strategies for alcohol, tobacco and illicit drugs. *Drug and Alcohol Review*, *25*(6), 611–624.

Tyndall, M. (2020). A safer drug supply: A pragmatic and ethical response to the overdose crisis. *CMAJ*, *192*(34), E986–E987.

Vakharia, S. P. (2024). *The Harm Reduction Gap: Helping Individuals Left Behind by Conventional Drug Prevention and Abstinence-only Addiction Treatment*. Taylor & Francis.

Western, B., & Simes, J. T. (2019). Drug use in the year after prison. *Social Science & Medicine*, *235*, 112357.

13

GUIDING PRINCIPLES OF THE BRIDGING THE TRANSITION FRAMEWORK

Trauma- and Violence-Informed Care

Nadine Wathen and Brenna Schmitt

The need for policy, practice, and research to be trauma- and violence-informed has never been so urgent. This is especially true in settings providing services for people facing the greatest barriers to care. Articulated in four principles, trauma- and violence-informed care (TVIC) provides a framework for examining current organizational policies, and individual practices, to orient all activities towards safety and equity. TVIC moves us beyond "trauma-informed" approaches to understand how both interpersonal and structural/systemic forms of violence influence how service users and providers are positioned, and the experiences they have in service settings. Using a case example relevant to interdisciplinary teams providing care to people experiencing housing precarity (tertiary prevention of homelessness), we articulate TVIC's four principles, emphasizing their application in practice, policy, research, and education.

Component of the Bridging the Transition Framework Addressed in this Chapter

TVIC is a guiding principle in research and practice supporting homelessness prevention and response (Figure 13.1). We provide an overview of TVIC and how it can be applied to support the daily life functioning, participation, and well-being of people at various points in the housing trajectory.

DOI: 10.4324/9781003541332-15

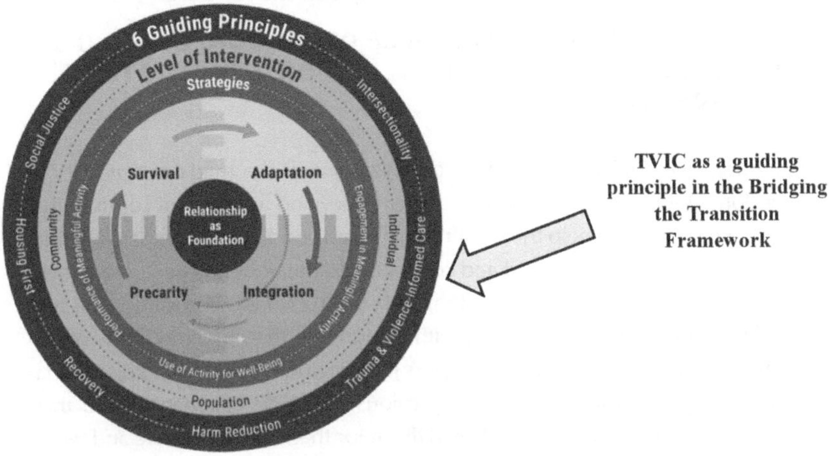

FIGURE 13.1 Trauma and Violence-Informed Care as a Guiding Principle.

How this Chapter Guides Practice and Research in Homelessness Prevention

TVIC has emerged as both a set of strategies and a values-based practice framework among organizations and individual practitioners providing care to people experiencing inequities, structural marginalization and poverty, stigma and discrimination, and, at the nexus of these, homelessness. Our conceptualization of TVIC builds on existing work in the area of trauma-informed practices, but, crucially, also focuses on the experiences and impacts of structural violence, and how stigma and discrimination operate in systems and services (Wathen & Varcoe, 2023; Ponic et al., 2016) to effectively block pathways to good care for marginalized people and groups. TVIC is also proving critical as a value under-pinning system-level change efforts specific to homelessness, as outlined in Box 13.1.

As we describe in more detail below, TVIC, as articulated and tested in EQUIP Healthcare (Browne & Varcoe, 2023), is one of three key dimensions of equity-oriented care, along with cultural safety/anti-racism and substance use health/harm reduction. We think of TVIC as a key "door" into equity-promoting policies and practices, with people entering this door also being provided strategies to enact all three key dimensions.

Introduction

In this chapter, we bring together our expertise and experience in teaching and learning about TVIC, in using it as a set of organizational and individual practice strategies, and in guiding research and knowledge mobilization in trauma- and violence-informed ways. One of us (BS) is a recent occupational

BOX 13.1 TVIC AS A CORE VALUE OF LONDON, ONTARIO'S WHOLE OF COMMUNITY SYSTEM RESPONSE TO HEALTH AND HOMELESSNESS

In 2023, over 200 people and 70 organizations in the medium-sized city of London, Ontario (Canada) came together to develop a "whole of community" system response "to help the most marginalized Londoners move safely inside, become stabilized, supported and connected to the right housing, and to help them stay housed" (City of London, n.d., para 2). TVIC is a core value and underlying principle of this work, with recognition that ongoing forms of systemic and structural violence in people's lives, including stigma and discrimination, along with their current and previous traumatic experiences and their ongoing impacts, make it especially difficult for them to get the care and wrap-around support they need to become and stay housed. TVIC education for direct service providers working in London's system has been made mandatory by the system's Workforce Development Table.

therapy graduate with prior experience working in research and social service contexts related to poverty and homelessness, who now practices in a context supporting people of diverse social and occupational identities. The other (NW) has taught, researched, and mobilized new knowledge about TVIC and equity-oriented care for decades, in the above contexts, and specific to gender-based violence and women's homelessness.

TVIC: A Primer

At its simplest, TVIC is about safety, compassion, and respect. To preserve this idea of simplicity, we have, in the EQUIP Healthcare research and implementation work (see www.equiphealthcare.ca), refined (Browne et al., 2024; Wathen et al., 2021) this key dimension of equity-oriented care into four principles that articulate how to enact safety, compassion, and respect through individual practices and organizational policies. The key evolution from previous iterations of trauma-informed practice (TIP) (Elliott et al., 2005; Hopper et al., 2010; Substance Abuse and Mental Health Services Administration, 2014; Strand et al., 2015) is, as noted in Figure 13.2, the focus on structural and systemic violence, and on actively countering discrimination and stigma across the care continuum, from intake and discharge/referral, to documentation, space planning, and service user or participant flow procedures. Every interaction, and every encounter they have with a service space, clinical and non-clinical staff, and service policies

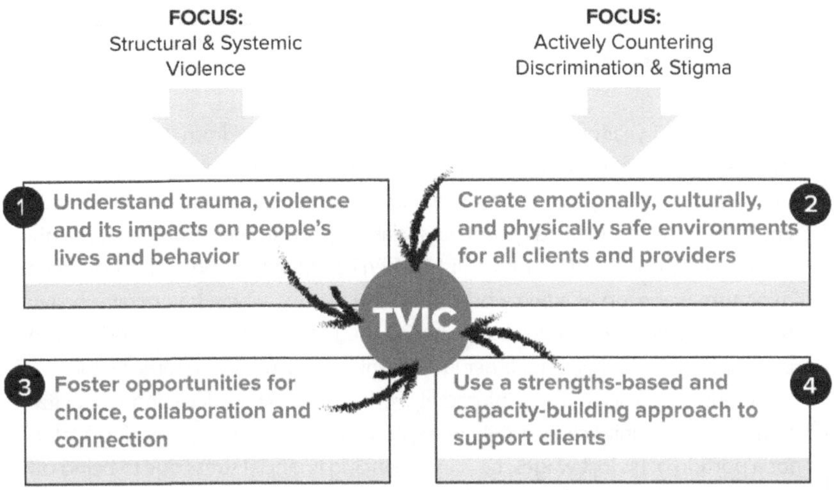

FIGURE 13.2 Principles of TVIC.

that impact them, is an opportunity to replicate prior bad experiences of care for those experiencing stigma, discrimination, and marginalization, or to actively counter these and break these cycles of poor care.

Thus, TVIC extends TIP by bringing an explicit focus to: (1) broad structural and social conditions that cause harm, such as policy-induced poverty and lack of affordable housing, ensuring we avoid seeing trauma as happening only "in people's minds"; (2) ongoing structural and interpersonal violence, including racism, sexism, ableism, ageism, substance use stigma, and other forms of discrimination, to avoid seeing trauma only as something that happened in the past; (3) institutional and systemic violence, including policies and practices that harm people and groups because they are designed to satisfy the needs of the system, rather than those of the person; and (4) the responsibility of organizations to set policies and assign resources such that providers can both provide safe and effective care, and themselves be well, rather than they or those they serve having to work around poor policies to ensure appropriate care and well-being.

Applying TVIC Principles

In the following section, we articulate the four TVIC principles through a practice lens using a composite case to bring them to life, including organizational strategies and how they shape individual provider practices. Following this, we will reflect on how the principles can be applied to homelessness research and the education of health and social service providers (Box 13.2).

BOX 13.2 MATEO

Mateo is a 33-year-old man who emigrated to Canada from Argentina four months ago to work and send money home to his family. Mateo has applied for permanent residency but is still awaiting status confirmation. He speaks little English and has had difficulty finding social supports in the community, mainly because they're only offered in English. When he arrived, Mateo was able to get a minimum-wage job as a line worker at a steel factory, where he operates heavy machinery. After two months using shelters then couch-surfing, he found a room in an apartment with several other immigrants who work at the same factory.

A month ago, Mateo was injured at work and is now undergoing rehabilitation at a community clinic. While workplace insurance is compensating Mateo for a portion of his lost wages, he is experiencing financial stress due to being off work, the high cost of living, and the need to send money back to his family. Mateo is concerned that he won't be able to pay his rent this month and that he will lose his housing.

Staff working with Mateo at the community clinic note that he has been uncooperative and expresses anger and confusion regarding his return-to-work plan, that he experiences flashbacks to the injury, and that he has generally made slow progress with recovery.

Principle 1: Understand the Impact of Trauma and Violence

TVIC Principle 1 requires that organizations and providers understand the nature and impact of trauma and violence, on a person and their interactions with care systems, including the role of structural violence in reinforcing cycles of trauma. A trauma lens prompts clinicians to consider how people may respond when (re)activated in care interactions (fight, flight, freeze, fawn), and how this can impact their ability to build trust and share details of their lives. This is especially true for those experiencing inequities, including poverty and homelessness. Previous poor care experiences, including those due to stigma and discrimination from providers, and policies that create additional barriers to care (e.g., sober-only care, or no flexibility around appointment times), make it especially difficult for people to feel confident in their care. Importantly, a person's confidence that the care they are receiving is trauma- and violence-informed and equity-oriented, and their feelings of self-efficacy, including being recognized as experts in their own lives, is key in the pathway to improving health outcomes (Ford-Gilboe et al., 2018).

Thus, TVIC asks organizations and individuals to know how trauma can present, but not assume that it will, for any specific service user or participant. Policies and practices should reflect the need to be flexible, understanding the prevalence of trauma, especially in highly marginalized groups, and ensure that providers are enabled and supported to work in these flexible and responsive ways. Strategies can be implemented before the first interaction even occurs. Providers can tailor which care options are presented to the person, acknowledging that meaningful activity and an individual's capacity to engage in it may be directly impacted by their trauma history and where they are in their recovery. For example, someone experiencing the physical, emotional, and mental shift that comes with transitioning out of homelessness may benefit from facilitation of basic self-care strategies as a first step, prior to setting longer-term goals.

Case Considerations

For Mateo and his health and social service providers, Principle 1 could be operationalized in several ways. When a provider is preparing to see Mateo for the first time and considering the behavioural and emotional challenges that have been flagged, she may consider some of the following: Mateo's still uncertain immigration status and his lack of awareness regarding Canadian health and social service systems, the difficulty he has experienced accessing community resources, his loneliness and isolation, his housing precarity, and the lack of effective communication he has experienced regarding his work and care.

Mateo's care team may consider how the intersection of financial distress, poor communication, and ongoing symptoms could lead to Mateo feeling overwhelmed, confused, and frustrated regarding the care he has received thus far. They may therefore approach him with empathy and respect and see if interpretation services are available, and if Mateo would want this. As providers get to know Mateo, this understanding may help to contextualize his frustration and capacity to engage in relational care planning.

Principle 2: Create Emotionally, Culturally, and Physically Safe Environments

Principle 2 is about ensuring physical, emotional, and cultural safety for those receiving and providing care. This starts with examining our own attitudes and how they influence what we think, say, and do. Implicit biases (Sukhera, 2023) can arise from beliefs (sometimes instilled or perpetuated through professional training) regarding certain groups, and can lead to a range of poor experiences for people, including having pain dismissed (common for women), having heavy substance use assumed, even when absent (common for Indigenous people), thinking people choose to be unemployed or use income support (common for many racialized and/or disabled people), and being unwilling to learn Canadian values and norms (common for racialized, especially Muslim, newcomers). These beliefs and assumptions can directly impact the degree to which compassion, respect, and care options are offered. From a service lens, this includes reflecting on the assumptions we make about certain people and/or activities and how this impacts our willingness to aid those in our care in pursuing/returning to them.

Promoting safety also means reflecting on organizational policies and how they may enable certain narratives about populations being served, and in turn how these narratives can reinforce trauma (e.g., abstinence/sobriety policies in hospitals, exclusion of those with diagnosed mental illness history from certain programmes, etc.). Much of this starts with eliminating the need to explicitly ask about trauma history. While discussing trauma and its implications may still be relevant in certain clinical settings, eliminating trauma screening/disclosure as necessary for consideration of trauma's impacts is key. TVIC is a universal baseline of service that acknowledges that disclosure is unnecessary to provide safety, compassion, and respect, and in fact may re-traumatize people and contribute to provider vicarious trauma and moral distress (Wathen & Varcoe, 2023).

From a practical standpoint, facilitating safety in care environments can begin with how a provider builds and maintains rapport with the service user or participant. Viewing them holistically and taking the time to try to empathize with their experiences and value their lived expertise can foster trust-building, especially for people who have encountered discrimination and inequity and have not previously experienced safe, compassionate, and respectful care. Embedding these qualities in communication among the care team through regular touchpoints and fact-based (non-judgemental) documentation facilitates care plan implementation and saves the person from having to relay their story repeatedly to different providers.

Promoting safety also means maintaining consent and confidentiality as pillars of the care interaction. This could mean setting aside time to share anticipatory guidance about the care process, and providing frequent opportunities to ask questions to ensure a service user or participant understands their rights and responsibilities within the care environment.

Case Considerations

When it comes to Mateo's care, his care providers should engage in reflexive practice to identify factors that might inadvertently influence their approach, including views on immigration, housing precarity, and social inclusion/

exclusion. It may also be useful to examine organizational policies and consider how they may impact Mateo's access to care. In devising a care plan, considerations for Mateo should go beyond his injury to include support to address his psychosocial barriers to recovery, including mental health, finances, and lack of community supports.

Given that Mateo does not speak English well, ensuring a professional interpreter is present (with his consent) is an integral first step for him to fully participate. In the first session, anticipatory guidance should be given, including specific activities, how long these are expected to take, his rights, and what is involved in referral processes. Through engaging in this conversation, the care team gives Mateo the opportunity to gain back a degree of control over his care.

Once decisions have been made about next steps, Mateo's team should also establish a robust communication system between all members of the care team, and any external resources (e.g., a Housing First Team), facilitating direct information-sharing and assuring that responsibility for care coordination does not fall to Mateo as his plan progresses.

Principles 3 and 4: Foster Opportunities for Choice, Collaboration, and Connection; and Use a Strengths-Based and Capacity-Building Approach

TVIC Principles 3 and 4 promote trust, collaboration, agency, and authentic choice in person-led care interactions and emphasize the importance of leveraging a person's strengths to build new capacities. Health and social service providers can enact this at several levels. First, they can consciously take action to understand the person's needs and preferences and provide realistic choices in care decision-making. Even in structured settings where options are limited, talking through these options and how they fit to the person's stated needs provides them agency and a feeling of control in their care.

Motivational interviewing strategies can help identify and leverage existing strengths to decide on areas of capacity development that support the care plan. This can include assessing readiness for change and encouraging people to practically think through goal attainment and consider what resources are available, and not, to meet stated goals (Kessler & Graham, 2015; Miller & Rollnick, 2023). For individuals transitioning out of homelessness who have been bounced between services, these strategies can help to counter isolation and build individual capacity for decision-making. Considering activities that provide meaning and fulfilment can help to re-establish personal identity and promote involvement in care, especially for those who have not had an opportunity to expand their meaningful activities and routines beyond survival.

Case Considerations

Mateo's team can promote choice and collaboration by establishing scheduled check-ins at which Mateo can provide feedback (if he wants to) regarding his care plan and progress and by facilitating ongoing conversation about Mateo's values, beliefs, and goals. Mateo's team can also work with him to identify barriers and facilitators to recovery and develop relevant care goals that are applicable to his home and work life through use of strategies like motivational interviewing, facilitated by a professional interpreter if needed. Connecting Mateo with additional supports (social work to assist with housing support, Spanish resources in the community, etc.) can also help him to build confidence and provide him with more agency both within the health and social care space and in his life more broadly.

TVIC Considerations for Research and Education

A Safety-First Approach to Generating and Sharing Knowledge

In early 2024, we [First author (NW) and Western University's Centre for Research on Health Equity and Social Inclusion (CRHESI)] held a day-long workshop to discuss with partners in London's Whole of Community System Response to Health and Homelessness (Box 13.1) how to launch research and evaluation, and, crucially, knowledge-sharing back to community, in TVIC ways. While strategies aligned in many ways with principles of action-oriented, community-based, and participatory research, participants highlighted the following additional considerations: (1) evaluation questions and designs must be developed collaboratively and address structural and systemic factors; (2) data should be used efficiently, effectively, and safely, with analysis and interpretation focused on the impact of structural factors on individuals and groups; (3) we need to shift from identifying problems to understanding and changing them; (4) research staff should be prepared to understand how trauma works (i.e., genetic, biological/physiological, and social factors) and how it can look in research interactions; and (5) when working with people with complex needs and barriers to health and housing stability, recognize that substance use is a continuum and there is a need to address related stigma as it often causes the most harm, including in how research is reported (CRHESI, 2024).

Pre- and In-Service Education

From an education perspective, efforts are being made to integrate equity, diversity, and inclusion more intentionally into curriculum content for health and social service providers in Canada. However, there remains a need for more explicit attention to TVIC concepts, along with systematic discussions to understand how to select and implement appropriate policies and practice strategies, tailored to person and setting. A key barrier to this integration is the wide scope required of some of these professions, obliging programmes to cover a lot of content within their allocated timeframes. For these professions, current programme accreditation standards focus on establishing a foundational knowledge base for emerging clinicians (Canadian Association of Occupational Therapists, 2022; Canadian Association of Schools of Nursing, 2020), meaning that while students gain some of the knowledge and understanding required to implement TVIC concepts, they receive minimal training regarding how to operationalize them in practice. Other accreditation standards, such as those for social work students, have begun to more explicitly integrate concepts like anti-racism and the impacts of colonialism into curricular frameworks (Canadian Association for Social Work Education, 2021).

Related steps include integrating Culture, Equity, and Justice as an overarching theme into professional competency frameworks. For example, the 2021 Competencies for Occupational Therapists in Canada prompts clinicians to promote equity and anti-oppressive behaviour in culturally safe, inclusive relationships, and contribute to equitable access to occupational participation and occupational therapy (ACOTRO, ACOTUP, & CAOT, 2021). Similarly, the 2017 Competency Profile for Physiotherapists in Canada prompts clinicians to practice in a way that fosters inclusion and considers the implications of diversity (CAPR, CCPUP, CPA, & PEAC, 2017). As Professional Competencies impact curriculum development, we anticipate that the structure of programmes will begin to shift in response to these types of additions.

Overall, while schools and the broader allied health and social service community are taking steps to more explicitly consider TVIC and equity ideas, there is still work to be done when it comes to preparing students for what this means in practice. Preparation for all new health and social service providers, and continuing professional development, requires more emphasis on understanding the pervasive impacts of trauma and structural violence and how providers can actively contribute to, or interrupt, experiences of sub-optimal care.

Conclusion

TVIC provides a values-based framework to guide organizations and individual providers to undertake safe, compassionate, and respectful care for all service users and participants, but especially those most marginalized by structural violence, stigma, and discrimination. It is both a call to action

(Wathen & Varcoe, 2023) and a set of practice and policy strategies that ensure that processes, programmes, spaces, and interactions are aligned to promote safety for all, trust and choice, and build on existing personal strengths, while bringing in related key dimensions and strategies for equity-oriented care specific to substance use health and anti-racism/cultural safety. TVIC principles are simple, but the work itself is not, as it requires examination and reflection of self, others, and how we interact.

References

ACOTRO, ACOTUP, & CAOT. (2021). *Competencies for Occupational Therapists in Canada*. https://www.coto.org/docs/default-source/competencies/competencies-for-occupational-therapists-in-canada-2021---final-en-web.pdf?sfvrsn=e4f10c52_2

Browne, A., & Varcoe, C. (2023). Taking organizational-level action: Creating a context for implementing TVIC in health care settings. In *Implementing Trauma- and Violence-Informed Care: A Handbook*, edited by C. Nadine Wathen & Colleen Varcoe (pp. 85–98). Toronto: University of Toronto Press.

Browne A.J., Varcoe C., Ford-Gilboe M., Wathen C.N., Wilson E., Bungay V., & Perrin, N. (2024). Using a health equity lens to measure patient experiences of care in diverse health care settings. *PLOS ONE 19*(6): e0297721. https://doi.org/10.1371/journal.pone.0297721

Canadian Association for Social Work Education. (2021). *Educational Policies and Accreditation Standards for Canadian Social Work Education*. https://caswe-acfts.ca/wp-content/uploads/2021/08/EPAS-2021-1.pdf

Canadian Association of Occupational Therapists. (2022). *Academic Accreditation Standards and Self-Study Guide*. https://caot.in1touch.org/uploaded/web/Accreditation/Academic%20Accreditation%20Standards%20and%20Self-Study%20Guide%20(2022)%20EN.pdf

Canadian Association of Schools of Nursing. (2020). *CASN Accreditation Standards and Framework*. https://accred.casn.ca/content/user_files/2023/10/EN-CASN-Accreditation-Standards-Aug-30-2022-plus-TRC.pdf

CAPR, CCPUP, CPA, & PEAC. (2017). *NPAG Competency Profile for Physiotherapists in Canada*. https://www.peac-aepc.ca/pdfs/Resources/Competency%20Profiles/Competency%20Profile%20for%20PTs%202017%20EN.pdf

City of London. (n.d.). *Whole of Community System Response to Health and Homelessness in London: A roadmap to help the most marginalized Londoners*. Retrieved November 22, 2024: https://london.ca/living-london/community-services/homeless-prevention-housing/whole-community-system-response-health

CRHESI - Centre for Research on Health Equity and Social Inclusion. (2024). *Trauma- & Violence-Informed & Equity Promoting Research & Knowledge Mobilization to Support London's Whole of Community System Response to Health & Homelessness*. Available: https://crhesi.uwo.ca/trauma-violence-informed-equity-promoting-research-knowledge-mobilization-to-support-londons-whole-of-community-system-response-to-health-homelessness-february-16-2024/

Elliott, D., Bjelajac, P., Fallot, R., Markoff, L., & Reed, B. (2005). Trauma-informed or trauma-denied: Principles for implementation of trauma-informed services for women. *Journal of Community Psychology*, *33*, 461–477. https://doi.org/10.1002/jcop.20063

Ford-Gilboe, M., Wathen, N., Varcoe, C., Herbert, C., Jackson, B., LaVoie, J., Pauly, B., Perrin, N., Smye, V., Wallace, B., Wong, S., Browne, A.J. (for the EQUIP

Research Team) (2018). How equity-oriented health care impacts health: Key mechanisms and implications for primary care practice and policy. *Milbank Quarterly*, *96*(4), 635–671. https://doi.org/10.1111/1468-0009.12349

Hopper, E. K., Bassuk, E. L., & Olivet, J. (2010). Shelter from the storm: Trauma-informed care in homelessness services settings. *The Open Health Services and Policy Journal*, *3*(1), 80–100.

Kessler, D., & Graham, F. (2015). The use of coaching in occupational therapy: An integrative review. *Australian Occupational Therapy Journal*, *62*(3), 160–176.

Miller, W. R., & Rollnick, S. (2023). *Motivational Interviewing: Helping People Change and Grow* (4th ed.). New York: The Guildford Press.

Ponic, P., Varcoe, C., & Smutylo, T. (2016). Trauma-(and violence-) informed approaches to supporting victims of violence: Policy and practice considerations. *Victims of Crime Research Digest*, *9*. Retrieved from http://www.justice.gc.ca/eng/rp-pr/cj-jp/victim/rd9-rr9/p2.html

Strand, V., Popescu M., Abramovitz R., & Richards S. (2015). Building agency capacity for trauma-informed evidence-based practice and field instruction. *Journal of Evidence-Informed Social Work*, 13(2), 179–197. https://doi.org/10.1080/23761407.2015.1014124

Substance Abuse and Mental Health Services Administration. (2014). SAMHSA's concept of trauma and guidance for a trauma-informed approach. Retrieved from https://ncsacw.samhsa.gov/userfiles/files/SAMHSA_Trauma.pdf

Sukhera, J. (2023). Leveraging implicit bias recognition and management curricula to advance: Trauma- and violence-informed care. In *Implementing Trauma- and Violence-Informed Care: A Handbook*, edited by C. Nadine Wathen & Colleen Varcoe (pp. 39–57). Toronto: University of Toronto Press.

Wathen, C.N., Schmitt, B., MacGregor, J.C.D. (2021). Measuring trauma- (and violence-) informed care: A scoping review. *Trauma, Violence & Abuse*, *24*(1), 261–277. https://doi.org/10.1177/15248380211029399

Wathen, C.N., Varcoe, C.M. (Eds.) (2023). *Implementing Trauma- and Violence-Informed Care: A Handbook*. Toronto: University of Toronto Press.

14

GUIDING PRINCIPLES OF THE BRIDGING THE TRANSITION FRAMEWORK

Intersectionality

Victoria Smye

This chapter provides an overview of **intersectionality**, its development and contribution as a critical social theory, and its usefulness as a theoretical framework and analytic tool to inform research, policy, and praxis. Applications of intersectionality in research are used to illustrate its usefulness in the homelessness and housing domain as a guiding principle for the Bridging the Transition Framework.

Component of the Bridging the Transition Framework Addressed in this Chapter

In this chapter, intersectionality is presented as a guiding principle of the Bridging the Transition Framework. Intersectionality is defined and described in relation to how it can be used to benefit people marginalized by inequity, for example, people living homelessness, through research, policy, and practice (see Figure 14.1).

How this Chapter Guides Practice and Research

Intersectionality is increasingly recognized as a 'generative' framework for addressing the complexities of housing precarity and homelessness as both individually experienced and institutionally shaped (MacDonald et al., 2024: p. 62). Grounded in critical feminist theoretical perspectives, intersectional analyses are useful in drawing attention to the dynamics of the intersections between homelessness and other aspects of social identity and different forms of oppression associated with social and structural

DOI: 10.4324/9781003541332-16

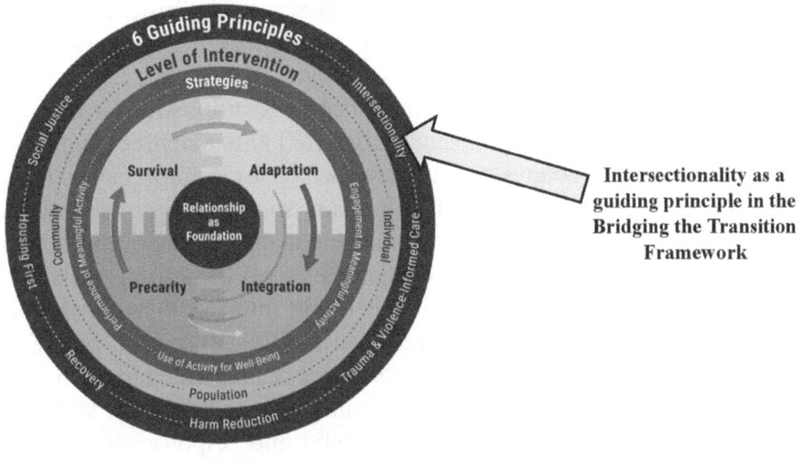

FIGURE 14.1 Intersectionality as a Guiding Principle.

contexts that can guide us in the pursuit of addressing the multiple inequities and intersecting stigmas associated with homelessness (Greene et al., 2013; Hanley et al., 2019; MacDonald et al., 2024; Schwan et al., 2020; Trochmann, 2021). Intersectionality can inform research, policies, and practices to support the well-being of people living in homelessness, including their transition to housing security. We cannot confront homelessness without simultaneously confronting ableism, racism, gender-based violence, and other interpersonal and systemic discriminations.

Introduction

Kimberlé Crenshaw, a Black legal scholar, is often cited as coining the term 'intersectionality' in a 1989 paper entitled, 'Demarginalizing the intersection of race and sex: A Black feminist critique of antidiscrimination doctrine, feminist theory and antiracist politics,' as a way to help explain the oppression of African-American women, those women whose lives were impacted by violence. Crenshaw applied intersectionality as an analytical tool to show how Black women were in a disadvantaged position when it came to how courts framed and interpreted the stories of plaintiffs: "For Crenshaw, intersectionality named the structural convergence among intersecting systems of power that created blind spots in anti-racist and feminist activism" (Collins, 2019, p. 26). The introduction of the construct of intersectionality also highlighted shifting relationships in academic and activist interpretive communities in the context of decolonization and neoliberalism – a shift at a time when the epistemological authority of the academy explaining the experiences of 'subordinated peoples' dominated – a position that was being challenged by subordinated groups (Collins, p. 124). Over time, socially structured categories of marginality grew, such as those related to gender, sexuality, class, race, and 'ableness,' and ceased to be considered separately. Instead, they were viewed as being produced by interrelated social forces of power and oppression (Andersen & Collins, 2020; Collins & Bilge, 2020; Collins et al., 2021).

Social identities/location (the groups people identify with, or belong to across categories of race, class, gender, age, etc.) and systems of oppression (larger forces and structures operating in society, for example, social norms, laws, and policies and systems of oppression such as racism, colonialism, heterosexism, class stratification, gender inequality, ageism, and ableism) intersect to create more or less disadvantage based on shifting social identity/location and context. Scholars in the field of intersectional epistemology acknowledge that people may experience multiple forms of power and oppression simultaneously and argue that recognizing and addressing these configurations of experience fosters more inclusive and equitable knowledge systems (Collins & Bilge, 2016; Nash, 2008) and responses to the same. Variations of intersectional scholarship can now be found across interdisciplinary fields as well as within more traditional disciplinary endeavors, and variations of intersectional practice can also be found within and outside the academy and, more recently, around the globe; a diverse range of practitioners both search for and propose ideas that will explain their experiences with the social problems around them (Collins, 2015, pp. 2–3).

Intersectionality

Intersectionality refers to the understanding that people experience inequities at the convergence of intersecting structural conditions, including systemic racism, poverty, homelessness, ableism, gender-based violence, and other unfair disadvantages, as well as social locations and identities such as Indigeneity, sexual orientation, immigration status, age, ability, religion, and so on (Hankivsky & Cormier, 2009). With its roots in a long history of Black feminist writing, Indigenous feminism, third world feminism, and queer and postcolonial theory, intersectionality has emerged as a widely respected, albeit variously defined research and policy paradigm (Hankivsky, 2012) and an analytic tool (Crenshaw, 1989, 1991; Collins, 2019; Collins & Bilge, 2020).

Understanding that the notion of intersectionality is taken up widely and with variability, Collins and Bilge (2020; p. 2) put forward the following definition as a general description of intersectionality:

> Intersectionality investigates how intersecting power relations influence social relations across diverse societies as well as individual experiences in everyday life. As an analytic tool, intersectionality views categories of race, class, gender, sexuality, class, nation, ability and age – among others – as interrelated and mutually shaping one another. Intersectionality is a way of understanding complexity in the world, in people, and in human experience.

Core concepts within the construct of intersectionality include: relationality, power relations, resistant knowledge, and reflexivity (Collins, 2019; Collins & Bilge, 2020).

Relationality

A recognition that race, gender, class, and other social identities and categories of analysis are interconnected and maintained through relational processes is a fundamental element of intersectionality; relationality is considered a central feature of theoretical analyses of social inequality and power relations, and as such, intersectionality (Collins, 2019, p. 226). As Oudshoorn et al. (2025) note, "the interconnectedness of how one group's privilege or success in that privilege is directly tied to the oppression or exploitation of another can be viewed in systems of access" (p. 7).

Power Relations

In the 1980s and 1990s, Patricia Hill Collins, a Black feminist scholar, focused on examining how the intersecting forces/systems of oppression/power relations are actually organized, what she described as a "matrix of domination." In her book, Collins (2000) describes four interrelated domains that organize power relations in society. This approach to an analysis of power informs us about how structural, disciplinary, hegemonic, and interpersonal domains of power shape human action. However, as Collins (2019) later articulates, her analysis of power relations does not emphasize 'domination,' rather it focuses attention on developing the concept of intellectual resistance as a two-pronged endeavor – one where resistance as a knowledge project is underpinned by critical analysis and also where intersectionality confronts epistemological challenges to its intellectual resistance, with critical social theory being a particular form of intellectual resistance (p. 10).

Resistance Knowledge/Resistant Knowledge Projects

Race, class, gender, sexuality, age, ability, ethnicity, nation – or whatever forces of oppression experienced by people marginalized by inequity – are not simply categories of difference; rather, they refer to resistant knowledge traditions of subordinated groups with a vested interest in resisting oppression, i.e., 'interpretive communities.' Resistant knowledge arises from the lived experience of "subordinated groups," such as those living with homelessness, with the aim of addressing social inequalities and social injustice propagated by racism, sexism, capitalism, colonialism, and similar systems of political domination and economic exploitation (Collins, 2019, p. 10). The naming of intersectionality reflects

Crenshaw's awareness of the challenges associated with engaging with "distinctive resistant knowledge projects" that also share a common space (Collins, 2019, p. 124), for example, homelessness alliances and anti-racist initiatives.

In linking power with knowledge, the construct of 'community' provides an important framework for understanding the interpretive communities that advance intersectionality's many resistance knowledge projects (Collins, 2015, p. 5). For example, community-led initiatives support the empowerment of communities marginalized by inequity to take ownership of solutions to homelessness, fostering collaboration and solidarity among diverse stakeholders. By centering the voices of people who have been most impacted, these initiatives ensure that interventions are responsive to the unique needs and experiences of people living in homelessness – community-based participatory research is one such model (MacDonald et al., 2024).

Intersectionality as a Critical Social Theory and Reflexivity

According to Collins (2019), although 'intersectionality as a critical social theory' is a work in progress (p. 9), it is inextricably interwoven with social change. To maintain a place within critical social theories, intersectionality must remain connected to resistive knowledge production projects and social justice movements (Collins, 2019; Collins & Bilge, 2020; Lovin, 2021) – it must remain attendant to the social world and its organization to advance reform and transformative change. In this vein, Collins notes the need for explicit and sustained processes of self-reflection regarding the interrelations between intersectionality's 'own critical analyses and social actions; an internal self-reflexive critical eye related to intersectional theorizing – an ongoing examination of its own constructs, premises, and practices through dialogical engagement with multiple 'interpretive communities,' 'critical theories' (e.g., critical race, feminist and postcolonial theories), and 'resistant knowledge projects'" (pp. 153; also cited in Lovin, 2021) – an engagement that will advance its potential utility as a tool of social justice and transformative change. Reflexivity is also required of individual researchers and activists engaged in this work to maintain their awareness of the power relations inherent in research processes, their assumptions and operating ideologies, and associated language – scrutinizing and disrupting power differentials and hegemonic forces and centering the voices of people subordinated by inequity is crucial to maintaining its integrity (Oudshoorn et al., 2025, p. 10).

Intersectionality-Based Policy Analysis Framework

With the aim of enhancing decision-making processes of a wide range of stakeholders, including those analysts working in health and health-related policy sectors, a team of researchers led an iterative, participatory process that culminated in the development of an Intersectionality-Based Policy Analysis (IBPA) Framework (Hankivsky, 2012; Hankivsky et al., 2014). The IBPA Framework was designed to explicate the "varied equity-implications of policy" and promote "equity-based improvements and social justice within an increasingly diverse and complex population base" (Hankivsky, 2012, p. 33), i.e., the IBPA framework utilizes a structured questioning process to consider problems and policies, while applying guiding principles of equity, social justice, power, intersectionality, and diversity of knowledge and input (Humphries et al., 2023; Hunting, 2012).

Intersectionality as a Guiding Principle: Homelessness and Housing Security

Emancipatory research approaches by diverse health disciplines support the exploration of intersectional identities and contextual nuances that govern the unique lived experiences of society's most vulnerable: people marginalized by inequity. An intersectionality framework is ideally suited to guide such transformational change, illuminating the reciprocal and compounding relationships between people and larger systems of power (Collins & Bilge, 2020; Sharif et al., 2022). For example, in our community-based participatory qualitative ethnographic study with Indigenous people living on or near the street in a large urban setting in Canada who were accessing Methadone Maintenance Treatment (MMT), we found that: (i) stigma and discrimination intersected with other disadvantages to profoundly shape people's lives and their access to and experiences with MMT; (ii) the policy context of MMT constrained people's lives, with significant consequences, and these experiences and consequences varied with people's social locations; and (iii) in concert with poverty and other disadvantages, these constraints contributed to housing instability and homelessness for many. Although harm reduction is based on the values of non-judgment and non-coercive approaches to service delivery and there are many positive outcomes associated with MMT, many of the participants in this study experienced 'harm' associated with "the intersectionality of disadvantages." This research underscored the importance of moving harm reduction approaches beyond a narrow concern with the harms directly related to drugs and drug use practices to address the harms associated with the determinants of drug use, such as *homelessness*, and the harms associated with drug and health policy (Smye et al., 2011, p. 6/12).

It is more recently that people have begun to consider how intersectionality applies to homelessness research and practice (e.g., Abramovich & Shelton, 2017; Cronley, 2020; Hanley et al., 2019; MacDonald et al., 2024; Rivers, 2023; Oudshoorn et al., 2025; Saewyc et al., 2017; Zufferey, 2016). Common explanations for why people experience homelessness include poverty, substance use, mental illness, and lack of affordable housing. However, these risks intersect with personal identities, including, for example, gender, race, and age, to create unique systems of oppression. As such, an intersectional lens offers a more critical and holistic theoretical framework through which to account for vulnerability within homelessness and offer solutions. Intersectionality is now considered an action-oriented theoretical framework used to guide critical inquiry and praxis, or practice (Collins, 2019; Collins & Bilge). The pragmatic, action-oriented nature of intersectionality is particularly useful when researchers conceptualize how people who navigate marginalization – on the basis of one or more dimension(s) of social location – experience larger social systems, such as healthcare, for example, women (Vohra-Gupta et al., 2023) and people living unhoused (e.g., MacDonald et al., 2024).

In their study, Cronley (2020) used intersectionality to help expose the possibility of racial bias in an instrument commonly used as a measure of vulnerability while homeless (VI-SPDAT). Even within this population highly marginalized by inequity, results suggest that structures of power and privilege based on gender and race continue to persist (Bowleg & Bauer, 2016; Bowleg et al., 2023). These structures create the risk of biases in instruments used to make decisions about critical service provision. As Cronley notes, if biases persist within the assessment and coordinated entry process, over time more Black people who are experiencing homelessness will be without housing for longer periods of time compared to their White counterparts, and Black women may face elevated risk for chronic trauma on the street (pp. 9–10).

Malik Rivers, a member of the National Alliance to End Homelessness in the US, argues for the use of an intersectional analysis in the realm of homelessness. As argued, racism, homophobia, and transphobia differentially impact the lives of Black, Indigenous, and People of Color and 2SLGBTQIA+ communities and need to be examined accordingly (Rivers, 2023). For example, in Canada, the 2020–2022 Nationally Coordinated Point-in-Time Counts notes that youth under 24 who identified as 2SLGBTQIA+ were more likely to report experiencing homelessness for the first time (61%, compared to 41% of non-2SLGBTQIA+ youth), pointing to the importance of understanding the unique intersecting social and structural factors that shape youth homelessness. In their study of homeless and street-involved Indigenous 2SLGBTQIA+ youth in British Columbia, Saewyc et al. (2017) advocated for services that are tailored to the unique circumstances and multiple identities of these youth. For example, they found cultural connectedness and safe connections as important to fostering better health for Indigenous youth; access to Elders and Two-spirited role models was suggested, and given youth experiences of unsafety and discrimination, the need for providers to unlearn racism and homophobia/biphobia/transphobia, as well as learning how to foster culturally safe practices and environments for Indigenous 2SLGBTQIA+ youth, was recommended. They also noted that professionals should be trained in 'trauma-informed' care, given the levels of trauma experienced by Indigenous 2SLGBTQIA+ youth experiencing homelessness (p. 35) (see Chapter 13 for more on trauma-informed care). In addition, researchers pointed to the need to address the multi-level forces of oppression shaping Indigenous youth homeless, for example, the importance of the federal government attending to the overrepresentation[1] of "Aboriginal" children in care – a feature of colonialism and neocolonialism.

In a study with migrant workers, Hanley et al. (2019) presented an intersectional analysis regarding how health intersects with the experience of housing insecurity and homelessness and argue for the importance of understanding the interplay of the unique social factors shaping homelessness to effectively advance solutions to support housing security. Similarly, in a recent study by MacDonald et al. (2024), intersectionality was found to be a powerful tool in relation to housing because of its potential to attend to the everyday lived experiences of housing insecurity, the interlocking systemic forms of oppression that create differentiated experiences of housing, and the specific contexts in which structural housing inequities are rooted (p. 62).

The intersectionality of homelessness reveals the complex web of social inequalities that perpetuate cycles of poverty and marginalization. By acknowledging and addressing the intersecting identities of people living within homelessness, we can develop more inclusive and effective solutions that uplift communities marginalized by inequity and more effectively support housing security and advance health equity. Although complex, a common criticism of intersectionality, it is also a more precise way of describing reality and thus is more likely to generate meaningful solutions. Intersectionality is a complexity-aware, socially conscious lens that provides a way to observe and analyze power relations and to address them; social change entails transforming power dynamics and social systems and structures. Through collective action, advocacy, and a commitment to social justice, we can strive toward a future where homelessness is not determined by one's identity, but by our collective resolve to create a more equitable society for all. In addition, community-determined solutions to homelessness are far more likely to yield positive results by focusing attention on the underlying socially grounded root causes of oppression and centering the voices of people marginalized by inequity (e.g., people experiencing homelessness) – particularly when we examine the multiple intersections of social location/identity and the multiple structures that give rise to inequity, such as colonialism, racism, patriarchy, capitalism, homophobia, etc.

Future Directions

Intersectionality has been used as a theoretical framework and an analytic lens in research, practice, and policy within and beyond academia to address social inequalities. For example, in research there exists a mixed method body of work that reflects the pragmatic opportunities of intersectional research (Grace, 2014). This mixing of methods to arrive at a more nuanced answer to a research question reflects the way intersectional scholars understand the social world as a mixing of normative social forces (Grace; Collins, 2019). Although used widely in qualitative studies, the uptake of intersectionality in mixed methods and quantitative studies is more recent (e.g., Bauer, 2014; Bauer et al., 2021; Bowleg, 2012; Bowleg, 2008; Green et al., 2017), including in the medical and life sciences. Pushing beyond traditional methods and focusing on outcome heterogeneity in quantitative research, Bauer and Scheim (2019a, 2019b), for example, examined the causal mechanisms underpinning intersectional disparities by employing intra-categorical and inter-categorical approaches to shared and differential constructs.

Intersectionality has also been deployed across the globe to illuminate structural violence experienced by different kinds of groups marginalized by inequity. For example, the findings of the research by Dean et al. (2022) suggest that syndemic[2]-informed approaches to care in the development of people-centered health systems are key to alleviating the burden of syndemic suffering associated with neglected tropical diseases (NTDs) and mental distress currently experienced by vulnerable populations in resource-limited settings (p. 20/25). Notably, the use and influence of intersectionality are growing.

Conclusion

Intersectionality is increasingly being used in health research for highlighting the interrelated and co-constructed nature of social locations and experiences for understanding differences in health needs and outcomes, for example, in nursing (e.g., Oudshoorn et al., 2025) and homelessness research (e.g., Cronley, 2020; Hanley, 2019; MacDonald et al., 2024; Saewyc et al., 2017). Today, Kimberlé Crenshaw's intersectional work spans legal, academic, public engagement, publishing, institution-building, and local and global activist contexts – intersectional theorizing has transcended academia (Lovin, 2021, p. 2/4). In this time of growing far-right populism and increased homelessness, I would argue that intersectionality, at minimum as a guiding principle, is critical to shedding light on the systems and structures or root causes of inequity and the solutions.

Notes

1 The term "Aboriginal" includes First Nations, Metis, and Inuit people living in Canada. It is language formalized in the Canadian constitution and was considered a preferred term until recently. However, it has a negative connotation due to its formalization in government policy. Indigenous is inclusive of First Nations,

Metis, and Inuit. It is also the language used in the United Nations Declaration on the Rights of indigenous Peoples and therefore understood internationally.

2 "Syndemics can be described as 'synergistically related' epidemics that cluster around harmful conditions. Syndemics occur where social and structural inequalities create increased physical and behavioural vulnerabilities to ill-health, resulting in the clustering of two or more diseases within a population" (Dean et al., 2022, p. 2/25).

References

Abramovich, A., & Shelton, J. (Eds.). (2017). *Where Am I Going to Go? Intersectional Approaches to Ending LGBTQ2S Youth Homelessness in Canada & the U.S.* Toronto: Canadian Observatory on Homelessness Press.

Andersen, M.L. & Collins, P.H., eds. (1992, 2020). *Race, Class & Gender*, 10th ed. Boston, MA: Cengage Learning.

Bauer, G. R. (2014). Incorporating intersectionality theory into population health research methodology: Challenges and the potential to advance health equity. *Social Science & Medicine, 110*, 10–17. doi:10.1016/j.socscimed.2014.03.022

Bauer, G.R., Churchill, S.M., Mahendran, M., Walwyn, C., Lizotte, D., Villa-Reuda, A.A. (2021). Intersectionality in quantitative research: A systematic review of its emergence and applications of theory and methods. *SSM-Population Health, 14*, 100798

Bauer, G. R., & Scheim, A. I. (2019a). Advancing quantitative intersectionality research methods: Intracategorical and intercategorical approaches to shared and differential constructs. *Social Science & Medicine, 226*, 260–262. https://doi.org/10.1016/j.socscimed.2019.03.018

Bauer, G. R., & Scheim, A. I. (2019b). Methods for analytic intercategorical intersectionality in quantitative research: Discrimination as a mediator of health inequalities. *Social Science & Medicine, 226*, 236–245. https://www.sciencedirect.com/science/article/pii/S0277953618306889?via%3Dihub

Bowleg, L. (2008). When Black + lesbian + woman ≠ Black lesbian woman: The methodological challenges of qualitative and quantitative intersectionality research. *Sex Roles: A Journal of Research, 59*(5–6), 312–325. https://doi.org/10.1007/s11199-008-9400-z

Bowleg, L. (2012). The problem with the phrase "women and minorities": Intersectionality, an important theoretical framework for public health. *American Journal of Public Health, 102*, 1267–1273. doi:10.2105/AJPH.2012.300750

Bowleg, L., & Bauer, G. (2016). Invited reflection: Quantifying intersectionality. *Psychology of Women Quarterly, 40*(3), 337–341. https://doi.org/10.1177/0361684316654282

Bowleg, L., Malekzadeh, A.N., AuBuchon, K.E., Ghabrial, M.A., Bauer, G.R. (2023). Rare exemplars and missed opportunities: Intersectionality within current sexual and gender diversity research and scholarship in psychology. *Current Opinion Psychology, 49*, 101511. doi: 10.1016/j.copsyc.2022.101511

Collins. P. & Bilge, S. (2016). *Intersectionality*. Malden, MA: Polity Press.

Collins, P.H. (2000). *Black Feminist Thought: Knowledge, Consciousness, and the Politics of Empowerment* (2nd ed). New York: Routledge.

Collins, P.H. (2015). Intersectionality's definitional dilemmas. *Annual Review of Sociology 41*,1–20. https://www.annualreviews.org/docserver/fulltext/soc/41/1/annurev-soc-073014-112142.pdf?expires=1738160576&id=id&accname=guest&checksum=F61926DC0592760928801C2BCA835552

Collins, P.H. (2019). *Intersectionality as Critical Social Theory*. Durham, NC: Duke University Press

Collins, P.H. & Bilge, S. (2020). *Intersectionality*. Cambridge: Polity Press.

Collins, P.H., da Silva, E.C.G., Ergun, E., Furseth, I., Bond, K.D., Martínez-Palacios, J. (2021). Intersectionality as critical social theory. *Contemporary Political Theory*, *20*(3):690–725. https://doi.org/10.1057/s41296-021-00490-0

Crenshaw, K. (1991). Mapping the margins: Intersectionality, identity politics, and violence against women of color. *Stanford Law Review*, *43*(6), 1241–1299. https://doi.org/10.2307/1229039

Crenshaw, Kimberle (1989). Demarginalizing the intersection of race and sex: A Black feminist critique of antidiscrimination doctrine, feminist theory and antiracist politics. *University of Chicago Legal Forum*, *1*(8). https://chicagounbound.uchicago.edu/cgi/viewcontent.cgi?article=1052&context=uclf

Cronley, C. (2020). Invisible intersectionality in measuring vulnerability among individuals experiencing homelessness – critically appraising the VI-SPDAT. *Journal of Social Distress and Homelessness*, *31*(1), 23–33. https://doi.org/10.1080/10530789.2020.1852502.

Dean, L., Theobald, S., Nallo, G., Bettee, A., Kollie, K., & Tolhurst, R. (2022). A syndemic born of war: Combining intersectionality and structural violence to explore the biosocial interactions of neglected tropical diseases, disability and mental distress in Liberia. *PLOS Global Public Health*, *2*(6):e0000551. https://journals.plos.org/globalpublichealth/article?id=10.1371/journal.pgph.0000551

Grace, D. (2014). *An Intersectionality-informed Mixed Methods Research: A Primer*. Vancouver, BC: Institute for Intersectionality Research and Policy, Simon Fraser University.

Green, M. A., Evans, C. R., & Subramanian, S. V. (2017). Can intersectionality theory enrich population health research? *Social Science & Medicine*, *178*, 214–216. https://doi.org/10.1016/j.socscimed.2017.02.029

Greene, S., Chambers, L., Masinde, K., & O'Brien-Teengs, D. (2013). A house is not a home: The housing experiences of African and Caribbean mothers living with HIV. *Housing Studies*, *28*(1), 116–134. https://doi.org/10.1080/02673037.2013.729269

Hankivsky, O. (2012). *An Intersectionality-Based Policy Analysis Framework*. Vancouver, BC: Institute for Intersectionality Research and Policy, Simon Fraser University.

Hankivsky, O. & Cormier, R. (2009). *Intersectionality: Moving Women's Health Research and Policy Forward*. Vancouver: Women's Health Research Network.

Hankivsky, O., Grace, D., Hunting, G., Giesbrecht, M., Fridkin, A., Rudrum, S., & Ferlatte, O, Clark, N. (2014, Dec 10). An intersectionality-based policy analysis framework: critical reflections on a methodology for advancing equity. *International Journal for Equity in Health*, *13* (119). doi: 10.1186/s12939-014-0119-x

Hanley, I., Ives, N., Lenet, J., Hordyk, S.R., Walsh, C.A., Soltane, S.B., & Este, D. (2019). Migrant women's health and housing security: an intersectional analysis. *International Journal of Migrant Health & Social Care*, *15*(1), 90–106. doi: 10.1108/IJMHSC-05-2018-0027

Hanley, J., Ives, N., Lenet, J., Hordyk, S. R., Walsh, C., Ben Soltane, S., & Este, D. (2019). Migrant women's health and housing insecurity: an intersectional analysis. *International Journal of Migration, Health and Social Care*, *15*(1), 90–106.

Humphries, D.L., Sodipo, M., Jackson, S.D. (2023). The intersectionality-based policy analysis framework: demonstrating utility through application to the pre-vaccine U.S. COVID-19 policy response. *Frontiers in Public Health*, *11*, 01–12 doi: 10.3389/fpubh.2023.1040851. PMID: 37655290; PMCID: PMC10466398

Hunting, G. (2012). *A call for a policy paradigm shift: an intersectionality-based analysis of FASD policy. An intersectionality-based policy analysis framework*. Institute for Intersectionality Research and Policy, 93–113.

Lovin, L. (2021). Intersectionality as a critical social theory. *Feminist Encounters: A Journal of Critical Studies in Culture and Politics*, *5*(2). 33.

MacDonald, K., Dorow, S., Klein, R. & Kochkina, O. (2024). Intersectionality in housing research: Early reflections from a community-based participatory research partnership. *Engaged Scholar Journal*, *10*(2), 62–82. https://doi.org/10.15402/esj.v10i2.70858

Nash, J. C. (2008). Re-Thinking Intersectionality. *Feminist Review*, *89*(1), 1–15. https://doi.org/10.1057/fr.2008.4

Oudshoorn, A., Rabiah-Mohammed, F., Ariba, O. Krywucky, A., Annor, B., Adu, J., Ndayisenga, J.P., Guerro, D., Reid, T.R., & Lindsay, S. (2025). Conducting intersectional analysis in nursing research. *Advances in Nursing Science*, *0*(0) 1–16.

Queen's University. (2019). *Indigenous terminology guide*. Available from: https://www.queensu.ca/indigenous/ways-knowing/terminology-guide

Rivers, M. (Feb., 2023). Intersectionality and homelessness: We need to take a deeper dive. Blog. https://endhomelessness.org/blog/intersectionality-and-homelessness-we-need-to-take-a-deeper-dive/

Saewyc, E., Mounsey, B., Tourand, J., Brunanski, D., Kirk, D., McNeil-Seymour, J., Shaughnessy, K., Tsuruda, S., & Clark.,N. (2017). Homeless & street-involved indigenous LGBTQ2S youth in British Columbia: Intersectionality, challenges, resilience & cues for action (Chapter 2, pp. 13–40). In *Where am I Going to Go? Intersectional Approaches to Ending LGBTQ2S Youth Homelessness in Canada & the US*, edited by A. Abramovitch & J. Shelton, Toronto: Canadian Observatory on Homelessness Press.

Schwan, K., Versteegh, A., Perri, M., Caplan, R., Baig, K., Dej, E., Jenkinson, J., Brais, H., Eiboff, F., & Pahlevan-Chaleshtari, T. (2020). *The State of Women's Housing Need & Homelessness in Canada: Literature Review*. Canadian Observatory on Homelessness Press https://www.homelesshub.ca/sites/default/files/attachments/state_womens_homelessness_10072020.pdf

Sharif, M. Z., García, J. J., Mitchell, U., Dellor, E. D., Bradford, N. J., & Truong, M. (2022). Racism and structural violence: Interconnected threats to health equity. *Frontiers in Public Health*, 9, 676783. https://doi.org/10.3389/fpubh.2021.676783

Smye, V., Browne, A.J., Varcoe, C. & Josewski, V. (2011). Harm reduction, methadone maintenance treatment and the root causes of health and social inequities: An intersectional lens in the Canadian context. *Harm Reduction Journal*, *8*(17), 7 doi:10.1186/1477-7517-8-17

Trochmann, M. (2021). Identities, intersectionality, and otherness: The social constructions of deservedness in American housing policy. *Administrative Theory & Praxis*, *43*(1), 97–116. https://doi.org/10.1080/10841806.2019.1700456

Vohra-Gupta, S., Petruzzi, L., Jones, C., & Cubbin, C. (2023). An intersectional approach to understanding barriers to healthcare for women. *Journal of Community Health*. *48*(1), 89–98. doi: 10.1007/s10900-022-01147-8

Zufferey, C. (2016). *Homelessness and Social Work: An Intersectional Approach*. Routledge Reports from the Field.

SECTION 3

Application of the Bridging the Transition Framework

15

APPLYING THE BRIDGING THE TRANSITION FRAMEWORK

Individual-Level Approaches

Lee Ann Westover

This chapter explores the application of Bridging the Transition Framework (referred here on as "The Framework") to support individuals through the spectrum of homelessness. Through two detailed case examples, the chapter illustrates how a treatment team can assist individuals in building essential skills, developing support networks, and regaining stability in their lives—with the goal not just of obtaining housing but also maintaining it long-term. It highlights the use of assessments, a harm reduction approach (Chapter 12), and principles of housing first (Chapter 10) to tailor personalized interventions that focus on clients' strengths to promote their autonomy and long-term success. By providing examples of how individual support strategies can guide personalized intervention for sustainable community reintegration, this chapter offers valuable guidance for providers who work with people experiencing homelessness.

Component of the Bridging the Transition Framework Addressed in this Chapter

The case examples presented here are illustrative of the individual nature of homelessness and how a multidisciplinary team can apply individual support strategies from the Framework into personalized intervention design from the first meeting of a client. As is emphasized in the Framework, mutual trust is at the foundation of the relationship. Housing first and harm reduction frameworks are also foundational to developing a trusting relationship with clients and patients. The following includes examples of how to apply those approaches as guiding principles for rapport-building. This chapter highlights how each member of a multidisciplinary team has an

DOI: 10.4324/9781003541332-18

important role in addressing individual cases, and how teams can coordinate to maintain fidelity to client-centered goals. Lastly, this chapter explores not just assessment and intervention, but also emphasizes that recovery (Chapter 11) takes time and is a very individual process.

How this Chapter Guides Practice and Research in Homelessness Prevention

This chapter will follow two people experiencing homelessness and their treatment teams as they implement the framework for intervention design with individual clients, instead of a population or community. The chapter serves as inspiration for practitioners, whose creativity and consistency will be required to assist their clients as they move through the stages of homelessness. The chapter aims to highlight relationship-building and fidelity to housing first and harm reduction models—which form part of the foundation of the Bridging the Transition Framework. It is also emphasized, herein, that the treatment team should always support a sense of agency in their clients, which will fuel their further successes.

Introduction

The objective of this chapter is to demonstrate how approaches and support strategies for individuals can be implemented in practice. The reader will explore case examples of two individuals as they move through the stages of homelessness. Their stories are fictionalized, but they are drawn from real people and real-life events in their lives.

Individual intervention guided by the Bridging the Transition Framework begins with the relationship as the foundation for meaningful work with people experiencing homelessness. The idea seems simple, but in practice the process takes a good deal of time and consistency on the part of the provider. Research demonstrates that people experiencing homelessness frequently are targets of harmful stigma and judgment from providers (Becker and Foli, 2022; Kaplan et al., 2020; Reilly et al., 2022). This can be as subtle as language choices and facial expressions or more obvious like criticism of failures and pressure to accomplish provider-generated goals. The resulting mistrust and avoidance of service providers has a strong negative impact on individuals experiencing homelessness. Before the real work can begin with an individual client, it is essential to take the time to build rapport. In short, relationships can be complicated, but fidelity to Bridging the Transition Framework and the guiding models at its foundation (harm reduction, housing first, intersectionality) can guide a service provider throughout the time they are working with an individual client. Two case examples presented here provide brief examples of how a multidisciplinary team can help a client progress through the stages of homelessness and also how individual providers' actions are a foundation for that work. The chapter describes the case of Desi, who is moving from the *survival* stage to *adaptation*, and Carmen as she moves from *integration* into *precarity* and back.

Desi: Survival and Adaptation

Desi in the Survival *Stage*

Desi, a 27-year-old man of Jamaican descent, has lived in shelters or on the street since he was 21. He attends an outpatient substance use treatment program geared toward people who are unhoused. Desi struggles with daily function in a number of domains, but does not make it to many appointments. Desi's substance use patterns are chaotic and risky, thus resulting in multiple overdoses from fentanyl-contaminated street drugs. While he has been resistant to individual intervention, he has lately begun to trust his counselor. He has recently been approved for supportive housing through his shelter and will be moving sometime in the next few months. With his counselor, Desi complains of anxiety, demonstrates poor hygiene, and resists making appointments with other disciplines on the team. Desi recently lost another of his many phones, although he stayed connected to his brother via social media. The team recognizes that he will need extra support through his transition into housing. Obtaining housing is an obviously positive event, but the period of transition into the new community can be rocky. This period of transition can last up to two years and often provides many challenges for people who are adapting from homelessness (Marshall et al., 2021). The team decided it was a good time to refresh their approach with Desi and help him identify new goals. Desi had reluctantly agreed to meet with a new provider, an occupational therapist on the interdisciplinary team, to learn about computers and strategies for improving short-term memory and organization to prevent losing another phone. Desi's concrete goals are an opening for rapport-building with other team members. If he meets success at the beginning, it is hoped he will be more likely to continue engaging.

The team understood Desi's resistance to meeting new people, so his provider had learned to keep initial sessions brief to accommodate his attention difficulties. Desi set his own goals for the day, and the provider refrained from asking too many probing questions. They practiced computer skills by logging into social media and played a memory game. Since he struggles to keep regular appointments, team members offered walk-in options in order to ensure that he was able to make progress in his session goals. He agreed to continue engaging in order to work toward longer term goals.

Assessment: Canadian Personal Recovery Outcome Measure (C-PROM)

After a few sessions, Desi agreed to participate in assessment. He was sensitive to being tested by providers who did not know him well, so it was essential to maintain transparency. Desi reviewed the document, assented to participate, and kept a copy of it after the session. The C-PROM was selected due to it serving as a thorough review of many areas of Desi's life (Barbic, 2018). The C-PROM serves as a framework to identify and discuss challenges in a number of life domains. Desi expressed surprise that there were no questions about drug use in the C-PROM, but the assessor clarified that managing substance use was his

QUESTIONNAIRE

NAME: Desi

Date: d/m/y 4 / 13 / 2024

Canadian Personal Recovery Outcome Measure (C-PROM)

Please take the time to fill in the following **questionnaire**.
There are 30 questions. The score for each question is as follows:

Based on your experiences in the **last week**, please indicate how often you have felt this way by selecting the option you most agree with.

0	1	2	3	4
None of the time	25% of the time	50% of the time	75% of the time	All of the time

QUESTIONS		RESPONSE				
1.	I am motivated to keep myself well	0	1	2	3	4
2.	I can access the health and social services that I need	0	1	2	3	4
3.	I can identify the early warning signs of becoming unwell	0	1	2	3	4
4.	I feel safe	0	1	2	3	4
5.	I am hopeful about my future	0	1	2	3	4
6.	I have an idea of who I want to become	0	1	2	3	4
7.	I am respected by others	0	1	2	3	4
8.	I know what helps me stay well	0	1	2	3	4
9.	I like myself	0	1	2	3	4
10.	I am driven by meaningful goals	0	1	2	3	4
11.	I am supported by family and friends	0	1	2	3	4
12.	I have a purpose in life	0	1	2	3	4
13.	I can be an advocate for myself	0	1	2	3	4
14.	I accomplish the goals I set out for myself	0	1	2	3	4
15.	I have fun	0	1	2	3	4

PROM 1 © Skye Barbic PhD 2018

FIGURE 15.1A Desi's C-PROM (Barbic et al. 2018) assessment findings.

choice and that it would probably be intertwined with other intervention areas. Desi identified other priorities of increasing his income, stress management, and getting ready to move into housing. The C-PROM identified goal areas that surprised Desi and that he agreed would be important (see Figures 15.1 and 15.1b).

The assessor linked these priorities to the Bridging the Transition Framework and discussed individual support strategies with Desi. Observe, below, how longer-term goals link to personal goals and framework components. Often, each goal can be served by a number of different strategies, and each strategy can address a number of goals. See Table 15.1 for Desi's initial intervention plan.

QUESTIONNAIRE

NAME: Desi

Date: d/m/y 4 / 13 / 2024

0	1	2	3	4
None of the Time	25% of the time	50% of the time	75% of the time	All of the time

QUESTIONS	RESPONSE				
16. I like the place that I live in (house, apartment, etc...)	0	1	2	3	**4**
17. I spend my day doing the things that I enjoy	0	1	2	3	**4**
18. I am confident	0	1	2	3	**4**
19. I sleep well	0	1	2	3	**4**
20. I have energy	0	1	2	3	**4**
21. I am happy	0	1	2	3	**4**
22. I have control over my life	0	1	2	3	**4**
23. I have new interests	0	1	2	3	**4**
24. I have good self-esteem	0	1	2	3	**4**
25. I have enough money to meet my basic needs	0	1	2	**3**	4
26. I feel a part of my community	0	1	2	3	**4**
27. I can manage stress	0	1	2	**3**	4
28. I contribute to my community	0	1	2	3	**4**
29. I am satisfied with my intimate relationships	0	1	2	**3**	4
30. I have peace of mind	0	1	2	3	**4**
TOTAL SCORE 113 /120	ADJUSTED SCORE = TOTAL SCORE / 4				

Scoring Instructions

1. Add up total score and divide by **4** to give you the ADJUSTED SCORE.
2. Based on the ADJUSTED score, mark an X on the ruler below corresponding to this number.

113 ÷ 4 = 28.5

0 1 2 3 4 5 6 7 8 9 10 11 12 13 14 15 16 17 18 19 20 21 22 23 24 25 26 27 28 29 30

RECOVERY

3. Return to the question on the scale that corresponds with the number on the ruler.
4. Begin conversation, assessment, and goal setting at this point.

PROM 2

FIGURE 15.1B Desi's C-PROM (Barbic et al. 2018) assessment findings.

TABLE 15.1 Desi's Initial Intervention Plan

Desi's Overarching, Longer-term Goals	*Desi's Personal Goal Areas*	*Bridging the Transition Approach*	*Bridging the Transition Individual Support Strategies*	*Personalized Interventions*
Feeling in control of one's life Maintaining tenancy Hope for the future Strategies to improve cognition and organization	Improving intimate relationships Leisure participation alone or with others	Developing positive social relationships	Use of person-centered counseling to elicit individualized strategies for developing positive social relationships during homelessness	Desi is not happy with his "friends" because he feels like people take advantage of him. His counselor will help him problem-solve current relationships. As he learns about healthy relationships, his counselor will help him identify the qualities in an ideal friend or romantic interest. Desi will participate in the social skills group to learn how to set boundaries and in the games group to practice conflict resolution strategies.
		Linking individuals to the broader community Engagement in meaningful activity	Identifying local opportunities for the person to join community groups, classes, and events that include primarily individuals from outside of the unhoused community Identifying strategies for establishing a routine and structure in one's day	The peer specialist will take Desi to the library to find out what classes and events are happening locally. He will also take Desi to a community clothing closet to get appropriate clothes for the events. OT will help Desi learn computer and mobile phone skills that will help him find more events and use an app to get directions. OT will also help Desi learn about internet safety. The office manager agreed to help Desi obtain the transport passes he is entitled to after participating in an individual or group session. When he is ready, his counselor will help Desi make an initial appointment with the clinic psychiatrist and help Desi express his concerns about psychiatric treatment.
	Increase income	Addressing poverty	Identifying strategies and supporting the person to engage in income generation strategies Uncovering possibilities for accessing benefits for which the person is eligible but not receiving	At the moment, Desi agrees he is not ready for employment and would benefit from working with OT to develop and implement organization and time management strategies. His counselor will help Desi call his shelter to learn what Desi needs to do to get ready to move. The peer specialist will help him obtain any materials he needs.

All of these interventions were designed with input and approval from Desi. While he does overdose regularly, he does not have a substance use goal at the moment. It is hoped that he will be able to discuss harm reduction strategies with nursing so he can increase his personal safety. The team is as transparent as possible through this process so Desi remains the agent of change—borrowed from harm reduction and housing first approaches.

By eventually engaging with the nurse, he was able to develop safer substance use habits, such as using fentanyl test strips and avoiding solitary use. By the time he moved, Desi felt confident in his ability to live independently.

Desi in the Adaptation *Stage*

A couple of weeks after moving into his apartment, Desi did not come to the clinic for a few days. The peer specialist visited his apartment. Desi appeared disheveled and downcast. Desi was struggling with increased substance use, boredom, and isolation. Without a phone or money for transportation, he felt trapped. Desi's situation reflects the challenges of adapting to housing.

The peer specialist came back later in the week and they discussed Desi's previous C-PROM results and updated his scores. Based on those scores, a crisis intervention plan was discussed with Desi and implemented by staff. See the excerpt presented in Table 15.2.

Over time, Desi regained stability. This meant that he was again able to make progress toward personal goals. He established a daily routine, learned about neighborhood resources, and began helping the building

TABLE 15.2 Desi's New Intervention Plan

Approach	*Individual Intervention Strategy*	*Personalized Interventions*
Addressing new health concerns and managing substance use Maintaining tenancy	Addressing new health concerns	Desi picked up more fentanyl test strips and refreshed his awareness of *harm reduction* strategies. The psychiatrist was able to meet with Desi via telehealth to address his anxiety with assistance from the peer specialist.
Incorporating peersupport	Incorporating individuals with lived experiences of homelessness into directservice within services designed to support persons who are unhoused.	Desi made it to a group session and talked about his challenges. Another client and neighbor that Desi respected offered to accompany him to the clinic every few days.

TABLE 15.3 Carmen's Strengths Assessment

Strengths Assessment		
Current Strengths	*Individual's Desires, Aspirations*	*Past Resources—Personal, Social, and Environmental*
Employment/Education/Specialized Knowledge		
"I am proud of how I cope mental illness and think I am resilient."	"I want to continue my education and find employment as a peer specialist."	"I have done lots of jobs and can adapt to different positions. I also have an education already."
Relationships		
"I have learned a lot about myself and I can finally say *no* to people. I like talking to people."	"I really hope there is time for me to be a better mom to my kids."	"I used to be really social and could get along with anyone."
Wellness/Health		
"I have learned a lot about how to live a healthy life and am excited to keep improving myself."	"I want to cook healthy foods that will give me energy. I also need to be doing cardio."	"I grew up with a garden and know a lot about plants. I think that might be fun to try again."

superintendent for a little income. After taking time to connect with appropriate care and support, and a few ups and downs, he was eventually able to begin adapting to community living and build a life he is proud of.

Carmen: Integration and Precarity

Carmen in the Integration *stage*

Carmen is a 44-year-old Latina woman who entered a housing first program a year ago. Carmen has experienced recurring periods of homelessness over the last 20 years. She has been diagnosed with bipolar disorder and has struggled with medication adherence until recently. Her first year in housing was challenging. Recently, with the support of a psychiatric nurse practitioner, she is consistently adhering to mental health treatment for the first time in her life. She recognizes that while she doesn't always feel like *herself*, her behavior is less chaotic and her daily life is more manageable. Carmen used substances primarily as a coping mechanism during her time in shelters. When she moved into her apartment her substance use largely ceased. She has become ready to address other parts of her life now that she feels more stable.

TABLE 15.4 A Part of Carmen's Intervention Plan Informed by the Bridging the Transition Framework

Carmen's Personal Priorities	*Bridging the Transition Approach*	*Bridging the Transition Individual Support Strategies*	*Relevant Personal Strengths from the Strengths Assessment*	*Personalized Interventions*
Health management	*Addressing new health concerns*	*Supporting individuals to access health care supports to manage new health* concerns and accompanying them to appointments if necessary	Awareness of health issues and how to address them Gardening and cooking skills	The OT will work with Carmen to find healthy recipes on her phone and teach her about internet safety. The peer specialist will work with Carmen to find local pantries. They also will begin to explore local community gardens where Carmen could meet new people and grow some of her own food.
Reconnect with family	*Building and* rediscovering meaningful relationships	*Identifying opportunities for engaging in activities with individuals in the* broader community *Supporting a person to reconnect with family and friends from their pasts if* desired and appropriate given their individual context	"I used to be really social and could get along with anyone."	Carmen has not been close with her children for a long time, so she works with her case manager and peer specialist to plan how she will reach out to them, as well as a crisis plan if they don't respond well and she needs extra support. If they respond positively, Carmen has recently found a church she likes and will invite them to church and then lunch after.
Explore peer specialist identification programs	*Finding meaningful* activities that informidentity *Addressing poverty*	*Identifying funding opportunities to decrease barriers to participation*	Strong motivation for education High school diploma, some college	Carmen will work with OT to continue development of computer and mobile phone skills by searching for peer specialist education programs. Carmen's case manager will help Carmen explore and apply for school funding. Her church has grants for parishioners who are going back to school. She was able to independently learn how to request a grant and will be able to do so independently.
Mobile phone and computer literacy	All of the above	Computer and mobile phone literacy is integrated in many daily activities and can be embedded in other interventions	Desire to learn about technology	For tasks that utilize computer and mobile phone skills, OT and peer specialist are available to help teach her skills, trouble-shoot, and—most importantly—teach about internet safety.

Assessment: The Strengths Assessment

To help Carmen formulate a plan, the peer specialist helped her complete the Strengths Assessment (Rapp & Goscha, 2011). This assessment will help her identify the resources she already has for goal accomplishment and her current priorities. See Table 15.3 for a summary of Carmen's Strengths Assessment.

Carmen's case manager at her housing program worked with Carmen and the clinical team to create an initial intervention plan, informed by Bridging the Transition Framework strategies. They worked with Carmen to make sure the interventions matched her goals and were achievable. See Table 15.4 for part of Carmen's intervention plan.

By following this plan, and adapting it as needed, Carmen was able to begin the process of reconnecting with her children and identify funding for an education program of her choice. She has more confidence in her computer and mobile skills. She is using social media to follow influencers in her chosen field, as well to look at her grandchild's baby pictures. She still reports occasional bouts of anxiety, but overall expresses great satisfaction with her progress.

Carmen in the Precarity *Stage*

Two years into her tenancy, Carmen faced an unexpected challenge: her landlord decided to sell the property, so she would need to find a new home. This sudden change represents Carmen's entry into the *Precarity* stage, which is marked by emotional upheaval, stress, and a sense of instability. Carmen's anxiety skyrocketed. She also began withdrawing from activities and struggling with sleep disturbances and nightmares. She stopped going to church but still prayed. She was overwhelmed by the fear of losing everything she had worked for and returning to homelessness. When the peer specialist and case manager learned of the eviction, they immediately went to Carmen's apartment to offer support. She burst into tears and was not able to effectively organize her thoughts. They offered reassurance, then the case manager and peer specialist worked with the team to develop an intervention plan to help Carmen through this crisis.

Intervention Using Bridging the Transition Framework Support Strategies

When staff couldn't reach Carmen by phone, they visited her apartment and found her in a distressed state—her apartment was messy, and she was using marijuana to cope with her anxiety. While marijuana use wasn't a primary concern, it represents a change in her pattern. The intervention began right away and focused on restabilization. They used Framework to identify appropriate approaches and potential individual support strategies, even though Carmen was not able to meaningfully participate at the moment. The main

TABLE 15.5 An Excerpt from Carmen's Crisis Plan

Bridging the Transition Approach	*Bridging the Transition Individual Support Strategies*	*Personalized Interventions*
Supporting mental well-being	Providing ongoing and frequent opportunities for support due to the level of distress that one may encounter at this time *Increase the availability of support using multiple means and methods*	Carmen, the peer specialist, and case manager make a plan for frequent apartment visits, texts, and phone calls to help Carmen navigate all of the stress surrounding this event. OT works with Carmen to learn mindfulness techniques and sensory strategies to help her manage stress.
Problem-solving around housing	Identify funding sources for new housing or the prevention of homelessness *Supporting the person to search housing listings and accessing housing vouchers and* emergency housing funds *Helping to identify and access safe emergency shelter options*	The case manager will ensure that Carmen's housing subsidies will continue if she changes apartments and find out how to enact the change. They also come up with a plan for Carmen to use her social strengths to network. She will speak to the office at her mental health clubhouse, get out the word at church, and inquire about listings from local businesses she frequents. Carmen will search for apartments online with help from OT, while emphasizing internet safety.
Incorporating peer support	Incorporating individuals with lived experience of homelessness into the direct support of the person at risk of losing their housing.	Support from the peer specialist is invaluable at this time, as the peer has lived experience of not just homelessness and mental health issues, but also of recovering stability and meaning in life. When Carmen finds potential apartments, the peer specialist will go with her to view them, help fill out paperwork, and identify potential scams.

goals of the interventions were to help Carmen reorient and regain focus, manage uncomfortable feelings, and participate in a plan to prevent a return to homelessness. By encouraging her to use her strengths, she can reconnect with her resilience. See Table 15.5 for an excerpt from Carmen's crisis plan.

With a lot of ongoing support, Carmen found a new apartment via a church parishioner and successfully transitioned into a new neighborhood. Throughout the process, she was able to rediscover her strengths, engage with her community, and rebuild her confidence. Over time, she reconnected with her social network and began to participate in more community activities. By the end of the year, Carmen was thriving again. Carmen's progress highlights the importance of a strengths-based approach in helping individuals move from the *precarity* stage to stable, fulfilling lives in the community.

Conclusion

Progression through the spectrum of homelessness is very individual. Because of the heterogeneity of clients, personalized interventions made specifically for the individual are *required*, not recommended. It may seem natural for a provider to launch into assessment and intervention design, but doing so without the relationship as foundation can sometimes do more harm than good. The client as the agent of change will be able to accomplish more than someone who is dependent on their providers. The Bridging the Transition Framework serves not only as a framework to create those client-led, personalized interventions, but also as a tool that supports multidisciplinary teams to effectively serve their clients.

References

Barbic, S. (2018) *The Canadian Personal Recovery Outcome Measure*. British Columbia Psychosocial Rehabilitation. https://www.psyrehab.ca/files/documents/ENGLISH%20VERSION.pdf

Becker, J.N. and Foli, K.J. (2022) "Health-seeking behaviours in the homeless population: A concept analysis," *Health & Social Care in the Community*, *30*(2), pp. e278–e286. https://doi.org/10.1111/hsc.13499

Kaplan, L.M. et al. (2020) "Barriers and solutions to advance care planning among homeless-experienced older adults," *Journal of Palliative Medicine*, *23*(10), pp. 1300–1306. https://doi.org/10.1089/jpm.2019.0550

Marshall, C.A. et al. (2021) "A systematic review of occupational therapy interventions in the transition from homelessness," *Scandinavian Journal of Occupational Therapy*, *28*(3), pp. 171–187. https://doi.org/10.1080/11038128.2020.1764094

Rapp, C.A. and Goscha, R.J. (2011) *The Strengths Model: A Recovery-oriented Approach to Mental Health Services*. 3rd ed. New York: Oxford University Press.

Reilly, J., Ho, I. and Williamson, A. (2022) "A systematic review of the effect of stigma on the health of people experiencing homelessness," *Health & Social Care in the Community*, *30*(6), pp. 2128–2141. https://doi.org/10.1111/hsc.13884

16

APPLYING THE BRIDGING THE TRANSITION FRAMEWORK

Community-Level Approaches

Andrea LeFlore

The Bridging the Transition Framework articulates community-level tools and strategies for organizational or regional impact. This chapter will present an in-depth case example where community assessment, engagement, and participatory research influenced a supportive housing organization to transform service provision and expand community-designed programming to meet member needs across the trajectory of unhoused to housing. Newly developed programming utilized emancipatory practices, co-designed with community members with lived expertise of homeless transition, to establish an Engagement Center, uniquely addressing the priorities of community members regardless of housing state. This community space intersects all organization programming and continues to evolve with ongoing community member input. This participatory process can be applied across homeless service settings to inform innovative and relevant program design.

Component of the Bridging the Transition Framework Addressed in this Chapter

This chapter will focus on describing an application of the Bridging the Transition Framework with a community across the trajectory of unhoused to housing. A case-based example for community-level interventions which emphasizes function, participation, and well-being of persons experiencing homelessness is presented.

DOI: 10.4324/9781003541332-19

How this Chapter Guides Practice and Research in Homelessness Prevention

This chapter outlines application of the Bridging the Transition Framework with a community organization in an urban setting where community members served as the co-facilitators of participatory research (including community assessment) and program development. With emerging research illuminating the complexities of housing transition after the traumas of homelessness, and opportunities to explore effective supports in housing, participatory approaches are warranted to build from the lived expertise of community members. The resulting establishment of new knowledge to inform programming allows for organizations to utilize otherwise untapped resources and the potential to design services with greater utility to the community using ongoing reflection and monitoring.

Introduction

This chapter will provide a case example of how the Bridging the Transition Framework can be applied with a community across the trajectory of unhoused to housing. Specifically, this chapter will outline an in-depth case example at ReVive® Center for Housing and Healing, a non-profit organization offering a continuum of programs from homeless street outreach to supportive housing in Chicago, IL, USA.

ReVive serves individuals experiencing housing insecurity in the near west side of Chicago through four programs and a community space that supports individuals experiencing or at risk of experiencing homelessness to rebuild lives. First, ReVive's Cressey House offers 28 units of congregate Permanent Supportive Housing (PSH), combining affordable housing and available supportive services since 1970 for individuals and families who have experienced chronic homelessness. Second, ReVive's Scattered Site Supportive Housing Program (SHP) supports 98 individuals at risk of homelessness or formerly homeless with supportive services through the Illinois Department of Human Services. The third program consists of 20 units within the SHP which became Scattered Site PSH units through a 2023 U.S. Housing and Urban Development (HUD) Supplemental Notice of Funding Opportunity (SNOFO) Leasing Grant. The supportive services team for ReVive's three housing programs includes onsite case management, occupational therapy, and array of community partner services to address housing, physical and mental health, employment, and community integration goals. Lastly, the 2023 HUD SNOFO also funded ReVive's establishment of a housing-focused interdisciplinary Street Outreach program, including case management, social work, occupational therapy, and a team of Peer Navigators with lived expertise of homelessness to provide tailored, intensive services for individuals experiencing unsheltered homelessness.

This chapter will describe the development of ReVive's innovative community space—a community Engagement Center—which is available to any interested community member. The Engagement Center was co-designed with ReVive community members through community-level assessment and intervention strategies, as outlined in the Bridging the Transition Framework, to address survival, adaptation, integration, and precarity. Interweaving each of these four processes into the low-barrier Engagement Center allows individuals experiencing homelessness to maintain stability through support systems as they move from unhoused to housing.

Community Assessment at ReVive

As ReVive sought to explore how to increase authentic engagement with supportive housing participants, the organization welcomed an Occupational Therapy Doctorate capstone student, this chapter's author, to design and implement a strengths-based, empowerment-focused, and accessible Participatory Community Assessment (PCA) that would identify and mobilize community member expertise to inform the development of relevant programs. The process focused on building social support networks, combating stigma and power dynamics, enhancing community integration, and improving quality of life. The PCA used a mixed-methods design for triangulation of findings with an iterative reflection process.

Upon review of available research on housing transition, this project was designed to distinctly build from community strengths and capacity, rather than focus on the needs and challenges. Homeless services often function in a consumer-based system: deficiency-oriented services with dependency-enabling environments that are funded to reinforce this system (Godoy-Vieira et al., 2018). Homeless services are generally designed to meet clear needs, such as food and shelter, rarely focusing on recognizing the potential of community members to design and influence their environments and services. This project recognized the impact of sustained societal stigma and marginalization and contrastingly the strengths within every community.

The Bridging the Transition Framework references asset-based development and community needs assessment (NA), which were integrated into the PCA design. This approach yielded a deeper understanding of ReVive community's structure and goals to tailor interventions and tackle change initiatives based on the community's readiness. In a community NA, the intent is to learn from the experts in the community within an organization, including both staff and community members served (Schensul, Berg & Nair, 2013). *Community* in this case example refers to ReVive as an organization serving a specific population (i.e., adults transitioning out of homelessness) with a common characteristic or shared space (Suarez-Balcazar, 2018).

ReVive's PCA built from three strengths-based NA approaches: (1) Asset/Capacity Building and NA Hybrid Framework, (2) Asset-Based Community Development (ABCD), and (3) Concerns Report Method, each emphasizing active and authentic partnership with community members (Altschuld, 2015; Kretzmann, & McKnight, 1993; Suarez-Balcazar, & Balcazar, 2016). These NA approaches guided ReVive through an applied research method with implications to directly inform practice and the community's situation. Community members define the community, the internal working team determines its key members, and assessment findings are interpreted by the community.

Based on these approaches, the following community assessment tools were selected for implementation in this order: (1) Capacity Inventory, (2) The World Café, and (3) Community-Engaged and Participatory Asset Mapping. During the Capacity Inventory, participants explored their own gifts, skills, passions, and "teachables" (J. McKnight, co-director of ABCD Institute, personal communication, August 9, 2018), sharing and combining their lists to understand their community's strengths (Kretzmann & McKnight, 1993). The World Café uses an appreciative inquiry approach with a café-ambience and rotating conversations on questions that are developed and prioritized by the community (Brown, Isaacs & World Café Community, 2005; Ludema, Cooperrider & Barrett, 2000). Questions are solutions-oriented; cross-pollination of ideas leads to action-oriented data to transform communities for social change. Asset Mapping then facilitates collective visual resource identification and sharing among community members, where participants document resources and spaces that supported their community participation (Kretzmann & McKnight, 1993).

These tools provide alternatives to writing-based strategies that are often not accessible for all individuals living in PSH. A series of Town Hall meetings followed the assessment phase to summarize and check findings with members, celebrate successes, and develop action plans for program development. Table 16.1 outlines the PCA Framework merging these concepts and tools.

Feedback forms adapted for accessibility, a rating form for user engagement, and a staff listening session were utilized for PCA process evaluation. Rating forms explored community members' perceived engagement throughout all aspects of the research process and power to influence organizational decision-making.

Community Impact

PCA findings, when presented to ReVive, led to an organizational decision to convert an existing Thrift Store into a community Engagement Center. PCA tools continue to be utilized for quality improvement and necessary adaptations to the Engagement Center space and programming. After four

TABLE 16.1 Participatory Community Assessment (PCA) Framework in Supportive Housing

Steps	*Activities*
1 Initiate university–community partnership; scope the context and plan for collaboration	• Engage in current programming to discover existing practices and routines • Build relationships with staff and community members • Conduct informal interviews and discussions • Learn about community's visions for the future and their view of strengths and needs; design a collective project vision
2 Develop a working team	• Deepen connections with community members • Establish a team of engaged community members and staff to participate in planning, implementing, and evaluating assessment methods personalized to the community • Continue to gain insight on organizational culture and context

3 Collect data	• Collectively set objectives and a timeline
	• Collaborate to determine assignments and responsibilities for team members based on member strengths and priorities
	• Preparatory community activities:
	  • Establish Community Vision
	  • SOAR Analysis (Strengths, Opportunities, Aspirations, Results)
	• Collect group data:
	  • Phase I: Capacity Inventory of key assets and resources among participants
	  • Phase II: World Café
	  • Phase III: Community-Engaged and Participatory Asset Mapping
	• Ongoing dialogue, reflection and debrief sessions, team meetings

4 Organize findings and analyze data	• Document assets and capacities in multimodal and accessible formats • Begin to build relationships with local community assets • Mutually engage in problem-solving solutions with the community • Prepare to present findings for decision-making and community use • Revisit Step 1 activities (e.g., vision, programming) in more detail

(*Continued*)

TABLE 16.1 (Continued)

Steps	*Activities*

5 Discuss findings and how to use results through Listening Session(s)	• Implement a series of Listening Session(s)
	  • Set priorities for action using Nominal Group Technique
	  • Reflect on and celebrate achievements and resources
	  • Translate findings into action plans with team
	• Engage the community in aligning actions with community vision
	• Set achievable, tangible goals for action items with barriers, supports, key people, and timelines

6 Implement action plans based on assessment findings with community-based planning	• Team makes decisions on programming toward positive change • Implement programming • Translate plans into real events and programs • Implement success mapping • Continue to assess community strengths and partnerships through use of assessment methods as relevant
7 Reflect and monitor planned activities	• Utilize formative and summative evaluation • Assess program functioning and document outcomes • Reflect and evaluate actions using praxis cycle
8 Recycle back to initial findings and revisit for action	• Reflect on project and restructure future activities for improvement • Revisit previous findings and progress toward organization goals • Conduct a follow-up World Café to collect feedback on progress and set goals for future

years of operation, ReVive received an Illinois Housing Development Authority grant to redesign the space for the center's purpose.

Development of the Engagement Center

In considering the design of ReVive's Engagement Center, PCA findings emphasized that many individuals in supportive housing valued wanting to help others still in survival and share their working knowledge from their transition experience, aligning with research on peer support (Barker & Maguire, 2017). Distinct from traditional drop-in spaces, community members developed the following vision for the Engagement Center: helping people thrive; meeting needs with respect; and inspiring, empowering, and lifting people up to believe in themselves. They designed the space for meaningful active daily engagement and community. Participants were not identified by their housing status to be triaged into a program; rather, the community space was designed for radical hospitality: to be low-barrier, trauma-informed, strengths-based, harm reduction and recovery-focused, diverse identity and intersectionality affirming, and relationship-focused with skilled onsite service providers available if and when community members identify a goal or priority. Conflicts are often inevitable in a space designed for authentic community engagement and belonging, particularly with the traumas and triggers from each person's experience. Center staff support crisis prevention and intervention, conflict resolution, and relationship redevelopment alongside trauma recovery processes. Safety guidelines communicating the requirements for using the space (i.e., no violence, stealing, use of weapons, etc.) and general community guidelines to create a healing space are clearly posted and regularly reviewed, particularly when needs arise. Participation agreements are utilized if and when guests may struggle with guidelines to ensure all who need and desire access to the center services can do so.

Center staff include case managers, occupational therapists, social workers, and most recently Peer Navigators with lived expertise. Onsite community partners are guided to embrace the same philosophy and all services are walk-in. These partners provide habitual specialty services, including substance use counseling, connections to medication-assisted recovery services, and quarterly HIV testing. An interdisciplinary inclusion health-model (Luchenski et al., 2018) medical care team (including a doctor, registered nurse, licensed clinical social worker, and community health worker) also provides services onsite with a free Over-The-Counter store, transportation assistance, and monthly Ear Nose and Throat clinics. Other partners include a mobile shower van, employment and bank services, and weekend specialty clinics, such as a free, annual, comprehensive onsite vision clinic.

When participants enter, they are greeted at the welcome table to identify preferred names, pronouns, and goals. Coffee and water are available, as well as prepared food from community partners. Guests can then engage with providers and build trusting relationships, which are often in the context of historic stigma by past providers and the broader community. Guests are also supported in available leisure and social group activities, including but not limited to board games, pool, targeted occupation-based groups (e.g., meal preparation, community engagement, wellness, job club), and even peer leader opportunities. This programmatic focus aligns with research findings on the need to combat the effects of pervasive boredom when unhoused, which often persist throughout housing transition (Marshall et al., 2019). ReVive's Engagement Center is a "one-stop shop" that prioritizes human dignity, identity redevelopment, peer mentorships, and social support network building.

The open-concept space offers choice and control over engagement activities and level of environmental sensory stimuli. The center additionally includes designated space for community meals, meal preparation, social engagement, quiet reading, individualized workspace with peers or service providers, a gardening space, community clothing pantry, guest storage, technology and games space, and a health center with exercise equipment. Laundry and shower facilities with policies designed for guest needs were secondarily added to the center design and programming space. The center also provides a structure for establishing meaningful routines as community members develop their own interests to engage in at the center, and the center supports broader community integration opportunities. Guests have engaged in community outings to the local zoo, museums, sports games, job fairs, and other community events, all maximizing use of available public transportation and scaffolding supports to promote independence and carryover outside of facilitated structured center opportunities. Welcoming pets and all ages, aligned with the center's low barrier pet policy and children policy, further promotes an inclusive environment for all to thrive.

Onsite service provider and community partner relationships are evaluated on a recurrent basis to explore opportunities to better facilitate interdisciplinary communication, equitable resource provision, and specific client support needs, as well as other dynamic needs that arise. The medical and occupational therapy team collaboration led to thoroughly integrated supports and capacity building for community members to effectively access and participate in primary and specialty health care services, along with increased engagement in health management as a daily occupation. The ReVive team first connects community members to the visiting medical team, supporting warm handoffs and trust building with the option to consent to team collaboration on their care. The medical team updates a shared Patient Appointments Tracker, where the occupational therapy team then provides the tailored level of supports for community members to engage in care. This involves determining the person's strengths, barriers, and disability or environmental factors influencing their ability to participate in their care. Some clients are independent with a day-before reminder and check-in on their plan and support needs. Others with cognitive impairment, routines with active substance use, significant fear of medical providers, and/or barriers due to lack of a stable living environment (such as regularly losing or having their phones, watches, or other temporal supports stolen due to rough sleeping) benefit from multifaceted interventions and supports to actively participate in their care to their maximal ability at a given time.

This partnership also supports clients' self-advocacy in their health care appointments, such as preparing topics in advance, and exploring pain management solutions with their surgical teams, as well as post-appointment advocacy if and when clients experience mistreatment within the health care system (such as racism, discrimination, or dismissive care). Occupational therapists can triage needs for adaptive equipment or accessibility modifications to their environment, as well as Letters of Medical Necessity for motorized wheelchairs or accessible housing units. Occupational therapists are especially instrumental in promoting physical health management and client carryover of medical recommendations after appointments. This follow-through on recommendations may be limited by barriers such as functional cognitive impairment, active substance use, motivation or readiness, and/or access barriers.

For community members in survival or precarity, the center offers a place to be seen as their true selves, and as trust develops, more private or apprehensive guests often begin to ask for supports such as housing resources. A team-based approach is utilized where occupational therapy often supports case managers when clients have disability- or accessibility-related barriers. Similarly, for guests in adaptation or integration, the service provider team addresses advocacy needs within supportive housing, such as need for in-unit accommodations or modifications under the Fair Housing Act (a U.S. policy). Occupational therapists are instrumental in this, as well as in addressing overall meaningful activity engagement to build new routines and support community members once housed. It is important that the center is not the only location for supportive service provision, given not all participants thrive in community spaces with such social demands.

ReVive's Engagement Center has served as a location for unhoused community members to maintain their center connections and supports alongside their new program's support team upon adaptation to housing. Members often return to the center when encountering challenges to reconnect with their trusted supporters for advocacy support to prevent precarity. The center offers a bridge between outreach and supportive housing teams, where participants report that once housed, transition can feel like they fall off a bridge from services. The center remains a welcoming center for anyone on that continuum, and a central location for any guest to access tailored supports, always with a focus on community and stability.

The Engagement Center has also been an epicenter for the development of varying levels of peer mentorships. Many individuals continue to support center development, starting with their engagement on the working teams of the PCA through to Center Advisory Board engagement. In the center's early development, before securing direct funding, many of these individuals and new community members began by obtaining the role of a Peer Leader, with a posted brief bio and picture and a list of ways they felt skilled and motivated to support their peer community in the center. These roles continue and often lead to desired volunteer engagement in assisting with food management, job connections, World Café table facilitators, and general peer supports, among others.

ReVive's most recent street outreach program involved establishing a team of four Peer Navigators, each working 10 hours per week, to serve as a bridge to other forms of employment and with pathways toward peer specialist certifications. This team is as diverse as the community members served, and an occupational therapy doctoral student developed a comprehensive Peer Navigator onboarding curriculum based on available research, which continues to be utilized. The Peer Navigator role benefits from uniquely tailored supports for individual skills and barriers to promote effective engagement in the worker role and provider wellness amidst a job distinctly close to the impact of vicarious trauma. Team cohesion and weekly supportive supervisory individual and group meetings, as well as using the occupational therapy skill set to address multifactorial considerations, such as Peer Navigator transportation barriers, technology skill development with documentation and data tracking, job accommodations, and connection to outside supports, are essential.

In almost two decades of engagement in homeless services, seeing center guests thrive and walk in the door with excitement, seeing peers and humanizing staff eager to socialize, shows that the Engagement Center concept is unique and could be a model uniquely designed and replicated to meet any community's needs based on individual PCA findings. Early visitors often describe that they finally found a place where they feel valued, where people care, and that they wish more spaces like this existed in communities. The greatest gift is witnessing community members transition to housing, building supportive connections and bridges along the way. While at a reduced frequency, guests often continue to return to the center to visit their support community, sharing their newfound life accomplishments and genuine encouragement to new guests walking a similar journey. All community members—housed, unhoused, or in precarity—are regularly engaged in reflection of center impact, feedback provision, and co-developing solutions based on formative evaluation, periodically utilizing a World Café event for this purpose. It is important, when designing any community's Engagement Center, that individuals with lived expertise from a variety of backgrounds and diverse identities are at the table to design, implement, and continually evaluate the program to build on the unique community strengths and target capacity building with local assets and priorities.

Conclusion

This chapter described a comprehensive case example of a formative participatory research process that transformed a community organization's programming. Through incorporation of Bridging the Transition Framework community-level strategies, findings informed tailored supports for the community that emerged through a capacity-building process. A PCA can support organizations to develop services specific to their community member-identified priorities. The Engagement Center offers a promising philosophy and program design for communities to implement for combatting historic deficit-oriented systems of care while prioritizing meaningful engagement and capacity building as community members rebuild their lives.

References

Altschuld, J.W. (2015) *Bridging the gap between asset/capacity building and needs assessment*. Las Angeles, CA: SAGE Publications.

Barker, S.L., & Maguire, N. (2017) Experts by experience: Peer support and its use with the homeless. *Community Mental Health Journal*, 53(5), 598–612. https://doi.org/10.1007/s10597-017-0102-2

Brown, J., Isaacs, D., & World Café Community. (2005) *The World Café. Shaping our futures through conversations that matter*. Berrett-Koehler Publishers. https://theworldcafe.com/world-cafe-book/

Godoy-Vieira, A., Soares, C.B., Cordeiro, L., & Campos, C.M.S. (2018) Inclusive and emancipatory approaches to occupational therapy practice in substance-use contexts. *Canadian Journal of Occupational Therapy*, *85*(4), 307–317.

Kretzmann, J., & McKnight, J. (1993) *Building communities from the inside out: A path toward finding and mobilizing a community*. Chicago, IL: ACTA Publications.

Luchenski, S., Maguire, N., Aldridge, R.W., Hayward, A., Story, A., Perri, P., ... & Hewett, N. (2018) What works in inclusion health: overview of effective interventions for marginalised and excluded populations. *The Lancet*, *391*(10117), 266–280.

Ludema, J.D., Cooperrider, D.L., & Barrett, F.J. (2000) Appreciative inquiry: The power of the unconditional positive question. In *Handbook of action research*, edited by P. Reason & H. Bradbury (pp. 189–199). Thousand Oaks, CA: Sage.

Marshall, C.A., Davidson, L., Li, A., Gewurtz, R., Roy, L., Barbic, S., ... & Lysaght, R. (2019) Boredom and meaningful activity in adults experiencing homelessness: A mixed-methods study. *Canadian Journal of Occupational Therapy*, *86*(5), 357–370.

Schensul, J.J., Berg, M.J., & Nair, S. (2013) Using ethnography in participatory community assessment. In *Methods for community-based participatory research for health*, edited by B.A. Israel, E. Eng, A.J. Schulz, & E.A. Parker (2nd Ed.). San Francisco, CA: Jossey-Bass.

Suarez-Balcazar, Y. (2018) Community needs assessment: Bringing real voices to the health care system. In *Patient navigation: Overcoming barriers to care*, edited by E.A. Calhoun, & A. Esparza (pp. 1–26). Chicago, IL: Springer.

Suarez-Balcazar, Y. & Balcazar, F. (2016) Functional analysis of community concerns in participatory action research. In *Handbook of methodological approaches to community-based research: Qualitative, quantitative, and mixed methods*, edited by L.A. Jason & D.S. Glenwick (pp. 314–322). New York: Oxford University Press.

17

APPLYING THE BRIDGING THE TRANSITION FRAMEWORK

Population-Level Approaches

Rebecca Gewurtz and Tom Regehr

Building on the population-level strategies for supporting function and participation in daily life presented in Chapter 8, this chapter explores examples of homelessness prevention and intervention at the population level by addressing structural factors through policy change, research, and advocacy. We highlight three key strategies to guide work at the population level: (1) identifying the problem, (2) building relationships, and (3) articulating a clear message. We then outline how these strategies supported efforts or created challenges in three different examples from our work in Ontario, Canada. These examples provide lessons learned for how to enact positive change at the population level utilizing the Bridging the Transition Framework. By reflecting on these experiences, we highlight the benefits and challenges of population-based work focused on addressing trauma-informed care, poverty prevention, and access to mental health and addiction services.

Component of the Bridging the Transition Framework Addressed in this Chapter

This chapter will focus on describing applications of the Bridging the Transition Framework at a population level. Three examples for supporting homelessness prevention and intervention by addressing structural factors through research and advocacy are presented: (1) the adoption of a trauma-informed approach, (2) a basic income pilot programme, and (3) a policy change at the provincial level to improve access to mental health and addiction services. Through these examples, we promote bold action and new ways of working at the population level.

DOI: 10.4324/9781003541332-20

How this Chapter Guides Practice and Research in Homelessness Prevention

In this chapter, we outline three case examples of population-level approaches to homelessness prevention and intervention through research and advocacy, a policy change, a bottom-up approach grounded in a grassroots vision, and a top-down approach led by the Ministry of Health (MOH) in Ontario, Canada. We build on the frameworks for anchoring discussions about housing precarity and homelessness prevention presented in Chapter 8, namely social determinants of health and mental health (Alegría, NeMoyer, Falgàs Bagué, Wang, & Alvarez, 2018). Health and social care practitioners, researchers, and advocates can draw on these examples to explore solutions that can improve access to housing, mental health and addiction services, health services, and income support for people in their communities, built on principles of trauma-informed care, social justice, and harm reduction. People with lived or living experience of being unhoused or precariously housed, health and social care leaders and practitioners, researchers, and advocates can draw on these approaches to advance solutions and increase the likelihood they are adopted by policymakers. Specifically, we note the need to innovate in this area by taking bold steps to try different solutions and evaluate associated outcomes because existing systems and structures (e.g. the status quo) have not made sufficient improvements in the lives of people who have experienced homelessness and housing precarity despite a range of advocacy efforts. As described in Chapter 8, work at the population level will require a paradigm shift and a social movement that holds policy and programme leaders accountable for their choices.

Introduction

The chapter will present examples of how the Bridging the Transition Framework can be applied at the population level, drawing on examples from policy, advocacy, and research in Ontario, Canada. Throughout, we have identified three key strategies for engaging in work at the population level (see Figure 17.1). Namely: (a) identify the problem, (b) build relationships, and (c) articulate a clear message. In our examples, these strategies will be highlighted as we reflect on what went well as we embarked on our efforts, and what fell short of affecting positive and enduring change to the experience of poverty, homelessness, and housing precarity.

Access to housing and homeless prevention are important social determinants of health (Raphael, Bryant, Mikkonen & Raphael, 2020) that typically revolve around efforts to improve income security and mental health and well-being at the population level (Smith-Carrier & Power, 2025). Our three examples revolve around policy programmes to improve access to and

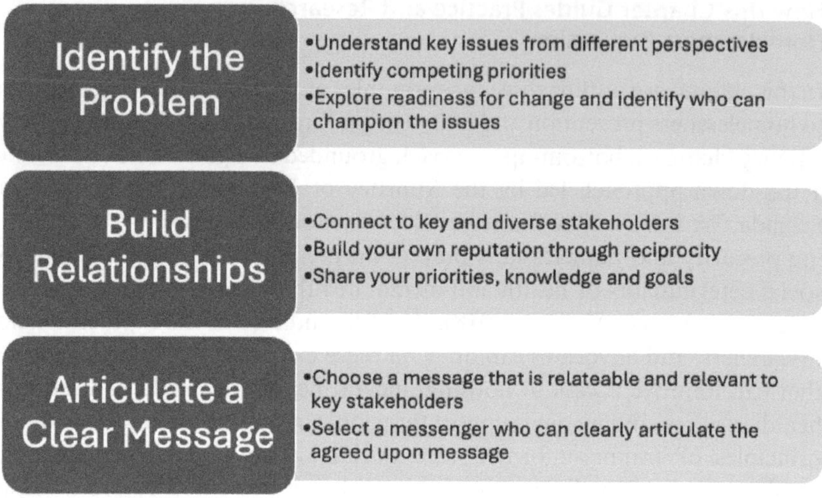

FIGURE 17.1 Case Examples.

delivery of mental health services at the population level, and income security. We begin by describing how a large healthcare institution was able to adopt a trauma-informed approach through grassroots advocacy and awareness building over a nine-year period. We then explore the impact of basic income programmes that have been promoted and trialled in Canada, starting with Ontario's basic income pilot project, which was intended to be rigorously evaluated but was instead cancelled prematurely. Our third example highlights how improved access to mental health, addiction, and other support services was taken up at a provincial level. Through these examples, we describe different entry points and how community partners, people with lived and living experience, and programme and political leaders can work together to take bold action, build positive change, and generate evidence that can be applied across jurisdictions. Although none of these examples specifically highlight efforts to increase affordable housing supply, which is desperately needed across Ontario and other jurisdictions in Canada and internationally (Kneebone & Wilkins, 2021), trauma-informed care, increased income, and better access to mental health and addiction services can improve the circumstances for homelessness prevention by improving tenancy sustainment and affordability (Oudshoorn, Dej, Parsons & Gaetz, 2020). Further, we highlight challenges and lessons learned for affecting enduring change.

Example 1 – Adopting a Trauma-Informed Approach at a Large Healthcare Institution

Experiences of trauma are pervasive among unhoused and precariously housed populations (Hopper, Bassuk & Olivet, 2010; Liu et al., 2021). However, in the early 2000s, trauma was not fully integrated into the vernacular of mental and addiction services (Harris & Fallot, 2001). In fact, at one leading organization in Canada (referred to by "the organization" hereafter), there was a lack of awareness and active resistance to adopting a trauma-informed approach. This example revolves around a nine-year process of gradual change that transformed the organization from being resistant to the idea of trauma as a cause or result of mental illness, addiction, and homelessness, to the adoption of a trauma-informed approach across the organization through grassroots advocacy and awareness building. Although the focus of this change was at the organizational level, this organization became a champion for change that influenced services across the province of Ontario, Canada, impacting access to services for many people who are precariously housed or unhoused.

In our example, Tom Regehr (the second author of this chapter) began his involvement with the organization as a member of the Citizens Advisory Group (CAG) after winning an award to acknowledge his own lived experience of trauma, addiction, homelessness, and recovery. This group consisted of representatives from across the province of Ontario, Canada, with a mandate to learn about the organization and provide input into its priorities, approaches, policies, and programmes. In this position, Tom took time to learn about the committee and its role and function within the larger organization and beyond, including who was listening to its members, who was able to champion change, and who was resistant to change. Tom volunteered for sub-committees and looked for opportunities to interact and engage with the members and leaders in meaningful ways. He focused on connecting everything back to the organization's mandate and priorities.

To raise awareness and acceptance of the role of trauma in the lives of people being served and studied within the organization, members of the committee often explicitly asked about trauma. This led to greater awareness. After a few years, there was a gradual opening and willingness to have trauma and trauma-related issues on the CAG agenda. People became more open and aware of the impact of trauma, and there were more champions related to trauma throughout the mental health, addiction, and housing sectors. Eventually, there was an effort to develop a handbook about becoming "trauma-informed". By this time, other voices in the field were promoting awareness of the role of trauma. Nine years of gradual change led to a trauma education day and a panel discussion about adopting a trauma-informed approach.

The three strategies for a population-level approach (see Figure 17.1) were used in this example. First, a problem was identified. At first, there was little openness to the role of trauma in the work of the organization. Gradually, trauma was clearly identified and recognized, both within and beyond the organization. Importantly, through deep engagement, relationships with the key decision-makers and champions developed. Tom and other members of the committee had opportunities to meet with key leaders within the organization and across the province. There was a collective coalescing around trauma as a priority within and beyond the organization, creating an opening for meaningful population-level change.

This example demonstrates how a clear and relatively simple message about adopting a trauma-informed approach in mental health and addiction services that connected directly to the mission of the organization and broader efforts across an entire region could eventually take hold. In this case, the message resonated with everyone involved, with a focus on improving client outcomes, drawing on research evidence. This message began to gain traction across the province as research and internationally renowned mental health and addiction advocates started pointing to the benefits of adopting this approach. It began to infiltrate all related services, including housing services, homelessness prevention efforts, and services for those who are unhoused (Lee, Kourgiantakis, Lyons, & Prescott-Cornejo, 2021).

The biggest challenge in this example was the slow and gradual process of change. Tom had to sustain the agenda of advancing trauma-informed care for almost a decade. New ideas and change were often resisted and dismissed at first. In reflecting on this experience, the scope of this population-level change was quite remarkable. It involved a large-scale culture change across an organization and a province, with widespread implications for mental health and addiction services. However, the success was due to sustained and collective effort, research, and advocacy coalescing around a consistent message at the population level.

Example 2 – Basic Income

People living with insufficient income to meet their basic needs often become stuck in a cycle of poverty fuelled, in part, by restrictive social assistance policies that can prevent individuals from saving money, limiting their earnings from employment, and thereby creating dependency (David et al., 2024; Smith-Carrier, 2017). This cycle can lead to an increased risk of housing precarity or homelessness, especially when it is occurring in a housing market that is increasingly unaffordable. Therefore, an important component of homelessness prevention includes adequate income (Oudshoorn et al., 2020).

In 2017, the provincial government in Ontario, Canada, did something bold to identify strategies to address the problem of poverty and the ineffectiveness of income support programmes – they announced an effort to innovate in the realm of poverty reduction by launching a basic income pilot project. A definition of basic income is provided in Chapter 8 based on the Consensus Statement on Basic Income Guarantee by the Basic Income Canada Network [BICN] (2023) that focuses on providing an income for everyone that is sufficient to cover basic needs and ensures that no one falls into poverty. The Ontario pilot was to be delivered over three years in three diverse cities across the province and be accompanied by a rigorous evaluation led by a team of researchers (Ferdosi, McDowell, Lewchuk & Ross, 2020; McDowell & Ferdosi, 2020). The central concept was to give people more money than what they would typically receive on income support programmes, with fewer requirements and rules, and study the impact it had on their lives (McDowell & Ferdosi, 2020). Although there was going to be a provincial election within the first year of the pilot project, leaders and advocates of the programme took steps to build relationships through non-partisan support and assurances that the programme would not be cancelled should a new government come into power (Smith-Carrier & Power, 2025).

The June 2018 provincial election brought in a new government that cancelled the pilot project after just over one year, citing affordability concerns (McDowell & Ferdosi, 2020; Smith-Carrier & Power, 2025). The cancellation of the programme and the associated evaluation initiative has prevented us from fully understanding what happens when we give people in poverty more money to pay for basic needs such as housing, food, and health. Some research teams, however, were still able to study the impact of this basic income programme on the lives of recipients. For example, one research team conducted a survey and qualitative interviews with recipients in Hamilton and Brantford (Ferdosi et al., 2020; Halpenny, 2023; McDowell & Ferdosi, 2020). Their findings highlight that recipients of basic income benefited in various ways from the increased income, including improvements in their health, their living standards, and their jobs and earning potential (McDowell & Ferdosi, 2020). Perhaps the most promising finding was that many recipients used the security associated with basic income benefits to further their education and training, in hopes of securing better, more stable employment opportunities in the future (Ferdosi et al., 2020). Many recipients specifically reported how the basic income benefits helped them secure better and more stable housing. Importantly, despite fears prior to the pilot that providing people with sufficient income would discourage them from seeking employment, there was not a massive retraction of labour market participation among participants in the pilot (Ferdosi et al., 2020). Those participants who did leave the labour market largely did so to attend school to increase their earning potential in the future.

This Ontario, Canada, example highlights the importance of building a broad base of support and how important social change requires non-partisan support and attention to articulating the problem and the message. The cancellation of the programme caused widespread chaos and distrust, and left many individuals across the province in unsustainable situations, forced to return to receiving assistance from existing and inadequate income support programmes, and return to accepting less income and more restrictions (McDowell & Ferdosi, 2020). This situation had real consequences for the lives of the recipients, including withdrawing from college programmes they had enrolled in to further their skills and improve their capacity to secure better paying and more secure employment (McDowell & Ferdosi, 2020). Others had to move into housing with lower rent (Ferdosi et al., 2020).

Governments across Canada and beyond have explored options for basic income to further their poverty reduction strategies, including Newfoundland and Labrador, Prince Edward Island (Smith-Carrier, 2023), and Quebec (Ragot, 2024). In addition to the provincial programmes, proposals are being advanced to develop a framework for a national basic income programme by expanding the Canada Workers Benefit (Koebel & Pohler, 2019). A National basic income programme in Canada would contribute to efforts to address the social determinants of health through improved access to adequate food, shelter, and income (Raphael, Bryan, & Mendly-Zambo, 2019).

The concept of basic income is gaining momentum across Canada, although progress is slow, stalled by political challenges, including the framing of poverty as an individual rather than a social problem (Smith-Carrier & On, 2021) and the misconception that basic income and addressing poverty is too expensive (Pereira, 2015; Smith-Carrier & Green, 2017) and would lead to a massive exit from the labour market (Ferdosi et al., 2020; McDowell & Ferdosi, 2020). The collective evidence associated with basic income highlights that additional money is typically used by recipients to create stability – build a foundation for securing better jobs, obtaining better housing for themselves and their family, and taking steps to improve their health and well-being. These findings highlight that basic income is consistent with a population approach to housing outlined in the Bridging the Transition Framework. It can cut across the challenges associated with the existing safety net to establish a standard for living, allowing for health and well-being, the pursuit of meaningful employment, and stable housing. Furthermore, its implementation can maintain the dignity of recipients while providing the security of an adequate income to secure stable and affordable housing.

Example 3 – Access to Mental Health and Addiction Services

This example is related to change within the MOH in Ontario, Canada, through the Minister's Advisory Group (MAG) on mental health and addiction. Housing and homelessness prevention was an indirect focus, given that MAG was formed with an ambitious two-year mandate to fully build and redirect actions around mental health and addictions, working closely with other provincial ministries. Evidence from across Canadian cities highlights this connection, with reported findings that substance use (61%) and mental illness (60%) are the most prevalent health challenges reported by individuals who are unhoused (Quayan, Love, & Hunter, 2024). Furthermore, housing affordability and precarity have been described as mental health issues for many Canadians (Raphael et al., 2020).

MAG met monthly, in person, for two days, with the provincial Minister of Health joining most of the time. The Minister was clear that this work to improve access to mental health and addiction services was a priority for his government and a legacy he wanted to leave behind. The central problem for the committee, however, was complex. Although it was well-accepted that people were having trouble accessing services when and where they needed them, this concern was not the committee's focus. It was one of the key issues the Minister wanted to address, but there were about 30 people involved with MAG, and each person in the group brought their own priorities and goals.

Given the diffused and high-level nature of provincial health policy in Canada, the key message of the committee needed to be nuanced. The Minister was very clear that he wanted transformative change towards improved access to services and ensuring services were available where and when needed. He had a vision that appropriate services and supports could be accessed seamlessly and that people could be steered to the services they needed at any point. To this end, a simple presentation was developed, entitled "One Woman's Story". It followed one woman's journey from childhood to adulthood as she experienced multiple traumas early in her life, from being a student with unmet needs, to interacting with the criminal justice system and becoming unhoused. The presentation highlighted the multiple missed opportunities when she could have been offered trauma-informed mental health services, preventing the complex cascade of events that led to her eventual incarceration and loss of housing. She could have received support in school, at work, or in her community. The Minister of Health started to invite people from the other ministries in Ontario to attend sessions, and everyone involved in this work heard the presentation, leading to a new report to guide the cross-ministerial work on mental health and addiction across the province of Ontario, focused on ensuring access to accessible supports.

There were many challenges associated with this work. The Minister of Health and his staff were supportive of the new approach, but the other interest holders, leaders, and decision-makers within government were not fully committed to the message. Despite efforts to build relationships, the hierarchical structure of government can make it challenging to ensure broad and enduring commitment. This lack of broad commitment became a challenge when new leadership became involved. This example illustrates that ideas and efforts for population change require broad acceptance and commitment for sustainability. This example also illustrates how personal narratives or case examples can help decision-makers understand the key population-level issues by making complex issues relevant and tangible.

Conclusion

Together, these examples highlight that supporting people throughout the cycle of homelessness and establishing secure and stable housing requires innovation at the population level. A population-level approach can focus on policy change or institutional change, driven by forces at the grassroots level or from innovative and progressive leaders who want to do things differently. However, these examples also warn us that sustained change and progress at the population level can be challenging to achieve. A change in government or a leadership change in an institution can reverse course and impede progress. Strategies for engaging in population-level change include identifying a problem, building relationships, and articulating a clear message. Sustained and enduring change requires broad acceptance and commitment to improve service delivery, access, and innovation to address social and population-level challenges and equities.

References

Alegría, M., NeMoyer, A., Falgàs Bagué, I., Wang, Y., & Alvarez, K. (2018) Social determinants of mental health: Where we are and where we need to go. *Current Psychiatry Reports*, 20(11), 95. https://doi.org/10.1007/s11920-018-0969-9

BICN. (2023) *Consensus statement on a basic income guarantee*. https://basicincomecanada.org/wp-content/uploads/2023/03/Consensus-Statement-February-2023.docx.pdf

David, K. M., Martin, B., McDowell, T., Ferdosi, M., Ederer, R., & Ma, A. (2024) "I Was Trusted for Once": Imagining more humane income supports through the Ontario basic income pilot. *Social Policy and Society*, 1–16. doi:10.1017/S1474746424000551

Ferdosi, M., McDowell, T, Lewchuk, W., & Ross, S. (2020) *Southern Ontario's basic income experience*. Hamilton Roundtable for Poverty Reduction, McMaster University Labour Studies & Hamilton Community Foundation. https://macsphere.mcmaster.ca/bitstream/11375/28173/1/southern-ontarios-basic-income-experience.pdf

Halpenny, C. (2023) "We need to take care of each other, and that's what this program was helping to do": Disabled women's experiences of the Ontario Basic Income Pilot. *Canadian Journal of Disability Studies*, *12*(3), 27–58. Retrieved from https://cjds.uwaterloo.ca/index.php/cjds/article/view/1033

Harris, M., & Fallot, R.D. (2001) Envisioning a trauma-informed service system: A vital paradigm shift. *New Directions for Mental Health Services*, 89, 3–22. https://doi.org/10.1002/yd.23320018903

Hopper, E. K., Bassuk, E. L., & Olivet, J. (2010) Shelter from the storm: Trauma-informed care in homelessness services settings. *The Open Health Services and Policy Journal*, *3*(2), 80–100.

Kneebone, R., & Wilkins, M. (2021) Local conditions and the prevalence of homelessness in Canada. *The School of Public Policy Publications*, *14*(28), 1–26. http://dx.doi.org/10.2139/ssrn.4032143

Koebel, K., & Pohler, D. (2019) Expanding the Canada Workers Benefit to design a guarantee basic income. *Canadian Public Policy*, *45*(3), 283–309. https://doi.org/10.3138/cpp.2019-016

Lee, E., Kourgiantakis, T., Lyons, O., & Prescott-Cornejo, A. (2021) A trauma-informed approach in Canadian mental health policies: A systematic mapping review. *Health Policy*, *125*(7), 899–914. https://doi.org/10.1016/j.healthpol.2021.04.008

Liu, M., Luong, L., Lachaud, J., Edalati, H., Reeves, A., & Hwang, S.W. (2021) Adverse childhood experiences and related outcomes among adults experiencing homelessness: A systematic review and meta-analysis. *The Lancet*, *6*(11), e836–e847. https://doi.org/10.1016 S2468-2667(21)00189-4

McDowell, T., & Ferdosi, M. (2020) The experiences of social assistance recipients on the Ontario Basic Income Pilot. *Canadian Review of Sociology/Revue canadienne de sociologie*, *57*, 681–707. https://doi.org/10.1111/cars.12306

Oudshoorn, A., Dej, E., Parsons, C., & Gaetz, S. (2020) Evolving an evidence-based model for homelessness prevention. *Health & Social Care in the Community*, *28*(5), 1754–1763. https://doi.org/10.1111/hsc.13000

Pereira, R. (2015) Universal basic income and the cost objection: What are we waiting for? *World Economic Review*, *5*, 1–21.

Quayan, S., Love, C., & Hunter, P. (2024) Everyone counts 2020–2022 – Results from the third nationally coordinated Point-in-Time counts of homelessness in Canada. *Infrastructure Canada*. https://housing-infrastructure.canada.ca/homelessness-sans-abri/reports-rapports/pit-counts-dp-2020-2022-results-resultats-eng.html

Raphael, D., Bryant, T., & Mendly-Zambo, Z. (2019) Canada considers a basic income guarantee: can it achieve health for all?, *Health Promotion International*, *34*(5), 1025–1031. https://doi.org/10.1093/heapro/day058

Ragot, S. (2024) The new Quebec basic income program: A useful set of policy directions for the Canadian Disability Benefit. *Osgoode Digital Commons*, *61*(2), 513–546. https://doi.org/10.60082/2817-5069.4020

Raphael, D., Bryant, T., Mikkonen, J. and Raphael, A. (2020) *Social Determinants of Health: The Canadian Facts*, 2nd Edition. Ontario Tech University Faculty of Health Sciences and Toronto: York University School of Health Policy and Management.

Smith-Carrier, T. (2023) Implementing a basic income means overcoming myths about the 'underserving poor'. *The Conversation*. https://theconversation.com/implementing-a-basic-income-means-overcoming-myths-about-the-undeserving-poor-218577?utm_source=clipboard&utm_medium=bylinecopy_url_button

Smith-Carrier, T. (2017) Reproducing social conditions of poverty: A critical feminist analysis of social assistance participation in Ontario, Canada. *Journal of Women, Politics & Policy*, *38*(4), 498–521. https://doi.org/10.1080/1554477X.2016.1268874

Smith-Carrier, T., & Green, S. (2017) Another low road to basic income? Mapping a pragmatic model for adopting a basic income in Canada. *Basic Income Studies*, *12*(2). https://doi.org/10.1515/bis-2016-0020

Smith-Carrier, T., & On, J. (2021) Debunking myths about poverty: Social actor representation of the participants of the canceled Ontario Basic Income Pilot Project. *Journal of Poverty*, *26*(6), 500–519. https://doi.org/10.1080/10875549.2021.1957070

Smith-Carrier, T., & Power, E. (2025) Structural violence and the social determinants of mental health: Exploring the experiences of participants on the Ontario Basic Income Pilot in Ontario, Canada. *Health & Social Care in the Community*, *2025*(1), 7816069. https://doi.org/10.1155/hsc/7816069

SECTION 4

Key Social Locations Related to Homelessness Prevention

18

KEY SOCIAL LOCATIONS RELEVANT TO HOMELESSNESS PREVENTION

A Structural and Systems Lens on Preventing Homelessness among Women and Gender-Diverse People in the Global North

Kaitlin Schwan

Research consistently shows that the causes, conditions, and pathways into homelessness for women, girls, and gender-diverse individuals differ significantly from those experienced by men. Gender fundamentally shapes access to safe, affordable housing, making it essential for homelessness prevention efforts by considering the distinct experiences of women and gender-diverse people rather than defaulting to a "gender-neutral" approach. While much of the existing research concentrates on individual or interpersonal causes of homelessness, this chapter shifts the focus to the structural and systemic drivers behind gendered homelessness. By examining these larger structural and system-based factors, the chapter provides researchers and practitioners with recommendations on policies, services, and interventions that challenge the foundational causes of homelessness among women and gender-diverse individuals in the Global North.

How this Chapter Guides Practice and Research in Homelessness Prevention

This chapter provides researchers and practitioners with a comprehensive analysis of effective homelessness prevention strategies for women and gender-diverse individuals, emphasizing the intersections of gender-based violence (GBV), socio-economic inequality, and systemic discrimination. It explores how these interconnected factors increase vulnerability to homelessness and offers evidence-based recommendations for preventive measures. Highlighting the importance of early intervention, targeted support

DOI: 10.4324/9781003541332-22

services, and systemic reforms, the chapter underscores the need for researchers and practitioners to adopt gender-responsive approaches to homelessness prevention.

Introduction

Research consistently demonstrates that the causes, conditions, and pathways into homelessness for women, girls, and gender-diverse individuals differ significantly from those of men (Bretherton, 2017; Savage, 2016). Gender matters—it plays a foundational role in shaping access to safe, affordable housing. Given this, it is vital that homelessness prevention efforts account for the unique realities and experiences of women and gender-diverse people (Mayock & Sheridan, 2012), rather than relying on a "gender-neutral" perspective (Savage, 2016). While much research and discussion on homelessness among women and gender-diverse individuals focuses on individual or interpersonal causes of homelessness (Schwan et al., 2020), with prevention efforts often concentrated in this area, this chapter shifts the focus to the *structural and systemic causes* of gendered homelessness. By doing so, it aims to broaden the framework for thinking about gendered homelessness prevention, and help researchers and practitioners expand the scope of their prevention efforts to address the deeper, underlying factors contributing to housing instability for these populations. To this end, this chapter explores the structural and system-based drivers of homelessness for women and gender-diverse people in the Global North, offering strategies for prevention at each of these levels. By equipping researchers and practitioners with the tools to address these diverse causes, the chapter seeks to support more effective policies, services, and practices that tackle the root causes of gendered homelessness.

Background: Homelessness among Women and Gender-Diverse People

Across the Global North, women, girls, and gender-diverse people face some of the most severe housing challenges and are often the most underserved in the homelessness sector (Pleace, 2016; Schwan et al., 2022). Those most affected include Black and racialized women, Indigenous women, gender-diverse individuals, women with disabilities, low-income women, LGBTQ2S+ people, sex workers, incarcerated women, newcomers, and both younger and older women (Schwan et al., 2021). However, existing estimates of women's homelessness and housing insecurity significantly underrepresent the true scale of the issue, partly because their experiences are often hidden (Pleace, 2016). This invisibility is echoed across Europe, the United States, Canada, and Australia, where women often remain in precarious or abusive housing arrangements due to lack of safe alternatives, making them statistically and politically invisible in homelessness counts (Baptista, 2010; Spinney, 2012). Women are also less likely to use mainstream shelters or other homelessness services—often due to access or safety issues—and instead rely on unstable and sometimes unsafe alternatives, such as staying with acquaintances or remaining in precarious living situations (Bretherton, 2017).

The homelessness sector has historically centered men's experiences, shaping policies and services in ways that overlook women's distinct needs (May, Cloke, & Johnsen, 2007; Van Berkum & Oudshoorn, 2015). This systemic invisibility means the number of unhoused women in Canada is vastly underestimated, leaving many without the support they require (Van Berkum & Oudshoorn, 2015; Pleace, 2016). Many homeless shelters designed for women and families are operating at or above capacity, with family shelter stays having risen significantly in recent years (Segaert, 2017). Similarly, shelters for women experiencing violence are also struggling with high occupancy rates in nearly every community, offering primarily short-term stays for women fleeing abuse, typically under three months (Statistics Canada, 2019b). According to the latest national data, 78% of shelters for women experiencing violence across Canada are short-term, with 428 out of 552 shelters providing temporary accommodations. One of the primary challenges women face when leaving abusive situations is the lack of affordable, long-term housing options (Statistics Canada, 2019b). Many existing systems are also failing to help women and girls transition out of homelessness, frequently leaving them trapped in cycles of violence, instability, and marginalization (Vecchio, 2019).

Despite these realities, housing policies rarely prioritize the unique challenges women and gender-diverse people face, leading to a critical shortage of women-centered, trauma-informed housing options (Nelson et al., 2023). In the absence of stable, safe, and affordable housing, women are often left to navigate emergency systems that are underfunded, overwhelmed, and unable to meet their needs (Baig et al., 2023). As a result, many women experiencing violence and extreme marginalization are turned away, highlighting the urgent need for housing solutions that address their specific circumstances (Vecchio, 2019).

Causes and Conditions of Homelessness for Women and Gender-Diverse People

To understand the gender-specific causes of homelessness, it's essential to examine both structural drivers and failures within public systems. The structural causes include socio-economic inequalities, such as poverty and GBV, which disproportionately affect women and contribute to housing instability. At the same time, systemic failures within public services—such as child welfare or the criminal justice system—further exacerbate these challenges, creating additional barriers to securing and maintaining stable housing.

Structural Causes of Gendered Homelessness

Across the literature, three primary structural causes of gendered homelessness emerge: (1) poverty and economic inequality, (2) GBV, and (3) gender-based discrimination in the housing market.

One of the primary structural drivers of gendered homelessness is pervasive poverty and economic inequality. Women often experience chronic housing affordability issues linked to low incomes, precarious employment, and the insufficiency of social assistance (Canadian Women's Foundation, 2022; Moyser & Burlock, 2018; Tunstall et al., 2013; Wolch & Dear, 1993). Women are more likely to be in non-permanent employment, receive lower wages than men, and pay higher rates for rental housing on average (Schwan et al., 2023a). In the Canadian context, research shows that racialized women earn significantly less than non-racialized men, highlighting the intersectional nature of economic disparity (Block, Galabuzi, & Tranjan, 2019).

The feminization of poverty makes it difficult for many women and women-led families to afford rent and basic necessities, trapping them in cycles of violence, housing precarity, and food insecurity (Schwan et al., 2023b). For example, in Canada, 28% of women-led, lone-parent family households are in core housing need, almost double the rate of male-led, lone-parent households (16%) (Canada Mortgage and Housing Corporation, 2019). Furthermore, 57% of renter households in core housing need are female-led families or singles (Pomeroy, 2021). The disproportionate burden of caregiving for children and other family members (Houle, Turcotte, & Wendt, 2017) also significantly impacts women's economic stability and ability to secure and maintain housing (Tunstall et al., 2013; Van Berkum & Oudshoorn, 2015; Vecchio, 2019). These dynamics are echoed globally. In the United Kingdom, austerity-driven cuts to social housing and benefits have disproportionately impacted single mothers and racialized women, contributing to sharp increases in hidden homelessness and housing precarity (Tunstall, Bevan, Bradshaw, Croucher, Duffy, Hunter, Jones, Rugg, Wallace, & Wilcox, 2013). In the United States, Black women face higher eviction rates due to intersecting structural disadvantages in income, race, and caregiving status (Desmond, 2016).

Poverty and socio-economic inequality are especially powerful structural drivers of women's homelessness in the context of the financialization of housing, which positions housing as commodity rather at the expense of its social function as a secure and dignified place to live (Farha et al., 2022). This process leads to rising housing prices and rental costs, which disproportionately affect women due to their existing economic disadvantages, including lower wages, precarious employment, and greater caregiving responsibilities that limit their earning potential (Schwan et al., 2021; Zell & McCullough, 2020). Consequently, financialization contributes to a loss of naturally occurring affordable housing (Farha et al., 2022), making it increasingly difficult for low-income women and women-led households, who are already overrepresented in core housing need (Statistics Canada, 2019a), to secure and maintain stable housing. Furthermore, the focus on profit generation can incentivize evictions, pushing marginalized women into homelessness or more precarious living situations, and can even exacerbate conditions leading to exploitative "sex-for-rent" or "labour-for-housing" arrangements as affordable options diminish (Schwan et al., 2023a). In essence, the financialization of housing intensifies the existing socio-economic vulnerabilities faced by women, making them more susceptible to housing instability and homelessness within a market driven by profit rather than human rights.

GBV is not merely an interpersonal issue but a profound structural cause of homelessness for women, deeply embedded in societal inequalities and systemic failures (Baig et al., 2023). The lack of safe and affordable housing itself acts as a structural barrier that can trap women in abusive situations or cause them to return to violence, as the fear of homelessness and the dangers associated with it often outweigh the risks of staying with an abuser (Watson, 2016). The inadequacy of emergency shelters and supports, with many violence against women (VAW) shelters being short-term, underfunded, and frequently operating at capacity, means that women escaping violence often have nowhere safe to go, pushing them into homelessness or back to their abusers (Schwan et al., 2021; Statistics Canada, 2019a; Vecchio, 2019). Even within the homelessness sector, co-ed shelters can be unsafe for women due to the risk of further violence (Bretherton, 2017; National Inquiry into Missing and Murdered Indigenous Women, 2019; Schwan et al., 2021). Globally, GBV is a leading cause of homelessness among women, with studies in Australia, South Africa, and the United States demonstrating that inadequate housing systems force survivors to choose between abuse and homelessness (Spinney, 2012; Baker et al., 2010). The fact that women who lose their homes due to male violence are sometimes categorized solely as "victims of domestic violence" rather than "homeless women" highlights a systemic failure to recognize the direct link between GBV and homelessness, hindering the development of comprehensive solutions (Tutty, 2015). In this way, GBV acts as a structural cause of homelessness by interacting with and being perpetuated by inadequacies and inequities within housing, social services, and societal attitudes toward gender and violence.

Gender-based discrimination in housing is also a significant structural driver of homelessness for women, manifesting in various forms throughout the housing system (Baig et al., 2023). Women, particularly those from equity-seeking groups such as Indigenous and racialized women, report experiencing significant levels of discrimination from landlords and property managers, including refusal to rent, illegal rent increases, and harassment, sometimes leading directly to housing loss or creating barriers to accessing new housing (Martin & Walia, 2019; Schwan et al., 2021). This discrimination can be based on gender alone or intersect with other factors like family status (single mothers), receipt of financial assistance, or race (Baker et al., 2010; Vecchio, 2019). Furthermore, women's housing security is often dependent on maintaining relationships, as breakups, sometimes due to violence or economic instability, are a primary reason for housing loss (Schwan et al., 2021). Even when experiencing intimate partner violence, women may face eviction due to landlord bias or zero-tolerance policies related to disturbances, effectively punishing survivors for the violence they endure (Buhler & Tang, 2019). In some egregious cases, landlords may even exploit women's vulnerability by demanding sexual favors in exchange for not evicting them (Martin & Walia, 2019). The fact that many women struggle to access legal advice and support when facing eviction further exacerbates the issue, leaving them with limited means to challenge discriminatory or unfair eviction processes (Schwan et al., 2021).

Public System Failures

Public systems in countries across the Global North, often designed with a facade of neutrality, are deeply implicated in perpetuating and exacerbating housing instability for marginalized women, girls, and gender-diverse people (Maki, 2017; Moffet-Bourassa, & F.-Dufour, 2024). In the Canadian context, for example, the Federal Housing Advocate has identified gendered homelessness as a pressing human rights issue in Canada due to the government's failure to eliminate homelessness among women and gender-diverse people (Office of the Federal Housing Advocate, 2023), demonstrating the systemic and longstanding nature of these issues.

One critical area is the child welfare system. In the United States, research has shown that former foster youth, especially young women and LGBTQ+ individuals, face elevated risks of homelessness due to systemic failures in transitional planning and support (Dworsky et al., 2013). Likewise, women exiting incarceration in Australia and the United Kingdom experience similar challenges in accessing safe housing, compounding their risk of recidivism (Baldry et al., 2006; Loucks, 2007). In the Canadian context, studies indicate that almost 60% of youth experiencing homelessness were involved with the child welfare system at some point in their lives, making them 193 times more likely to report such involvement than youth in the general population (Nichols et al., 2017). For mothers, child apprehension is often an event that contributes to and precipitates housing instability and homelessness (Van Berkum & Oudshoorn, 2015). The fear of child apprehension due to mandatory reporting policies in some VAW or homelessness services may also deter women with children from accessing these supports (Maki, 2017; Martin & Walia, 2019). These policies and practices can exacerbate child-parent separation and contribute to intergenerational homelessness (Gaetz et al., 2016; Schwan et al., 2020).

The criminal justice system also plays a significant role. Research indicates a bidirectional relationship between criminal justice involvement and homelessness for women and gender-diverse people (Schwan et al., 2020), where engagement with the justice system can increase housing instability, and housing precarity can result in greater encounters with law enforcement. In the Canadian context, a third of gender-diverse people (33%) report that the criminal justice system contributed to their housing instability and homelessness, and 56% have had encounters with law enforcement (Schwan et al., 2021). Women interacting with the criminal justice system often carry histories of trauma, including intimate partner or family violence, which are major drivers of homelessness (Martin & Walia, 2019). The lack of housing support services and discharge planning in correctional facilities exacerbates the issue, leaving women released without adequate housing options. Due to extreme poverty or exclusion from services, many women and gender-diverse individuals may resort to survival activities that are criminalized, further complicating their ability to escape homelessness (Henchuk & Bopp, 2007). Indigenous women are particularly impacted, facing disproportionately harsh sentences and limited access to reintegration support, perpetuating a cycle of incarceration and homelessness, with barriers to stable housing due to criminal records (Martin & Walia, 2019).

Even within the homelessness and VAW sectors, policies and practices can inadvertently create housing precarity or deepen exclusion. Shelter policies related to substance use, pets, and adult children can be discriminatory. The prioritization of chronic homelessness, often interpreted as chronically homeless emergency shelter users (where women and gender-diverse people are underrepresented), can inadvertently exclude many women experiencing situational vulnerability from accessing Homelessness Partnering Strategy funding (Baig et al., 2023; Schwan et al., 2020). Moreover, there is a lack of equitable investment in emergency homeless shelters and shelter beds for women across the country, with the majority of beds being designated for men or co-ed, which many women and gender-diverse people avoid due to safety concerns (Schwan et al., 2020). Accessibility is also a concern, with a Disabled Women's Network of Canada study reporting that only 75% of homeless shelters have a wheelchair accessible entrance, and even fewer offer other accessibility features like sign language or braille (Alimi, Singh, & Brayton, 2018).

Preventing Homelessness among Women and Gender-Diverse People: A Structural and Systems Approach

The prevention of homelessness among women and gender-diverse individuals demands a structural and systems-based approach that addresses the root causes of housing instability. In this context, it is essential to address the intersection of gender, poverty, systemic barriers, and inadequate policies that disproportionately impact these groups. While there is significant need for individual-level interventions, the real challenge lies in shifting the broader policy landscape to ensure equitable access to housing, income support, and public systems. This requires comprehensive changes that prioritize the dignity and rights of women and gender-diverse people, especially those facing compounded forms of discrimination.

Among many other changes needed, the following are some places to start for structural and system change that researchers and practitioners can focus on to advocate for and create real impact.

Priority Action 1: Addressing Gendered Poverty

To tackle gendered poverty effectively, the federal government must significantly increase investment in income support programs and undertake a rights-based gender equity analysis to eliminate access barriers. This means adjusting income support rates to reflect the true cost of living, particularly for women and gender-diverse individuals who experience disproportionate poverty. Such interventions can draw on innovation in Nordic countries—like Sweden, Norway, and Denmark—which, through integrated universal welfare models, labor-market and childcare policies supportive of women, and housing-led approaches, show lower overall homelessness rates, including among women (Benjaminsen & Dyb, 2008; Benjaminsen & Andrade, 2015).

Researchers Can:

- Focus on gathering intersectional and disaggregated data on poverty, exploring how overlapping forms of discrimination create unique economic barriers for diverse groups of women and gender-diverse individuals.
- Investigate the root causes of gendered poverty, assessing how different income support models perform in alleviating housing instability and economic insecurity.

Practitioners Can:

- Advocate for higher income support rates and greater accessibility to social assistance programs across all levels of government.

- Support women and gender-diverse individuals in navigating the often-complex income support systems, offering both direct assistance and advocacy to remove systemic barriers.
- Track and document how inadequate income levels lead to housing insecurity and hidden homelessness, providing essential evidence to drive policy changes.

Priority Action 2: Transforming Public Systems

Federal, regional, and municipal governments must undertake comprehensive reforms of public systems, including child welfare, criminal justice, healthcare, and the VAW sector, to ensure these systems uphold the right to housing and do not create pathways into homelessness for women and gender-diverse people. This includes cross-departmental collaboration and the development of integrated service delivery frameworks. Models of cross-sector collaboration in Finland's Housing First framework offer insights into how gender-sensitive system transformation can reduce housing instability for women (Pleace et al., 2016).

Researchers Can:

- Conduct rights-based inquiries and Gender-Based Analysis Plus audits to identify systemic failures and discriminatory practices within public systems that contribute to housing instability.
- Investigate the intersections between individuals' experiences in public systems and their housing outcomes to pinpoint critical intervention points.
- Evaluate the effectiveness of trauma-informed and harm reduction approaches within these systems to understand how they can prevent homelessness.

Practitioners Can:

- Implement trauma-informed, violence-informed, and harm reduction approaches in service delivery, recognizing the high rates of trauma and violence experienced by women and gender-diverse individuals facing housing insecurity.
- Foster collaboration across different sectors to enhance service coordination.
- Advocate for policy changes that prioritize housing stability, ensuring that public systems do not perpetuate housing precarity.

Priority Action 3: Curb the Financialization of Housing and Prevent Evictions

The federal government, alongside lower levels of government, must actively intervene to regulate the financialization of housing, including measures to curb excessive rent increases, regulate financial actors like Real Estate Investment Trusts, and strengthen tenant protection laws across all provinces and territories. Adopting national standards for residential tenancies is also crucial. Inspiration can be drawn from innovation around the globe, including Germany, where rent control and tenant protections have curbed some of the harmful effects of financialization, offering useful models for resisting market-driven housing precarity (Kohl, 2017).
Researchers Can:

- Investigate the gendered impacts of housing financialization on affordability, security of tenure, and the prevalence of hidden homelessness for women and gender-diverse people.
- Study the effectiveness of eviction prevention strategies and analyze housing policies to identify discriminatory aspects, providing a basis for equitable reforms.

Practitioners Can:

- Provide direct support to women and gender-diverse individuals facing eviction, assisting with legal processes and connecting them to resources.
- Document housing precarity and advocate for eviction prevention policies that prioritize financial assistance and stronger tenant protections, aiming to prevent homelessness.

Priority Action 4: Invest in Affordable Housing That Is Equitably Accessible for Women and Gender-Diverse People

The federal government must make significant and sustained investments in a diverse range of deeply affordable housing options, including social housing, non-profit housing, and supportive housing, that are safe, accessible, and meet the specific and intersectional needs of women and gender-diverse people. This requires redesigning capital programs to substantially increase access for women-led and women-focused organizations. Australia's Common Ground and women-led housing initiatives in Vienna offer promising examples of how inclusive housing design can address gender-specific safety and accessibility needs (Flatau et al., 2008; Tsenkova, 2009).

Researchers Can:

- Conduct participatory research with diverse women and gender-diverse people to identify their specific housing needs and barriers to accessing safe and affordable housing.
- Evaluate the accessibility and inclusivity of existing affordable housing programs to ensure equitable access for these populations.
- Develop innovative, gender-sensitive housing models to meet the diverse needs of women and gender-diverse individuals.

Practitioners Can:

- Advocate for sustained investment in affordable housing options and collaborate with lived experts to ensure that housing environments are gender-affirming, non-discriminatory, and trauma-informed.
- Support women-led and women-focused housing providers to build their capacity to develop and manage affordable housing projects, ensuring they meet the specific needs of these communities.

Conclusion

Addressing homelessness among women and gender-diverse individuals requires a comprehensive, structural, and systems-based approach that goes beyond individual interventions. The unique challenges faced by these groups are shaped by deep-rooted socio-economic inequalities, GBV, and systemic failures within public systems. By focusing on the intersections of these issues, we can begin to dismantle the barriers that contribute to gender-based housing instability.

References

Alimi, S., Singh, S. & Brayton, B. (2018) Parliamentary brief: A brief prepared for the Standing Committee on the Status of Women in Canada (FEWO) for their study of the system of shelters and transition houses in Canada.

Baker, C. K., Billhardt, K. A., Warren, J., Rollins, C., & Glass, N. E. (2010) Domestic violence, housing instability, and homelessness: A review of housing policies and program practices for meeting the needs of survivors. *Aggression and Violent Behavior*, 15(6), pp. 430–439.

Baig, K., Schwan, K., … Bayes, S. (2023) *An intersectional feminist housing agenda for Canada – A briefing guide for Canada's Housing Minister*. Toronto, ON: Women's National Housing & Homelessness Network.

Baldry, E., McDonnell, D., Maplestone, P. & Peeters, M. (2006) Ex-prisoners, homelessness and the state in Australia. *The Australian and New Zealand Journal of Criminology*, 39(1), pp. 20–33.

Baptista, I. (2010) *Women and homelessness*. European Observatory on Homelessness, FEANTSA.

Benjaminsen, L., & Dyb, E. (2008) The effectiveness of homeless policies – Variations among the Scandinavian countries. *European Journal of Homelessness*, 2, pp. 45–70.

Benjaminsen, L., & Andrade, S. B. (2015) Testing a typology of homelessness across welfare regimes: Shelter use in Denmark and the USA. *Housing Studies*, 30(6), pp. 858–876

Block, S., Galabuzi, G.E. & Tranjan, R. (2019) *Canada's colour coded income inequality* (Report No. 978-1-77125-478-6). Canadian Centre for Policy Alternatives.

Bretherton, J. (2017) Reconsidering gender in homelessness. *European Journal of Homelessness*, 11(1), pp. 1–21.

Buhler, S., & Tang, R. (2019) Navigating power and claiming justice: Tenant experiences at Saskatchewan's Housing Law Tribunal. *Windsor Yearbook of Access to Justice*, 36, pp. 210–230.

Canada Mortgage and Housing Corporation (2019) *Core housing need data — By the numbers*. CMHC – SCHL.

Canadian Women's Foundation (2022) *Fact sheet: Women and poverty in Canada*. Ottawa, ON: CWF.

Desmond, M. (2016) *Evicted: Poverty and profit in the American city*. New York: Crown Publishing Group.

Dworsky, A., Napolitano, L. & Courtney, M. (2013) Homelessness during the transition from foster care to adulthood. *American Journal of Public Health*, 103(S2), pp. S318–S323.

Farha, L., Freeman, S., Gabarre de Sus, M., Perucca, J. & McMurty, A. (2022) *The shift directives – From financialized to human rights-based housing*. Ottawa, ON: The Shift.

Flatau, P., Conroy, E., Spooner, C., Edwards, R., Eardley, T. & Forbes, C. (2008) *Effective housing support for the homeless: Evidence for practice*. Australian Housing and Urban Research Institute, AHURI Final Report No. 119.

Gaetz, S., Dej, E., Richter, T. & Redman, M. (2016) *The state of homelessness in Canada 2016*. Toronto: The Canadian Observatory on Homelessness Press.

Henchuk, C. & Bopp, J. (2007) *A little kindness would go a long way in a study of women's homelessness in the Yukon*. Yukon Status of Women Council.

Houle, P., Turcotte, M. & Wendt, M. (2017) Changes in parents' participation in domestic tasks and care for children from 1986 to 2015. *Spotlight on Canadians: Results from the General Social Survey*, Statistics Canada Catalogue no. 89-652-X2017001.

Kohl, S. (2017) The power of institutional legacies: How nineteenth-century housing associations shaped twentieth-century housing regimes in Germany and the United States. *European Journal of Sociology*, *58*(2), pp. 271–306.

Loucks, N. (2007) *No one knows: Offenders with learning difficulties and learning disabilities – The prevalence and associated needs of offenders with learning difficulties and learning disabilities*. London: Prison Reform Trust.

Maki, K. (2017) *Housing, homelessness, and violence against women: A discussion paper*. Women's Shelters Canada.

Martin, C.M. & Walia, H. (2019) *Red women rising: Indigenous women survivors in Vancouver's downtown eastside*. Downtown Eastside Women's Centre.

May, J., Cloke, P. & Johnsen, S. (2007) Alternative cartographies of homelessness: Rendering visible British women's experiences of "visible" homelessness. *Gender, Place & Culture*, 14(2), pp. 121–140.

Mayock, P., & Sheridan, S. (2012) Women's homelessness and domestic violence: (Re)assessing the evidence. *European Journal of Homelessness*, 6(2), pp. 75–99.

Moffet-Bourassa, M., & F.-Dufour, I. (2024) Women's homelessness and the justice system: A study of desistance and social (re) integration among Canadian women who used or did not use criminal activities to survive. *Criminal Justice and Behavior*, 51(9), pp. 1433–1449.
Moyser, M. & Burlock, A. (2018) *Time use: total work burden, unpaid work, and leisure*. Statistics Canada.
National Inquiry into Missing and Murdered Indigenous Women and Girls (NIMMIWG) (2019) *Reclaiming power and place: The final report of the National Inquiry into Missing and Murdered Indigenous Women and Girls*. Vol. 1a.
Nelson, A., Malenfant, J., Schwan, K. & Watchorn, M. (2023) *Literature review & practice scan – Housing need & homelessness amongst gender-diverse people in Canada*. Toronto, ON: Women's National Housing & Homelessness Network.
Nichols, N., Schwan, K., Gaetz, S., Redman, M., French, D., Kidd, S. & O'Grady, B. (2017) *Child welfare and youth homelessness in Canada: A proposal for action*.
Office of the Federal Housing Advocate (2023) *Federal housing advocate requests review into the failure to eliminate homelessness amongst women and gender-diverse people*. Ottawa, ON: Canadian Human Rights Commission.
Pleace, N. (2016) Exclusion by definition: The under-representation of women in European homelessness statistics. In *Women's homelessness in Europe*, edited by P. Mayock & J. Bretherton, pp. 105–126. London: Palgrave Macmillan.
Pleace, N., Culhane, D., Granfelt, R. & Knutagård, M. (2016) *The Finnish homelessness strategy: An international review*. Helsinki: Ministry of the Environment.
Pomeroy, S. (2021) *Toward evidence-based policy: Assessing the CMHC rental housing finance initiative (RCFI)*. Ottawa, ON: Carleton University, Centre for Urban Research and Education.
Savage, M. (2016) Gendering women's homelessness. *Irish Journal of Applied Social Studies*, 16(2), pp. 43–64.
Schwan, K., Baig, K., Smyth, E., Nelson, A. & Biss, M. (2023a) *Submission to the National Housing Council's Review Panel on the Role of Corporate Investment in Housing – Gendered evictions in financialized housing markets across Canada*. Ottawa, ON: National Right to Housing Network.
Schwan, K., Baig, K., Smyth, E., Nelson, A., Biss, M. & Raza, M. (2023b) *Submission to the Standing Committee on human resources, skills, and social development and the status of persons with disabilities (HUMA) review of financialization*. Ottawa, ON: National Right to Housing Network.
Schwan, K., Nelson, A., Marks, H., Dej, E. et al. (2022) *The crisis ends with us: Request for a review into the systemic denial of the equal right to housing of women and gender-diverse people in Canada*. Toronto, ON: Women's National Housing & Homelessness Network.
Schwan, K., Vaccaro, M., Reid, L. & Ali, N. (2021) *Implementation of the right to housing for women, girls, and gender diverse people*. Prepared for the Canadian Human Rights Commission. Toronto, ON: Women's National Housing & Homelessness Network.
Schwan, K., Versteegh, A., Perri, M., Caplan, R., Baig, K., Dej, E., Jenkinson, J., Brais, H., Eiboff, F. & Pahlevan Chaleshtari, T. (2020) *The state of women's housing need & homelessness in Canada: Literature review*, edited by A. Hache, A. Nelson, E. Kratochvil & J. Malenfant. Toronto, ON: Canadian Observatory on Homelessness Press.
Segaert, A. (2017) *The national shelter study: Emergency shelter use in Canada 2005–2014*. Homelessness Partnering Secretariat, Employment and Social Development Canada.

Spinney, A. (2012) *Home and safe? Policy and practice innovations to prevent women and children who have experienced domestic and family violence from becoming homeless.* Australian Housing and Urban Research Institute.

Statistics Canada. (2019a) *First results from the Canadian Housing Survey, 2018.* Ottawa: Statistics Canada Catalogue.

Statistics Canada. (2019b) *Canadian residential facilities for victims of abuse, 2017/2018.* Ottawa: Statistics Canada Catalogue.

Tsenkova, S. (2009) *Housing policy reforms in post-socialist Europe: Lost in transition.* Heidelberg: Physica-Verlag.

Tunstall, R., Bevan, M., Bradshaw, J., Croucher, K., Duffy, S., Hunter, C., Jones, A., Rugg, J., Wallace, A. & Wilcox, S. (2013) *The links between housing and poverty: An evidence review.* York: Joseph Rowntree Foundation.

Tutty, L. (2015) Addressing the safety and trauma issues of abused women: A cross-Canada study of YWCA shelters. *Journal of International Women's Studies*, 16(3), pp. 101–116.

Van Berkum, A. & Oudshoorn, A. (2015) *Best practice guidelines for ending women's and girls' homelessness.* Ottawa, ON: Homelessness Partnering Strategy.

Vecchio, K. (2019) *Surviving abuse and building resilience – A study of Canada's systems of shelters and transition houses serving women and children affected by violence.* Report of the Standing Committee on the Status of Women.

Watson, J. (2016) Gender-based violence and young homeless women: Femininity, embodiment and vicarious physical capital. *The Sociological Review*, 64(2), pp. 256–273.

Wolch, J.R. & Dear, M. J. (1993) *Malign neglect: Homelessness in an American city.* San Francisco, CA: Jossey-Bass.

Zell, S. & McCullough, S. (2020) *Housing research report: Evictions and eviction prevention in Canada.* Ottawa, ON: Canada Mortgage and Housing Corporation.

19

KEY SOCIAL LOCATIONS RELEVANT TO HOMELESSNESS PREVENTION

Homelessness among 2SLGBTQIA+ Persons

John Ecker

2SLGBTQIA+ (Two-Spirit, Lesbian, Gay, Bisexual, Transgender, Queer or Questioning, Intersex, Asexual, and additional gender identities and sexual orientations) people who experience homelessness have unique needs and thus require tailored responses. This chapter reviews what is known about 2SLGBTQIA+ homelessness across the lifespan and identifies potential strategies for homelessness prevention. To understand the scope of the issue, this chapter begins with discussing the prevalence and measurement of 2SLGBTQIA+ homelessness. The chapter then focuses on the unique pathways into homelessness, service use experiences, and exits out of homelessness for 2SLGBTQIA+ people across the lifespan. It concludes with a review of the housing and support needs of 2SLGBTQIA+ people. Within each section, homelessness prevention considerations are identified. The chapter demonstrates that to universally prevent homelessness from occurring or re-occurring, the unique needs of 2SLGBTQIA+ individuals must be acknowledged and addressed.

How this Chapter Guides Practice and Research in Homelessness Prevention

This chapter provides an overview of considerations for homelessness prevention specifically among 2SLGBTQIA+ persons. 2SLGBTQIA+ persons are identified as a group that would benefit from selected prevention efforts, as discrimination is a driver of their homelessness (Gaetz & Dej, 2017). Despite calls to have targeted prevention efforts, there has been little focus

DOI: 10.4324/9781003541332-23

on what 2SLGBTQIA+ homelessness prevention could look like at a policy and programme level. One previous review by Abramovich (2016) identifies what this could look like for 2SLGBQIA+ youth, but there has yet to be a similar review for 2SLGBTQIA+ adults and older adults. This chapter takes a lifespan approach on the issue and reviews the literature base on homelessness among 2SLGBTQIA+ youth to older adults. It identifies practical strategies and considerations that policy makers, programme developers, programme operators, and researchers can take to address prevention efforts for 2SLGBTQIA+ individuals.

This chapter particularly aligns with the sixth guiding principle of the Bridging the Transition Framework – Intersectionality (Marshall et al., 2023). It also recognizes the importance of relationships, both professional and peer, as vital to exiting homelessness. Furthermore, the chapter addresses the four processes of leaving homelessness, with a particular emphasis on survival and adaptation strategies 2SLGBTQIA+ people use when experiencing and exiting homelessness.

Introduction

Homelessness among 2SLGBTQIA+ people has gained more attention in the research literature. It is well substantiated that 2SLGBTQIA+ youth disproportionately experience homelessness compared to non-2SLGBTQIA+ youth and that they have unique pathways into homelessness (Abramovich, 2012; Ecker, 2016). Recent research has shed light on the experiences of homelessness among 2SLGBTQIA+ people across the lifespan (e.g., Ecker, Aubry, & Sylvestre, 2019; Fraser, Chisholm, & Pierse, 2021).

Despite this growing body of evidence, many global homelessness strategies, including Canada's strategy entitled "Reaching Home", do not mention 2SLGBTQIA+ individuals within its policy directives (Infrastructure Canada, 2024). In order to truly prevent homelessness, tailored measures must be co-developed that address the interplay of structural, systemic, and individuals and relational factors that cause homelessness (Gaetz, Donaldson, Richter, & Gulliver, 2013). In the case of 2SLGBTQIA+ people, this means acknowledging the impact of homophobia, biphobia, and transphobia on entries into homelessness, experiences while homeless, and exits out of homelessness.

This chapter begins by providing an overview of the prevalence and measurement of homelessness among 2SLGBTQIA+ persons. It then reviews pathways into homelessness, service use experiences, and exits out of homelessness among 2SLGBTQIA+ persons across the lifespan, along with outcomes and descriptions of housing programmes for 2SLGBTQIA+ individuals. Within each section, policy recommendations focused on the prevention of 2SLGBTQIA+ homelessness are discussed.

Prevalence and Measurement

Estimates of homelessness are largely based on annual emergency shelter usage and the enumeration of homelessness on a single night [i.e., Point-in-Time (PiT) counts]. Both of these counts include a measurement of gender that extends beyond the gender binary (e.g., cisgender man, cisgender woman, transgender man, transgender woman, non-binary); however, PiT counts are often the only enumeration effort that inquires about a person's gender identity and sexual orientation. It is important to have questions on gender identity and sexual orientation because it provides an indication of the scale of the population in the country and locally within each municipality. This data can then build the case for targeted funding and policy development (Abramovich, 2016).

PiT counts are mandated in Canada and the United States. In the United States, participants are asked questions about their gender identity, but not their sexual orientation. Since 2018, Reaching Home has included mandatory PiT count survey questions on gender identity and sexual orientation (Infrastructure Canada, 2024). Both questions have expansive response options. Gender options are: man, woman, Two-Spirit, trans woman, trans man, non-binary (genderqueer), not listed (specify), don't know, and decline to answer. Sexual orientation options are: straight/heterosexual, gay, lesbian, bisexual, Two-Spirit, pansexual, asexual, queer, questioning, not listed (specify), don't know, and decline to answer. Even though these questions are mandatory, participants do have the option to decline to respond.

Results from the United States show that approximately 1 percent of respondents identified as non-binary, questioning, transgender, more than one gender, a culturally specific identity (e.g., Two-Spirit), or reported a different identity (US Department of Housing and Urban Development, 2025). Results from Canada's most recent PiT count show that 13 percent of all respondents identified as 2SLGBTQIA+ (Infrastructure Canada, 2024). The report notes that this is in comparison to 4 percent of the general population in Canada identifying as 2SLGBTQIA+. Of 2SLGBTQIA+ respondents, the majority identified as bisexual (46 percent), with 12 percent identifying as gay and 9 percent identifying as pansexual (Infrastructure Canada, 2024). Age breakdowns were also presented. Twenty-six percent of youth (ages 13–24) identified as 2SLGBTQIA+. The proportion decreased with age, as 13 percent of adults (ages 25–49), 7 percent of older adults (ages 50–64), and 6 percent of seniors (ages 65 and older) identified as 2SLGBTQIA+. These results provide evidence that 2SLGBTQIA+ people, particularly youth, are disproportionately impacted by homelessness.

Although these descriptive statistics from PiT counts are important to have, they may be underestimations. PiT counts are limited by the reliance on self-report data. 2SLGBTQIA+ individuals may not feel comfortable disclosing their gender identity and/or sexual orientation with PiT count surveyors (Abramovich, 2019). PiT count respondents may also be in different stages in the development of their gender identity and/or sexual orientation and be hesitant to disclose due to feelings of stigmatization (Savin-Williams & Ream, 2007). Further, hidden homelessness [i.e., those who are at risk homelessness, temporarily staying with family and friends; (Gaetz et al., 2013)] is often not accurately assessed within PiT counts. This is particularly salient among 2SLGBTQIA+ individuals, as some may not feel comfortable accessing emergency shelters due to fears of discrimination, harassment, and violence (Ecker et al., 2019).

On the research side, data on gender identity and sexual orientation within studies focused on homelessness is variable. Reviews of the literature on 2SLGBTQIA+ youth and adult homelessness found that there is not standardized approach on how data on gender identity and sexual orientation are collected (Ecker, 2016; Ecker et al., 2019). There are also inconsistencies with how data are analysed. For example, transgender participants may not be separated out from 2SLGBTQIA+ participants (Abramovich, 2019). This variance in measurement and analysis can lead to inaccurate conclusions on the needs of 2SLGBTQIA+ individuals. There has also been a lack of focus on the intersecting identities of 2SLGBTQIA+ individuals when conducting analyses (Ecker et al., 2019). Therefore, research focused on 2SLGBTQIA+ individuals experiencing homelessness must take these methodological considerations into account before developing their research activities.

Considerations for prevention:

- Although the risk of undercounting is high, having a standardized process to collect data on the prevalence of 2SLGBTQIA+ homelessness will help inform programming, policy making, finding, and research (Ecker et al., 2019).
- Given the overrepresentation of 2SLGBTQIA+ people, particularly youth, among those experiencing homelessness, targeted policies at the municipal, regional, and national level need to be developed to address the root causes of 2SLGBTQIA+ homelessness – biphobia, homophobia, and transphobia (Abramovich, 2016). This includes investments in public education on 2SLGBTQIA+ inclusion and early identification measures for 2SLGBTQIA+ people at risk of homelessness.
- Researchers should look to the PiT count questions when developing questions on gender identity and sexual orientation and should vet analysis plans with 2SLGBTQIA+ researchers. This will help contribute to the literature base on 2SLGBTQIA+ homelessness.

Entries into Homelessness

Homophobia, biphobia, and transphobia are at the root of entries into homelessness among 2SLGBTQIA+ individuals, particularly youth. Research consistently finds that familial rejection due to one's gender identity and/or sexual orientation is the primary driver for homelessness among 2SLGBTQIA+ youth (Abramovich, 2012; Ecker, 2016). 2SLGBTQIA+ youth have been found to enter homelessness earlier than non-2SLGBTQIA+ youth (Ecker, 2016) and experience longer episodes of homelessness (Choi, Wilson, Shelton, & Gates, 2015). Discrimination from landlords and unsafe shelter environments can limit access to housing and supports once a 2SLGBTQIA+ young person becomes homeless, which further exacerbates their homelessness experience (Abramovich, 2016).

2SLGBTQIA+ adults also note the impact of homophobia, biphobia, and transphobia. Results from small qualitative studies find that some 2SLGBTQIA+ adults first experience homelessness during childhood and their early adult years (Ecker et al., 2020; Fraser et al., 2021). This indicates the importance of early interventions to prevent young 2SLGBTQIA+ adults from remaining or re-entering homelessness as they enter adulthood. Focusing on housing, discrimination from landlords limits access to housing opportunities for 2SLBGTQIA+ adults (Ecker et al., 2020; Fraser et al., 2021) and is particularly impactful for transgender individuals (Levy et al., 2017). Previous research has shown that lesbian, gay, and bisexual couples were significantly less likely than heterosexual couples to receive positive responses to e-mail inquiries about online rental housing advertisements (Friedman et al., 2013).

Other factors contributing to entries into homelessness among 2SLGBTQIA+ adults are intimate partner violence (Cusack et al., 2022), substance use (Ecker et al., 2020), and being unable to afford private market rent (Ecker et al., 2020). Unaffordability is particularly impactful for 2SLGBTQIA+ individuals, as they have higher odds of living in poverty compared to non-2SLGBTQIA+ individuals (Romero et al., 2020). 2SLGBTQIA+ people of colour and transgender people experience even higher rates of poverty compared to non-2SLGBTQIA+ individuals (Romero et al., 2020). This may be directly related to employment discrimination, as a large American study found that 90 percent of transgender and gender nonconforming individuals reported experiencing harassment or mistreatment on the job (Grant et al., 2011).

Considerations for prevention:

- Targeted early intervention plans need to be developed for 2SLGBTQIA+ youth (Abramovich, 2016). This could include school-based interventions such as the Upstream Project (Sohn & Gaetz, 2020) and the community-based Family and Natural Supports programme (Borato, Gaetz,

& McMillan, 2020). In schools, Genders & Sexualities Alliance Networks (formerly Gay-Straight Alliances) could be included within Upstream programmes to identify 2SLGBTQIA+ youth who may be at risk of homelessness. The families of these youth could then be referred to a Family and Natural Supports programme, with a major focus on educating parents on 2SLGBTQIA+ issues.

- As some people, particularly youth, will not be able to safely reconnect with family, it is imperative that 2SLGBTQIA+ individuals have access to safe and affirming emergency shelter and housing options (Abramovich, 2016).
- To address housing discrimination, greater consequences for discriminatory landlords must be developed and implemented. One strategy is to create mandatory training for landlords and housing developers funded through government programmes, such as the National Housing Strategy (Ecker, 2024). Relatedly, legal clinics could educate and support 2SLGBTQIA+ people to file human rights complaints against landlords when discrimination occurs (Ecker, 2024).
- Income insecurity could be addressed via universal basic income (UBI) (Kerman, 2021). UBI may be particularly impactful for transgender individuals given the multiple forms of discrimination they experience.

Service Use Experiences

2SLGBTQIA+ individuals across the lifespan report feeling unsafe in the emergency shelter system (Abramovich, 2016; Bardwell, 2019; Carr et al., 2025; Ecker et al., 2022). 2SLGBTQIA+ people can experience verbal and physical assault from other residents, and encounter homophobic, biphobic, and transphobic staff members (Abramovich, 2016; Ecker et al., 2022). 2SLGBTQIA+ people who have used emergency shelters report applying identity management techniques, meaning that they were cautious about disclosing their sexual orientation and/or gender identity with other residents and staff (Ecker et al., 2022; Fraser, Chisholm, & Pierse, 2024a). Because of these pressures, some 2SLGBTQIA+ people may avoid the shelter system and attempt to find alternative accommodation or sleep rough (Abramovich, 2016).

Emergency shelters can be particularly dangerous and harmful for transgender individuals. Transgender people across the lifespan report being misgendered by staff and other residents (Abramovich, 2016; Bardwell, 2019) and can experience violence from other residents (Ecker et al., 2022). In spite of this knowledge, there are few, if any, emergency shelters in operation that are specific to transgender people experiencing homelessness (Carr et al., 2025).

The experiences of 2SLGBTQIA+ people in emergency shelters are directly related to heteronormative and gendered policies. For example, emergency shelters often operate on the gender binary (i.e., shelters specific to men and shelters specific to women). This divide can be distressing for transgender people, as they may not feel comfortable accessing such segregated services (Carr et al., 2025) or are denied access to shelters based on their gender identity (Abramovich, 2016); however, some municipalities now have policies that protect the rights of transgender individuals to access the emergency shelter that aligns with their gender identity (Ecker et al., 2019).

To cope with the biphobic, homophobic, and transphobic nature of emergency shelters, some 2SLGBTQIA+ people report finding community among other 2SLGBTQIA+ people experiencing homelessness (Ecker et al., 2022; Fraser et al., 2024a) or non-2SLGBTQIA+ residents who identify as allies (Ecker et al., 2022). 2SLGBTQIA+ adults report advocating for 2SLGBTQIA+ rights in the shelter system and developing networks among other 2SLGBTQIA+ residents and staff (Ecker et al., 2022; Fraser et al., 2024b). This is particularly true for transgender adults, and it is often required out of necessity and survival. Several studies highlight the mutual aid that transgender adults provide to one another. This includes offering information about the shelter system and the rights of transgender adults to express their gender identity in the system (Billies, 2015; England, 2022) and providing temporary accommodation to other transgender individuals so they do not have to access the shelter system (England, 2022). These forms of support are critical, but also highlight the need for more services specific to transgender adults experiencing homelessness.

Considerations for prevention:

- Housing and shelter standards need to be co-developed and continuously reviewed to meet the needs of 2SLGBTQIA+ individuals (Abramovich, 2016). This includes gender-inclusive intake processes, gender-inclusive washroom and sleeping accommodation policies, and guidelines for mandatory and ongoing training for staff. Welcoming shelters could reduce street-based homelessness among 2SLGBTQIA+ people and potentially increase access to the supports offered in the shelter system. Access to services in the shelter system has been identified as a facilitator to exiting out of homelessness for 2SLGBTQIA+ adults (Ecker, 2024).
- Co-developing social programming with and for 2SLGBTQIA+ people experiencing homelessness (Ecker, 2017; Ecker et al., 2022). This can provide formal opportunities for 2SLGBTQIA+ people to come together and build social connections within and outside of the emergency shelter system. The building of social networks can help 2SLGBTQIA+ people address potential social isolation concerns when they move into housing.
- Developing ally training workshops for non-2SLGBTQIA+ residents could help to foster a sense of inclusivity in emergency shelters (Ecker et al., 2022). A 2SLGBTQIA+ ally is someone who is united with 2SLGBTQIA+ people and advocates for their inclusion and protection of their rights (Eichler, 2010).

Exits Out of Homelessness

Few studies have examined exits out of homelessness among 2SLGBTQIA+ individuals. Having access to supportive staff, particularly those who also identify as 2SLGBTQIA+, and strong friend networks positively impacted 2SLGBTQIA+ adults' ability to exit out of homelessness (Matthews et al., 2019; Ecker, 2024; Fraser, Chisholm, & Pierse, 2024b). In some cases, 2SLGBTIA+ adults moved into temporary housing locations (e.g., couch surfing) with their supportive friends rather than permanent housing (Matthews et al., 2019). As noted above, staying temporarily with friends is particularly common among transgender and gender non-confirming adults (England, 2022). In other cases, 2SLGBTQIA+ individuals report wanting to focus on other areas of their life outside of housing, including alcohol and substance use or focusing on their gender transition (Ecker, 2024).

Barriers to exiting out of homelessness for 2SLGBTQIA+ people are largely tied to biphobia, homophobia, and transphobia. For example, 2SLGBTQIA+ people experiencing homelessness report discrimination from landlords in the private market (Ecker, 2024). This limits access to housing opportunities and can be distressing for 2SLGBTQIA+ people (Ecker, 2024). Once housed, some 2SLGBTQIA+ people report not feeling safe in their housing due to harassment within one's neighbourhood (Ecker, 2024).

Considerations for prevention:

- 2SLGBTQIA+ housing options need to be developed (Abramovich, 2016; Ecker, 2024). This includes permanent supportive housing programmes and Housing First programmes. Dedicated housing to 2SLGBTQIA+ individuals may increase housing stability and reduce re-entries into homelessness because of the inclusiveness of the housing.
- Housing First may be particularly suitable for 2SLGBTQIA+ adults, as it is a person-directed programme that recognizes the importance of individual choice in housing. 2SLGBTQIA+ people will need to be supported to select housing in 2SLGBTQIA+ affirming areas with 2SLGBTQIA+ supportive landlord (Ecker, 2024).
- Permanent supportive housing in congregate environments could also benefit 2SLGBTQIA+ people as residents will feel more open to disclose their 2SLGBTQIA+ identity and build community with other 2SLGBTQIA+ residents (Ecker, 2017).

Housing Programmes for 2SLGBTQIA+ Individuals across the Lifespan

Some studies have examined the housing preferences of 2SLGBTQIA+ people and outcomes of 2SLGBTIA+ housing programmes (Abramovich &

Kimura, 2021; Dopp et al., 2022; Ecker, 2017; Nolan, 2006). The scholarship is largely focused on the needs of older adults as they move from independent living to supported living environments (e.g., assisted living housing, long-term care housing); however, two studies focused on 2SLGBTQIA+ youth transitional housing programmes and two studies focused on the housing needs of 2SLGBTQIA+ adults.

Two transitional housing programmes for 2SLGBTQIA+ youth have been evaluated. Nolan (2006) evaluated a transitional housing programme with capacity for 10 2SLGBTQIA+ youth in New York City, United States. The average length of stay was 10 and a half months, but 40 percent of residents stayed for a year or more. The most common living situations after leaving the programme were shared accommodation (47 percent) and independent housing (20 percent). Abramovich and Kimura (2021) evaluated a transitional housing programme with capacity for 25 2SLGBTQIA+ youth in Toronto, Canada. They found that 2SLGBTQIA+ residents felt safe in the programme and that this feeling of safety was much higher compared to previous experiences in non-2SLGBTQIA+ programmes. Each evaluation noted the importance of having 2SLGBTQIA+ staff as part of the programme.

Dopp et al. (2022) focused on the development of supportive housing for 2SLGBTQIA+ adults with homelessness and criminal justice histories. They recommended that supportive housing should offer comprehensive services that address individuals' interrelated needs, including 2SLGBTQIA+-specific services such as support with identity development, family reunification, and interpersonal relationships. They also recommend that staff of supportive housing for 2SLGBTQIA+ individuals reflect the identities of residents. Ecker (2017) in his study of 2SLGBTQIA+ adults with current and previous experiences of homelessness reports similar results. Participants in the study wanted a range of housing options specific to 2SLGBTQIA+ adults, including emergency shelters, supportive congregate housing, and supportive independent housing. Some participants preferred to live in housing specific to the 2SLGBTQIA+ community, while others did not. Neighbourhood location was important for some participants, as they wanted to live in a safe and 2SLGBTQIA+-friendly space. Support needs included substance use, mental health, and trauma-specific services that take an intersectional approach. Staff should also reflect the communities that they work with. These findings reflect the values of the Bridging the Transition Framework, as it emphasizes the importance of individual interventions, but also how they fit within the community and broader population.

The housing needs of older 2SLGBTQIA+ adults are slightly different. Safety in housing is often a major concern (King & Stoneman, 2017). Older 2SLGBTQIA+ adults report fears of encountering homophobia, biphobia, and transphobia in housing arrangements, with some older adults feeling forced to go "back into the closet" (King & Stoneman, 2017). To address this, housing options for 2SLGBTQIA+ older adults must have inclusive policies, programming specific to 2SLGBTQIA+ residents, and celebrations of 2SLGBTQIA+ people and history (Redden et al., 2023).

Like results from Ecker (2017), some older 2SLGBTQIA+ adults do not request access to 2SLGBTQIA+-specific housing, indicating the need for housing options that are not "one-size-fits-all" (Redden et al., 2023; Rosenwohl-Mack et al., 2022). This is particularly true for racialized 2SLGBTQIA+ older adults, as they may experience from racism other residents, including 2SLGBTQIA+ older adults, and could benefit from specific services that reflect their intersecting identities (Chen et al., 2022).

Considerations for prevention:

- To co-develop, implement, and sustain inclusive housing programming that will promote housing stability among residents, several steps should be taken:
  - The majority of staff members should identify as 2SLGBTQIA+ (Dopp et al., 2022; Ecker, 2017).
  - Include programming that addresses gender identity and sexual orientation (Abramovich, 2016). This could include developing in-house resources or partnering with community agencies.
  - Develop programming that addresses the intersectional identities of residents (Abramovich, 2016; Ecker, 2017). This could include programming that is specific to Indigenous 2SLGBTQIA+ individuals, racialized 2SLGBTQIA+ individuals, and newcomer 2SLGBQTIA+ individuals (Abramovich, 2016). Relatedly, housing programmes must address unique factors related to residents across the lifespan (Ecker, 2017). For example, younger people will have different needs than older adults.

Conclusion

Preventing entries and re-entries into homelessness requires comprehensive policy and programme responses. Although affordable and adequate housing is the panacea to homelessness, how this housing looks requires deeper examination. This chapter has highlighted the unique and diverse housing and support needs of 2SLGBTQIA+ people across the lifespan and aligns with the Bridging the Transition to Housing Framework – Intersectionality (Marshall et al., 2023). There is an emerging understanding of the scope of 2SLGBTQIA+ homelessness in Canada, which has identified the need for targeted policy development at the municipal, regional, and national levels. Early interventions are needed to address 2SLGBTQIA+ youth homelessness, with a focus on school- and family-based interventions when it is safe to include the family. The protection of the rights of 2SLGBTQIA+ individuals must be reinforced, as this review has highlighted the detrimental impact of housing discrimination as it relates to exiting homelessness. This review also highlighted the importance for emergency shelter and housing programmes to protect 2SLGBTQIA+ individuals through inclusive policies, well-trained staff, and social programming. To truly prevent homelessness from occurring or re-occurring, the unique needs of 2SLGBTQIA+ individuals must be acknowledged and addressed.

References

Abramovich, I.A. (2012) No safe place to go: LGBTQ youth homeless in Canada – Reviewing the literature. *Canadian Journal of Family and Youth*, *4*(1), 29–51.

Abramovich, A. (2016) Preventing, reducing and ending LGBTQ2S youth homelessness: The need for targeted strategies. *Social Inclusion*, *4*(4), 86–96. https://doi.org/10.17645/si.v4i4.669

Abramovich, A. (2019) *Creating LGBTQ2S Inclusive, Affirming, and Safe PiT Counts*. Toronto: Canadian Observatory on Homelessness and CAMH. Retrieved from: https://www.homelesshub.ca/sites/default/files/attachments/LGBTQ2S-PiT-Count.pdf

Abramovich, A. & Kimura, L. (2021) Outcomes for youth living in Canada's first LGBTQ2S transitional housing program. *Journal of Homosexuality*, *68*(8), 1242–1259.

Bardwell, G. (2019) The impact of risk environments on LGBTQ2S adults experiencing homelessness in a midsized Canadian city. *Journal of Gay & Lesbian Social Services: The Quarterly Journal of Community & Clinical Practice*, *31*(1), 53–64. https://doi.org/10.1080/10538720.2019.1548327

Billies M (2015) Low income LGBTGNC (Gender Nonconforming) struggles over shelters as public space. *ACME: An International E-Journal for Critical Geographies*, *14*(4), 989–1007.

Borato, M., Gaetz, S., and McMillan, L. (2020) *Family and Natural Supports: A Program Framework*. Toronto, ON: Canadian Observatory on Homelessness Press.

Carr, H., Cooper, A., England, E., Matthews, P., Taylor, G., & Tunåker, C. (2025) Queer utopias of housing and homelessness, *Housing Studies*, https://doi.org/10.1080/02673037.2022.2146067

Chen, J., McLaren, H., Jones, M., & Shams, L. (2022) The aging experiences of LGBTQ ethnic minority older adults: A systematic review. *Gerontologist*, *62*(3), e162–e177.

Choi, S.K., Wilson, B.D.M., Shelton, J., & Gates, G.J. (2015) *Serving our Youth 2015: The Needs and Experiences of Lesbian, Gay, Bisexual, Transgender, and Questioning Youth Experiencing Homelessness*. UCLA: The Williams Institute. Retrieved from: https://escholarship.org/uc/item/1pd9886n

Cusack, M., Montgomery, A.E., & Byrne, T. (2022) Examining the intersection of housing instability and violence among LGBTQ adults. *Journal of Homosexuality*, *70*(12), 2943–2954. https://doi.org/10.1080/00918369.2022.2085936

Dopp, A.R., McKenna, S., Gilbert, M., & Hunter, S.B. (2022) Supportive housing for sexual and gender minority individuals with criminal justice histories:

Challenges and opportunities identified by providers and clients. *Housing Policy Debate*, *34*(1), 108–131. https://doi.org/10.1080/10511482.2022.2055615

Ecker, J. (2016) Queer, young, and homeless: A review of the literature. *Child & Youth Services*, *37*(4), 325–361. https://doi.org/10.1080/0145935X.2016.1151781.

Ecker, J. (2017) LGBTQ2S adult housing needs assessment. Retrieved from: https://homelesshub.ca/resource/lgbtq2s-adulthousing-needs-assessment

Ecker, J. (2024) Facilitators and barriers to attaining housing among 2SLGBTQ+ adults with experiences of homelessness. *Journal of Gay & Lesbian Social Services*, *36*(2), 247–272. https://doi.org/10.1080/10538720.2023.2251132

Ecker, J., Aubry, T., & Sylvestre, J. (2019) A review of the literature on LGBTQ adults who experience homelessness. *Journal of Homosexuality*, *66*(3), 297–323. https://doi.org/10.1080/00918369.2017.1413277

Ecker, J., Aubry, T., & Sylvestre, J. (2020) Pathways into homelessness among LGBTQ2S adults. *Journal of Homosexuality*, *67*(11), 1625–1643.

Ecker, J., Aubry, T., & Sylvestre, J. (2022) Experiences of LGBTQ adults who have accessed emergency shelters in a large urban city in Canada. *Social Work in Public Health*, *37*(2), 168–185. https://doi.org/10.1080/19371918.2021.1976345

Eichler, M.A. (2010) Joining the family: Experiences of being and becoming ally activists of LGBTQ people. *Journal of Transformative Education*, *8*(2), 89–102.

England, E. (2022) 'Homelessness is a queer experience': Utopianism and mutual aid as survival strategies for homeless trans people. *Housing Studies*, *40*(7), 1585–1602. https://doi.org/10.1080/02673037.2022.2108381

Fraser, B., Chisholm, E., & Pierse, N. (2021) "You're so powerless": Takatāpui/LGBTQI+ people's experiences before becoming homeless in Aotearoa New Zealand. *PLOS ONE*, *16*(12). https://doi.org/10.1371/journal.pone.0259799

Fraser, B., Chisholm, E., & Pierse, N. (2024a) "There's no room for falling apart:" Takatāpui/LGBTIQ + people's experiences of homelessness in Aotearoa New Zealand. *Sexual and Gender Diversity in Social Services*, *36*(3), 379–406, https://doi.org/10.1080/10538720.2023.2253431

Fraser, B., Chisholm, E., & Pierse, N. (2024b) "Eventually it just hit like a tonne of bricks": Life after homelessness amongst Takatāpui/LGBTIQ+ people in Aotearoa New Zealand. *International Journal on Homelessness*, *4*(2), 42–61.

Friedman, S., Reynolds, A., Scovill, S., Brassier, F. R., Campbell, R., & Ballou, M. (2013) *An Estimate of Housing Discrimination Against Same-Sex Couples*. Washington, DC: U.S. Department of Housing and Urban Development, Office of Policy Development and Research.

Gaetz, S., Donaldson, J., Richter, T., Gulliver, T. (2013) *The State of Homelessness in Canada 2013*. Toronto: Canadian Homelessness Research Network Press.

Gaetz, S. & Dej, E. (2017) *A New Direction: A Framework for Homelessness Prevention*. Toronto: Canadian Observatory on Homelessness Press.

Grant, J. M., Mottet, L.A., Tanis, J., Harrison, J., Herman, J.L., & Keisling, M. (2011) *Injustice at Every Turn: A Report of the National Transgender Discrimination Survey*. Washington, DC: National Center for Transgender Equality and National Gay and Lesbian Task Force.

Infrastructure Canada. (2024) Reaching Home: Canada's Homelessness Strategy Directives. Retrieved from: https://housing-infrastructure.canada.ca/homelessness-sans-abri/directives-eng.html

Kerman, N. (2021) The role of Universal Basic Income in preventing and ending homelessness. *International Journal on Homelessness*, *1*(1), 3–13.

King, A. & Stoneman, P. (2017) Understanding SAFE Housing – putting older LGBT* people's concerns, preferences and experiences of housing in England in a sociological context. *Housing, Care and Support*, *20*(3), 89–99.

Levy, D. K., Wissoker, D., Aranda, C. L., Howell, B., Pitingolo, R., Sewell, S., & Santos, R. (2017) *A Paired-testing Pilot Study of Housing Discrimination Against Same-Sex Couples and Transgender Individuals*. Washington, DC: Urban Institute. Retrieved from http://www.urban.org/research/publication/paired-testing-pilot-study-housing-discrimination-against-same-sex-couples-and-transgender-individuals/view/full_report

Marshall, C., Gewurtz, R., Barbic, S., Roy, L., Cooke, A. & Lysaght, R. (2023) *Bridging the Transition to Housing: A Social Justice Framework to Guide the Practice of Occupational Therapists and other Professionals who Support Individuals with Experiences of Homelessness* (2nd Edition). 10.13140/RG.2.2.24013.41443.

Matthews, P., Poyner, C., & Kjellgren, R. (2019) Lesbian, gay, bisexual, transgender and queer experiences of homelessness and identity. *International Journal of Housing Policy*, *19*(2), 232–253. https://doi.org/10.1080/19491247.2018.1519341

Nolan, T. C. (2006) Outcomes for a transitional living program serving LGBTQ youth in New York City. *Child Welfare*, *85*(2), 385–406.

Redden, M., Gahagan, J., Kia, H., Humble, A.M., Stinchcombe, A., Manning, E., Ecker, J., de Vries, B., Gambold, L.L., Oliver, B., & Thomas, R. (2023) Housing as a determinant of health for older LGBT Canadians: Focus group findings from a national housing study. *Housing and Society*, *50*(1), 113–137, https://doi.org/10.1080/08882746.2021.1905996

Romero, A.P., Goldberg, S.K., & Vasquez, L.A. (2020) *LGBT People and Housing Affordability, Discrimination, and Homelessness*. Los Angeles: UCLA School of Law, Williams Institute.

Rosenwohl-Mack, A., Smith, D., Greene, M., Skultety, K., Deutsch, M., Dubbin, L., Flatt, J.D. (2022) Building H.O.U.S.E (Healthy Outcomes Using a Supportive Environment): Exploring the role of affordable and inclusive housing for LGBTQIA+ older adults. *International Journal of Environmental Research Public Health*. *19*, 1699. https://doi.org/10.3390/ijerph19031699

Savin-Williams, R.C. & Ream, G.L. (2007) Prevalence and stability of sexual orientation components during adolescence and young adulthood. *Archives of Sexual Behavior*, *36*(3), 385–394.

Sohn, Jacqueline and Gaetz, Stephen. (2020) *The Upstream Project Canada: An Early Intervention Strategy to Prevent Youth Homelessness & School Disengagement*. Toronto: Canadian Observatory on Homelessness Press.

US Department of Housing and Urban Development. (2025) *CoC Homeless Populations and Subpopulations Reports*. Retrieved from: https://www.hudexchange.info/programs/coc/coc-homeless-populations-and-subpopulations-reports/?filter_Year=&filter_Scope=NatlTerrDC&filter_State=&filter_CoC=&program=CoC&group=PopSub

20

KEY SOCIAL LOCATIONS RELEVANT TO HOMELESSNESS PREVENTION

Homelessness among Racialized Persons

Oyedeji Ayonrinde and Bhavana Varma

Racialized individuals, particularly visible minority populations, face significant discrimination through seeking and sustaining housing against a backdrop of historical, political, policy, and race-related factors. New migrant populations with less inter-generational rootedness are also vulnerable to unstable housing. In some countries experiencing historical colonization for example, Australia, Canada, South Africa, and the United States, Indigenous populations have been displaced from their ancestral lands and may find themselves living in reservation areas, less viable agricultural land, or high-density neighborhoods of urban centers. This chapter discusses the interplay of multiple historical, social, and political determinants in the experiences of homelessness among racialized persons.

How this Chapter Guides Practice and Research in Homelessness Prevention

Historical, socioeconomic, policy, and political factors can contribute significantly to homelessness among racialized individuals. This chapter highlights the interplay between historical processes such as the eviction of racialized individuals from traditional land and territories, the destruction of communities by settler populations, and the economic impact of gentrification on housing for diverse populations. The influence of poverty on one's ability to rent or buy property is explored from the lens of the multiple systemic and structural determinants behind economic disparities including racism. The chapter encourages scholars and policymakers to carefully observe,

DOI: 10.4324/9781003541332-24

recognize, and advocate for housing equity for racialized people, factoring in the harmful, intended, and unintended consequences of policies, legislation, and access to resources over many decades, and in some cases, centuries.

Introduction

In many high- and middle-income countries, racialized individuals experience homelessness at disproportionately higher rates than non-racialized populations. This pattern is well-documented in Canada, the United States, the United Kingdom, Australia, and beyond (OECD, 2025). These disparities, however, are not coincidental; they are the result of layered structural, systemic, and historical forces that have shaped access to housing, income, education, and healthcare. These forces, often rooted in colonialism, racism, and policy failures, have created deep and persistent inequities for Black, Indigenous, and other racialized communities.

The experiences of homelessness among racialized people cannot be separated from the broader social determinants of health and well-being. Factors such as poverty, incarceration, unemployment, and housing policy affect all populations, but are often magnified for those who are racialized due to systemic bias and discrimination (Banaji, Fiske and Massey, 2021). For example, policies that may appear neutral may have racialized consequences, such as reduced access to public services, culturally inappropriate support systems, or biased risk assessments that influence shelter access or housing placements (Cronley, 2020).

While early research on homelessness emphasized individual pathologies—mental illness, substance use, or family breakdown—such approaches frequently ignored the role of race and racism as critical determinants (Bhugra and Ayonrinde, 2010). Even when racial disparities were observed, they were often attributed to income differences alone, without acknowledging the racialized nature of poverty itself or the historic displacement of racialized communities (Fowle, 2022). Similarly, in the United States, people of color account for more than half of all individuals experiencing homelessness despite comprising a much smaller proportion of the population (Fowle, 2022). These patterns persist because systems—including housing, child welfare, criminal justice, and healthcare—continue to reinforce racial inequities, both through intentional policy design and unconscious bias.

This chapter explores the multiple, intersecting drivers of homelessness among racialized people, emphasizing the importance of addressing systemic racism and historical trauma in research, policies, and practice. It builds on foundational understandings of racialization, colonial displacement, and institutional discrimination, while offering examples from Canada and other nations with colonial histories. Through this lens, we aim to challenge colorblind frameworks that obscure racial inequities and to advocate for anti-racist, equity-based responses to homelessness. In so doing, the chapter seeks to provide researchers, service providers, and policymakers with a deeper understanding of the structural roots of homelessness in racialized communities—and with it, a pathway toward more just and effective housing policy and practice.

Understanding Race and Racialization

Race is a non-biological, socially constructed concept that classifies individuals based on perceived physical traits—such as skin tone or facial features—often assumed to signify inherited differences (Templeton, 1998). These constructs have historically served to establish and reinforce hierarchies of power. Whether under the banners of colonialism, slavery, or apartheid, race has been used, historically and in contemporary society, as a justification for discrimination, dispossession, and social exclusion. Over time, dominant groups have employed racial paradigms to assign meaning, entitlement, and roles to both in-groups and out-groups. While human populations exhibit considerable genetic variation, research has shown that there is greater genetic diversity within so-called racial groups than between them (Duello et al., 2021). As such, the term "race" lacks biological validity. For this reason, the term "racialized" has been used in this chapter to better capture the socio-political processes that classify and marginalize people based on perceived differences.

To be racialized is to be placed into categories that carry unequal weight in terms of power, opportunity, and treatment. The term also underscores that this categorization is an action imposed by social structures—not an innate trait. Racialized individuals are those who, through social processes, are "othered" in ways that result in discrimination and inequity. Racialization manifests through racism, which operates on multiple levels (Jarvis et al., 2023):

1 *Micro-level racism* includes interpersonal experiences such as overt discrimination and microaggressions—subtle insults, misrecognition, or unwarranted scrutiny based on physical appearance, accent, or cultural practices.
2 *Meso-level racism* refers to institutional policies and practices that disadvantage racialized groups—such as discriminatory lending practices, school policies, or housing regulations.
3 *Macro-level or structural racism* is embedded in the fabric of society, shaping who has access to wealth, housing, education, and political influence. It is reproduced through laws, norms, and institutions that may appear neutral but disproportionately harm racialized populations.

These forms of racism interact with and reinforce one another. For example, a racialized individual might experience microaggressions while applying for housing, encounter biased credit scoring algorithms (meso-level), and simultaneously face systemic exclusion from affordable housing due to zoning laws or political disinvestment in racialized neighborhoods (macro-level).

A lesser-discussed, but equally harmful, expression of racism is epistemic injustice (Fricker, 2007; Carel and Kidd, 2014). That is, the devaluing or dismissal of knowledge held by racialized people. This can manifest in housing systems where policy decisions are made without consulting racialized communities, or when academic and policy research ignores alternative worldviews or culturally rooted understandings of home, community, and wellness.

Taken together, these mechanisms demonstrate that homelessness among racialized people is not solely a result of individual hardship, but entrenched exclusionary systems. Without an understanding of racialization and its impacts, policy responses to homelessness risk being ineffective—or worse, perpetuating the very harms they aim to address.

Racial Discrimination and Housing Systems

In the context of housing, the effects of racialization are particularly stark. Racialized individuals are often denied equal access to rentals, mortgages, or housing programs, and their experiences with landlords, service providers, or financial institutions are frequently shaped by bias—whether overt or unconscious (Korver-Glenn, 2018). Even when policy frameworks appear to be neutral, their implementation often reflects societal prejudices, thereby producing racialized outcomes. Understanding these processes is essential to unpacking the overrepresentation of racialized and Indigenous populations in homelessness. It also sets the stage in this chapter, which explores the historical, policy-based, and health-related factors that contribute to this inequity.

Historical and Systemic Roots of Housing Inequities

Housing inequity among racialized populations is not a recent phenomenon. It is deeply rooted in colonial, political, and economic histories that have systematically excluded Black, Indigenous, and other racialized communities from access to land, property, and secure housing. Across countries with histories of colonization—including Canada, the United States, Australia, and the United Kingdom—racialized groups have faced dispossession, displacement, and disinvestment over generations.

Colonial Legacies and Land Dispossession

The historical displacement of Indigenous peoples in Canada, Australia, and the United States exemplifies the foundational role of colonialism in housing precarity. Indigenous populations were forcibly removed from their traditional lands and relocated to reserves, often on marginal or less viable land (Kandasamy and McDonnell, 2025). In Canada, this process was compounded by residential schools, the "Sixties Scoop," and systemic barriers to land ownership, contributing to intergenerational trauma and economic exclusion (Government of Canada, 2024). In apartheid-era South Africa, Indigenous Black communities were segregated and forced into townships through state-enforced land seizure. Similar practices were seen in the United States, where thriving Black neighborhoods were razed under the guise of "urban renewal." See Box 20.1 for historical examples of cases where intentional destruction or displacement of racialized communities has occurred in multiple international locations, thereby leading to and perpetuating homelessness.

Gentrification and Economic Displacement

While overt acts of state violence are well-documented, gentrification represents a more insidious form of displacement. As urban neighborhoods undergo redevelopment, long-standing communities—often racialized—are priced out of their homes. Displacement occurs without formal eviction but with the same result: loss of housing security and community connection. In cities like Chicago, Toronto, and London, racialized neighborhoods are systematically targeted for redevelopment, often without corresponding investments in affordable housing (Zuk et al. 2015)

"Colorblind" Policy and the Myth of Equal Access

Historically, housing policy has often been framed through a "colorblind" lens, emphasizing income or need without addressing race. This approach obscures how racialized individuals are disproportionately impacted by housing shortages, credit access, and policy enforcement. Arguably, colorblindness erases the very inequities it claims to treat equally, resulting in a lack of targeted intervention for those most affected.

Discriminatory housing practices have been overtly codified in the past. In the UK, it was common to see rental advertisements stating "No Blacks, No Irish, No Dogs" (Solanke, 2018, Hickman and Ryan, 2020). In the United States, redlining policies by banks and governments denied Black families mortgages and devalued homes in Black neighborhoods. Although these practices are now illegal, their legacy continues to shape patterns of segregation, underinvestment, and homelessness.

Structural Drivers of Homelessness for Racialized Groups

Overrepresentation of racialized and Indigenous homeless individuals is not coincidental. It reflects a complex interplay of systemic inequities, discriminatory policies, and socioeconomic marginalization creating and sustaining housing precarity. While factors like poverty, unemployment, and incarceration affect many populations, their impact is amplified for racialized communities through compounding systems of disadvantage.

Poverty and Economic Disparity

Poverty is a core driver of homelessness, and racialized groups are significantly more likely to live in poverty due to systemic barriers in employment, education, and income mobility. In many countries, racialized individuals (including migrants) earn significantly less than their non-racialized counterparts (Cholbi, 2023). These disparities can persist across generations (Box 20.1).

BOX 20.1 CASE STUDIES: THE INTENTIONAL DESTRUCTION OR DISPLACEMENT OF RACIALIZED COMMUNITIES

***Africville, Canada*:** A Black Canadian settlement near Halifax, Nova Scotia, was systematically neglected by municipal authorities. Basic infrastructure like clean water, sewage, and waste disposal was denied. In the 1960s, the city forcibly evicted residents and demolished the community under the pretext of "slum clearance." Africville is now recognized as a stark example of state-sanctioned anti-Black racism in urban policy (Canadian Museum for Human Rights, 2024; UNESCO Canadian Commission, 2024).

***Black Wall Street, USA*:** The Greenwood neighborhood in Tulsa, Oklahoma, was one of the most prosperous Black communities in the early 20th century. In 1921, white mobs attacked, looted, and burned over 1,400 homes and businesses, leaving nearly 10,000 people homeless. The massacre, ignored in public discourse for decades, highlights how violence and economic sabotage were used to prevent Black economic mobility and home ownership (Library of Congress, 2024).

***Romani Gypsies, Europe*:** Romani communities have faced racial, structural, and systemic exclusion from stable housing in a number of European countries such as Hungary, France, and the UK. Often living in migratory communities and subjected to eviction, segregation, and denial of public housing, Romani individuals experience some of the highest rates of homelessness in Europe (Cioarta, 2023).

Poverty limits the ability to afford rent, secure housing loans, or recover from financial setbacks. For many, this results in unstable housing, overcrowding, or homelessness as well as difficulty with the law.

Incarceration and Housing Instability

Incarceration is both a cause and consequence of homelessness. Individuals with criminal records face discrimination in the housing market and are often excluded from public housing. This is especially problematic given the racial disparities in incarceration rates. For instance, in Canada, 32% of federal inmates are Indigenous, while making up only 5% of the population (Public Safety Canada, 2023). While in the United States, Black men are six times more likely than white to be incarcerated (Bushway et al., 2022). High rates of incarceration in Indigenous populations is manifest in New Zealand, where 50% of incarcerated individuals are Māori (New Zealand Ministry of Justice, 2023), and in Australia, with 36% being Aboriginal and Torres Strait Islander peoples (Australia Bureau of Statistics, 2024).

These disparities often reflect systemic bias in law enforcement and sentencing practices. Once released, individuals face multiple barriers to reintegration, with recidivism and increased risk of homelessness.

Child Welfare as a Pipeline to Homelessness

Child welfare systems play a critical role in youth homelessness, particularly for Black and Indigenous children (Alberton et al., 2020). Many youth who "age out" of care are exposed to structural and systemic challenges facing unemployment and unstable housing. In Canada for instance, 53.7% of children in foster care are Indigenous, though they represent only 7.6% of the child population (Statistics Canada, 2024) and Black children account for 14% of child welfare investigations, despite being a smaller portion of the population. These disproportionalities may stem from systemic racism, cultural misunderstanding, and historic or intergenerational trauma (Bombay et al. 2009). Overall, transition from care to independence is especially precarious for racialized youth, making them highly vulnerable to homelessness.

Racialized Migrants and Newcomers: Policy Failures and Structural Exclusion

Racialized newcomers, refugees, and asylum seekers face distinct challenges that exacerbate their risk of homelessness. These challenges are rooted not only in the difficulties of migration and settlement but also in systemic racism, bureaucratic exclusion, and policies that create housing precarity (Lukes et al., 2018).

Systemic Oppression in Host Countries

In high-income countries such as Canada, the UK, and Australia, racialized migrants may enter systems not designed for their inclusion. Lack of access to social benefits, inadequate labor protections, and restrictive immigration policies combine to produce structural precarity. In Canada, for example, refugee claimants are often denied access to provincial health and housing programs due to gaps in federal-provincial coordination (Paquet, 2025).

Some policies that delay work permits or restrict eligibility for shelter funding directly contribute to migrant homelessness. Black refugees and asylum seekers—particularly from African countries—have been disproportionately impacted by these exclusions (Ombudsman Toronto, 2024). Across the European Union, 31% of respondents of African descents reported encountering racial discrimination while trying to rent or buy property (OECD, 2025). In the UK, homelessness associated with immigration resource policies has been described as "destitution by design" (Watts-Cobbe et al., 2024), characterized by government strategies that intentionally limit support to asylum seekers in order to deter migration. These policies result in long wait times for housing, inadequate financial support, and geographic dispersion to remote areas with limited infrastructure and community support. Such systems disproportionately affect racialized claimants and reinforce segregation and marginalization.

Language, Documentation, and Legal Barriers

Some new migrants navigate unfamiliar linguistic bureaucracy with applications for housing subsidies, immigration hearings, causing insurmountable barriers and difficulty asserting their rights. This serves to exclude racialized newcomers, as immigration status is a critical gatekeeper in which persons without legal status or citizenship may be considered ineligible for subsidized housing, public benefits, or shelter services (Lukes et al. 2018). This legalized form of exclusion disproportionately impacts asylum seeker and refugees, including racialized individuals under emergency immigration pathways.

Intersectional Vulnerabilities

Many racialized migrants experience multiple intersecting layers of marginalization. For instance, a racialized single parent seeking asylum as a survivor of trauma may face a combination of: racial discrimination in housing markets, cultural and gender-based isolation, ineligibility for certain benefits due to immigration status, and inadequate support from mainstream services. Without an intersectional lens, public policy and service delivery frameworks may fail to capture the complexity of these lived realities. See Chapter 14 for a discussion of the guiding principle of intersectionality in the Bridging the Transition Framework.

Discrimination in Housing Access: Market Bias and Systemic Gatekeeping

Discrimination in housing remains one of the most pervasive, yet under-acknowledged, barriers facing racialized populations. From rental rejections to biased mortgage approvals, racialized individuals routinely encounter systemic and interpersonal obstacles that restrict access to safe, affordable, and stable housing. These discriminatory practices, rooted in both historic exclusion and bias, undermine housing equity and contribute to insecure housing.

Racism in Rental and Housing Markets

For many racialized individuals, racism in the rental market is not an exception, but an expectation. Landlords may, for instance, reject applicants with non-Anglo names, express concern about "cultural fit," impose stricter credit checks, or request more documentation from racialized renters. Sometimes, language such as "quiet tenants preferred" can codify exclusion. This form of subtle or overt gatekeeping can restrict housing choices and lead to layers of disadvantage in underserved neighborhoods (OECD, 2025).

Mortgage Denials and Lending Discrimination

Beyond rental housing, access to home ownership remains inequitable. Racialized individuals face higher rates of mortgage rejection, even when controlling for income and creditworthiness (Faber, 2018). This is a direct legacy of redlining, a practice that historically excluded non-white applicants from property ownership through racially coded lending maps (Zenou and Boccard, 2000). While redlining is no longer legal, its impacts are still visible in devaluation of homes in historically Black or Indigenous neighborhoods; reluctance of financial institutions to lend in "high-risk" (often racialized) communities; and concentrated wealth gaps between white and non-white households, rooted in unequal access to home equity. Discrimination in lending sustains intergenerational poverty and limits the wealth-building potential of racialized families.

Shelter Access and Service Denials

Discrimination extends beyond the private housing market into public services. Racialized individuals—particularly those who are migrants or refugees—are more likely to face barriers in shelter systems. These may include a lack of culturally safe spaces, denial of entry due to perceived risk or racialized stigma, and inequitable application of shelter policies, such as curfews or identification requirements. In 2023, the City of Toronto in Canada faced widespread criticism for excluding refugee claimants, many of whom were Black, from the city's shelter system (Ombudsman Toronto, 2024; Ricketts, 2024). In this case, policies intended to prioritize "local" residents functioned as de facto racial exclusions. These practices violate equity and expose racialized individuals to life-threatening conditions.

Algorithmic Bias and Technological Discrimination

Conscious and unconscious bias in the housing market can directly contribute to homelessness. Rental applications, mortgage approvals, and shelter access are susceptible to bias against racialized people. Even tools meant to create equity, such as technology-based housing vulnerability assessments, may be flawed. In the USA, Blattner and Nelson (2021) observed that AI-based assessments under-ranked Black and Latino clients as "less vulnerable," despite higher risk factors.

With increasing reliance on technology, a new frontier of discrimination is emerging: algorithmic bias, where vulnerability assessments powered by machine learning are used to make housing decisions. Although AI was introduced to make housing decisions more "objective," it risks entrenching systemic exclusion when not developed with an anti-racist lens. As machine learning expands globally in housing systems, lessons from the United States highlight the urgent need for ethical oversight, community involvement, and equity-based design (Rosen, Garboden and Cossyleon, 2021).

Structural Solutions to Discriminatory Practices and Policy

Addressing housing discrimination requires more than awareness. It requires intervention at policy, institutional, and service levels, such as:

a Enforcing anti-discrimination laws in rental and mortgage markets;
b Investing in culturally specific housing options;
c Training housing providers in anti-racism and unconscious bias;
d Involving racialized communities in co-designing shelter and housing programs; and
e Auditing algorithmic tools for racial and socioeconomic fairness.

Health and Social Consequences of Racism

Housing is not only a basic human need—it is a cornerstone of health and well-being. The links between housing precarity and poor health outcomes are well-documented (Rana et al., 2025), but for racialized populations, these consequences are intensified by intersecting social determinants and systemic exclusion. Oftentimes, barriers are compounded by underfunding of public services in racialized communities and limited access to appropriate care.

Health Disparities

Studies have shown stark health disparities among homeless individuals from racialized and Indigenous backgrounds (Richard, 2023). In Canada, for example, Indigenous people experiencing homelessness are more likely to experience post-traumatic stress disorder, substance use disorder, and infectious diseases (Bingham et al., 2019). Equitable healthcare responses to homelessness must recognize the trauma associated with colonial violence, forced displacement, and systemic discrimination, which often manifests with both psychological and physical sequelae.

A tragic consequence of structural racism in housing and healthcare is premature death. In Australia, Tuson et al. (2024) observed that 30% of people who died while homeless were Indigenous Australians. The average age of death for Indigenous people experiencing homelessness was 49.1 years, compared to 51.3 years for non-Indigenous homeless individuals—significantly lower than national averages. Though homeless and racialized individuals experience earlier trajectories of chronic illness and death, national data on homeless mortality rates disaggregated by race remains limited and obscures the full scope of health inequities.

Environmental Racism

Environmental racism—the disproportionate exposure of racialized communities to polluted or hazardous environments—also plays a role in housing-related health risks (Waldron, 2021). This ecological and environmental form of systemic racism can manifest in the location of water, land and air polluting industries such as toxic waste sites, landfills, and incinerators. These harmful activities near racialized communities result in greater health risks and environmental degradation (Beard et al. 2024). For instance, in Nova Scotia, Canada industrial wastewater into traditional and sacred Indigenous water not only destroyed the African-Nova Scotian and Mi'kmaq communities' fishing livelihoods but also desecrated spiritual land, with higher rates of cancer observed in the community (Waldron, 2021). Less affluent racialized communities are more likely to be near polluted industrial zones or waste sites or in substandard housing with poor sanitation and ventilation.

Conclusion

Racialized individuals face persistent and disproportionate barriers to safe, stable housing. These inequities are deeply embedded in systems shaped by colonialism, racism, and economic exclusion. From child welfare and incarceration, to health disparities and housing discrimination, the structural drivers of homelessness intersect and compound across generations. Addressing homelessness among racialized communities demands more than service delivery—it requires a shift in how policies are made, how data is gathered, and how histories are acknowledged. Equity in housing is not achievable without an intentional and sustained commitment to anti-racist action, structural reform, and culturally grounded supports.

References

Alberton, A. M., Angell, G. B., Gorey, K. M. and Grenier, S. (2020) Homelessness among Indigenous peoples in Canada: The impacts of child welfare involvement and educational achievement. *Children and Youth Services Review*, *111*, p.104846.

Australia Bureau of Statistics (2024) https://www.abs.gov.au/statistics/people/crime-and-justice/prisoners-australia/latest-release#:~:text=The%20age%2Dstandardised%20imprisonment%20rate,had%20experienced%20prior%20adult%20imprisonment

Banaji, M. R., Fiske, S. T. and Massey, D. S. (2021) Systemic racism: Individuals and interactions, institutions and society. *Cognitive Research: Principles and Implications*, *6*(1), p.82.

Beard, S., Freeman, K., Velasco, M. L., Boyd, W., Chamberlain, T., Latoni, A., Lasko, D., Lunn, R. M., O'Fallon, L., Packenham, J., Smarr, M. M., Arnette, R., Cavalier-Keck, C., Keck, J., Muhammad, N., Wilson, O., Wilson, B., Wilson, A., & Dixon, D. (2024) Racism as a public health issue in environmental health disparities and environmental justice: Working toward solutions. *Environmental Health: A Global Access Science Source*, *23*(1), 8. https://doi.org/10.1186/s12940-024-01052-8

Bhugra, D. and Ayonrinde, O. (2010) Racism, racial life events and mental ill health. In R. Bhattacharya, S. Cross, and D. Bhugra (Eds.), *Clinical topics in cultural psychiatry* (pp. 39–51). Royal College of Psychiatrists.

Bingham, B., Moniruzzaman, A., Patterson, M., Distasio, J., Sareen, J., O'Neil, J. and Somers, J. M. (2019) Indigenous and non-Indigenous people experiencing homelessness and mental illness in two Canadian cities: A retrospective analysis and implications for culturally informed action. *BMJ Open*, *9*(4), p.e024748.

Blattner, L. and Nelson, S. (2021) How costly is noise? Data and disparities in consumer credit. *arXiv* preprint arXiv:2105.07554.

Bombay, A., Matheson, K. and Anisman, H. (2009) Intergenerational trauma: Convergence of multiple processes among First Nations peoples in Canada. *International Journal of Indigenous Health*, *5*(3), pp.6–47.

Bushway, S., Cabreros, I., Paige, J. W., Schwam, D., & Wenger, J. B. (2022) Barred from employment: More than half of unemployed men in their 30s had a criminal history of arrest. *Science Advances*, *8*, eabj6992. https://doi.org/10.1126/sciadv.abj6992

Canadian Museum for Human Rights (2024) https://humanrights.ca/story/story-africville (accessed March 1, 2025).

Carel, H., and Kidd, I. J. (2014) Epistemic injustice in healthcare: A philosophical analysis. *Medicine, Health Care and Philosophy*, *17*, pp. 529–540.

Cholbi, M. (2023) Why racialized poverty matters–and the way forward. In *The Routledge Handbook of Philosophy and Poverty* (pp. 406–416). Routledge.

Cioarta, I. (2023) *Exploring the Phenomenon of Roma Homelessness in the UK*. Institute for Social Policy, Housing, Equalities Research, Heriot-Watt University. https://www.hw.ac.uk/news/articles/2023/roma-people-living-in-the-uk-are.htm#:~:text=Roma%20people%20living%20in%20the%20UK%20are%20disproportionately%20facing%20overcrowding,-Published%3A%204%20Aug&text=New%20research%20published%20by%20Heriot,overcrowded%20and%20severely%20substandard%20housing

Cronley, C. (2020) Invisible intersectionality in measuring vulnerability among individuals experiencing homelessness – critically appraising the VI-SPDAT. *Journal of Social Distress and Homelessness*, *31*(1), pp. 23–33. https://doi.org/10.1080/10530789.2020.1852502

Duello, T. M., Rivedal, S., Wickland, C., & Weller, A. (2021) Race and genetics versus 'race' in genetics: A systematic review of the use of African ancestry in genetic studies. *Evolution, Medicine, and Public Health*, *9*(1), pp. 232–245. https://doi.org/10.1093/emph/eoab018

Faber, J. W. (2018) Segregation and the geography of creditworthiness: Racial inequality in a recovered mortgage market. *Housing Policy Debate*, *28*(2), pp. 215–247.

Fowle, M. Z. (2022) Racialized homelessness: A review of historical and contemporary causes of racial disparities in homelessness. *Housing Policy Debate*, *32*(6), pp. 940–967. https://doi.org/10.1080/10511482.2022.2026995

Fricker, M. (2007) *Epistemic Injustice: Power and the Ethics of Knowing*. Oxford University Press. https://doi.org/10.1093/acprof:oso/9780198237907.001.0001, accessed 28 Apr. 2025.

Government of Canada, Indian Residential Schools (2024). https://www.rcaanc-cirnac.gc.ca/eng/1625663008357/1625663325319 (accessed March 1 2025)

Hickman, M. J. and Ryan, L. (2020) The 'Irish question': Marginalizations at the nexus of sociology of migration and ethnic and racial studies in Britain. *Ethnic and Racial Studies*, *43*(16), pp. 96–114. https://doi.org/10.1080/01419870.2020.1722194

Jarvis, G. E., Andermann, L., Ayonrinde, O. A., Beder, M., Cénat, J. M., Ben-Cheikh, I., Fung, K., Gajaria, A., Gómez-Carrillo, A., Guzder, J., Hanafi, S., Kassam, A., Kronick, R., Lashley, M., Lewis-Fernández, R., McMahon, A., Measham, T., Nadeau, L., Rousseau, C., Sadek, J., … Kirmayer, L. J. (2023) Taking action on racism and structural violence in psychiatric training and clinical practice. *Canadian Journal of Psychiatry. Revue canadienne de psychiatrie*, 68(10), pp. 780–808. https://doi.org/10.1177/07067437231166985

Kandasamy, N. and McDonnell, M. (2025) Powerful stories: Indigenous and refugee Histories of dispossession and displacement in settler colonies. *Journal of Intercultural Studies*, pp. 1–19. https://doi.org/10.1080/07256868.2024.2437984

Korver-Glenn, E. (2018) Compounding inequalities: How racial stereotypes and discrimination accumulate across the stages of housing exchange. *American Sociological Review*, *83*(4), pp. 627–656.

Library of Congress (2024) https://guides.loc.gov/this-month-in-business-history/june/black-wall-street-destroyed (accessed March 1 2025).

Lukes, S., de Noronha, N. and Finney, N. (2018) Slippery discrimination: A review of the drivers of migrant and minority housing disadvantage. *Journal of Ethnic and Migration Studies*, *45*(17), pp. 3188–3206. https://doi.org/10.1080/1369183X.2018.1480996

New Zealand Ministry of Justice (2023) https://www.justice.govt.nz/justice-sector-policy/key-initiatives/key-initiatives-archive/hapaitia-te-oranga-tangata/

Organization for Economic Co-Operation and Development (2025) *Monitoring and Assessing the Impact of National Action Plans Against Racism*. Paris: OECD Publishing, https://doi.org/10.1787/13e32676-en

Ombudsman Toronto. (2024) *Report an Investigation into the City's Decision to Stop Allowing Refugee Claimants into Base Shelter System Beds*, December 10. https://www.toronto.ca/legdocs/mmis/2024/cc/bgrd/backgroundfile-251504.pdf (accessed 28 April, 2025).

Paquet, M. and Schertzer, R. (2025) A complex intergovernmental problem: Why Asylum seekers challenge Canada's immigration system. *Publius: The Journal of Federalism*, p.pjaf009.

Public Safety Canada. Overrepresentation (Indigenous Offenders) (2023) https://www.publicsafety.gc.ca/cnt/trnsprnc/brfng-mtrls/prlmntry-bndrs/20230720/12-en.aspx

Rana, K., Kent, J. L. and Page, A. (2025) Housing inequalities and health outcomes among migrant and refugee populations in high-income countries: A mixed-methods systematic review. *BMC Public Health*, *25*(1), p.1098.

Richard, M. K. (2023) Race matters in addressing homelessness: A scoping review and call for critical research. *American Journal of Community Psychology*, *72*(3–4), pp. 464–485.

Ricketts, J. (2024) Contextualizing black (dis) placement in Ontario through systems of housing, homelessness and incarceration. *Journal of Canadian Studies*, *58*(3), pp. 650–675.

Rosen, E., Garboden, P. M. and Cossyleon, J. E. (2021) Racial discrimination in housing: How landlords use algorithms and home visits to screen tenants. *American Sociological Review*, *86*(5), pp. 787–822.

Solanke, I. (2018) The stigma of being Black in Britain. *Identities*, *25*(1), pp. 49–54. https://doi.org/10.1080/1070289X.2017.1412143

Statistics Canada (2024) Indigenous foster children living in private households: Rates and sociodemographic characteristics of foster children and their households. https://www150.statcan.gc.ca/n1/pub/41-20-0002/412000022024001-eng.htm

Templeton, A. R. (1998) Human races: S genetic and evolutionary perspective. *American Anthropologist*, *100*(3), pp. 632–650.

Tuson, M, Vallesi, S, Wood, L. (2024) Tracking deaths of people who have experienced homelessness: A dynamic cohort study in an Australian city. *BMJ Open*, *14*, e081260. https://doi.org/10.1136/bmjopen-2023-081260

UNESCO Canadian Commission (2024) https://en.ccunesco.ca/about-ccunesco/press/2024/10/africville-unesco-places-of-history-and-memory (accessed March 1, 2025)

Waldron, I. R. (2021) *There's something in the water: Environmental racism in Indigenous & Black communities*. Fernwood Publishing.

Watts-Cobbe, B., McMordie, L., Bramley, G., Sims, R., Young, G. and Rayment, M. (2024) Destitution by design. https://pure.hw.ac.uk/ws/portalfiles/portal/141149624/DESIGNED_MASTER_Fair_Way_Scotland_Evaluation_End_of_Year_2_Report_FINAL_Sept_10th_copy.pdf

Zenou, Y. and Boccard, N. (2000) Racial discrimination and redlining in cities. *Journal of Urban Economics*, *48*(2), pp. 260–285.

Zuk, M., Bierbaum, A. H., Chapple, K., Gorska, K., Loukaitou-Sideris, A., Ong, P. and Thomas, T. (2015 August) Gentrification, displacement and the role of public investment: A literature review. In *Federal Reserve Bank of San Francisco* (Vol. 79).

21

KEY SOCIAL LOCATIONS RELEVANT TO HOMELESSNESS PREVENTION

Homelessness among Youth

Jeff Karabanow and Andrea Titterness

This chapter is a discussion on how homeless youth experience the process of exiting homelessness during the developmental period of emerging adulthood (EA). Attention will focus on similarities and differences in how mainstream youth progress through EA compared to youth who have experienced homelessness. Additionally, the process in which youth disengage from homelessness will be described and how youth interact with this process while navigating the complexities of EA. It will be suggested that support provided to homeless youth should be both trauma and developmentally informed. By opening the discussion of how EA and exiting homelessness intersect, this chapter will help inform future studies on this topic in an effort to better understand the lived experiences of this population through a developmentally appropriate lens.

How this Chapter Guides Practice and Research in Homelessness Prevention

This discussion highlights the experience of homeless youth as they engage in the process of exiting homelessness, but through the lens of the developmental stage of emerging adulthood (EA), which includes youth between the ages of 18–25 years. The characteristics of EA present unique challenges to individuals as they exit homelessness. Viewing the exiting process through this developmental lens provides insight into ways in which supports can be tailored to provide a more wholistic approach to supporting emerging adults as they engage with exiting homelessness.

DOI: 10.4324/9781003541332-25

Introduction

Youth comprise a growing proportion of the homeless population (Gaetz et al., 2013) and includes those between 13 and 24 years of age (Government of Canada, 2020, 2022); the average age of youth in the vast majority of studies is 19.8–21.8 years old (Gaetz et al., 2016; Schwan et al., 2018). This discussion focuses on youth between 18 and 24 years because this range has been the primary focus of the authors' investigations and falls within the age range of EA. EA is a developmental stage characterized by exploration of personal identity, instability, feeling in-between, focusing on oneself, and the feeling of possibility (Arnett, 2007). Our previous work has explored the intersection of EA and individuals exiting homelessness (Karabanow et al., 2016), and the current discussion elucidates this relationship further within the process of exiting homelessness described by Karabanow (2008). Attention will first focus on factors that contribute to emerging adults entering homelessness (Karabanow et al., 2025). The experiences of emerging adults who are exiting homelessness will then be provided (Karabanow et al., 2016), followed by a discussion on how core components of EA overlap with a process of exiting homeless that is described by Karabanow (2008). Finally, suggestions on how support can be tailored, in a *trauma-informed* manner (see Chapter 13 for more details on trauma-informed care), to emerging adults exiting homelessness during EA will be described.

Emerging Adulthood

Originally conceptualized by Arnett (2000), EA encompasses the ages of 18–25 and has unique characteristics from adolescence and young adulthood. The challenges faced by emerging adults are exploration (e.g., identity, career, relationships, etc.) and change (Arnett, 2000) and is characterized by instability, self-focus, feeling in-between, and feelings of possibility (Arnett, 2007, 2004). Adolescents typically live with families of origin, attend school, and are immersed in peer culture. Much of this normativity ends as individuals progress into EA, during which there is great heterogeneity in life course as individuals pursue a variety of avenues (e.g., attending school, starting employment). Personality growth is more rapid during adolescence, particularly within the context of a stable family (Syed and Seiffge-Krenke, 2013), and stable identity is established in early adulthood (Eriksson et al., 2020). Within EA, however, there is fluidity in identity between that which started during adolescence and is solidified in early adulthood, which is exactly why this period is so heterogeneous (Arnett et al., 2014; Arnett, 2007; Wood et al., 2018). Healthy family/caregiver and peer support, positive adjustment within the school system, higher socioeconomic status (SES), and control over emotions contribute to successful navigation through EA (O'Connor et al., 2011), most of which are often absent for youth who experience homelessness. Throughout the chapter, we will explore ways in which individuals who are homeless experience EA, noting similarities and differences to youth who are stably housed.

Factors Contributing to Entering Homelessness for Emerging Adults

As noted in the Bridging the Transition Framework outlined in Chapter 1, the pathways to homelessness can be as complicated as pathways of exiting homelessness. The following section will review factors that contribute to homeless in the emerging adult period, with a specific emphasis on trauma amongst homeless youth.

Experiencing trauma is common amongst many youth experiencing homelessness. Experiencing trauma contributes to youth homelessness (Coates and McKenzie-Mohr, 2010; Davies and Allen, 2017; Karabanow et al., 2025; Martijn and Sharpe, 2006). Many youth experienced poverty; physical, sexual, and/or emotional abuse; and poor experiences with child welfare (Karabanow, 2004; Karabanow et al., 2007, 2018). Foster care was often precarious and unsupportive, with high rates of neglect and maltreatment (Bender et al., 2015). Homelessness was often seen as a safer option than living in homes of origin or navigating the foster care system (Karabanow, 2006). Trauma continued to pervade the lived experience of youth throughout the stages of exiting homelessness (Karabanow et al., 2025) and increased the likelihood of victimization when homeless (Kim et al., 2018). Trauma can result in feelings of marginalization, hopelessness, and alienation, along with poor mental health in youth experiencing homelessness (Karabanow et al., 2025). Therefore, emerging adults who are homeless may be in a fragile state from the beginning of the homelessness cycle (see Chapter 5 for the four processes of existing homelessness) and likely continue experiencing trauma.

Emerging adults who are homeless also face challenges, including a lack of stable housing, which creates constant uncertainty and strain on mental health (Government of Canada, 2020), and barriers to education and employment (Bakken, 2023; Malenfant et al., 2020). They often experience isolation, lack of social support, and limited access to healthcare (Labelle et al., 2020; Pitcher et al., 2019), which exacerbates mental health struggles and trauma from past experiences. This combination of immediate survival needs and long-term planning challenges leaves many young adults stuck in a cycle of instability, making it difficult to break free and achieve self-sufficiency.

Navigating EA and Homelessness

Individuals who experience homelessness during EA may have endured at least one adverse childhood event (ACE) and many meet the diagnostic criteria for multiple mental health conditions (e.g., anxiety, depression) (Dawson-Rose et al., 2020). Homeless youth who experienced abuse in childhood are more likely to have substance use disorders (Ararso et al., 2021; Dawson-Rose et al., 2020) and to engage in substance use and risky behaviors (e.g., sex) within social networks established on the streets (Wenzel et al., 2012). Furthermore, obtaining financial stability and independence was paramount for populations of individuals who experienced homelessness (Bowen et al., 2021), yet ACEs predict economic instability for emerging adults (Tucker et al., 2022). Emerging adults who experience homelessness often report a sense of alienation and marginalization within the mainstream culture, including from police, service providers, and family (Budescu et al., 2021). Therefore, emerging adults experiencing homelessness encounter isolation, mental health challenges, substance use disorders, and community networks that can be both supportive and harmful, all while managing the complexities associated with EA.

Process of Exiting Homelessness for Emerging Adults

Karabanow (2008) investigated the lived experiences of youth who were homeless as they engaged with the process of exiting homelessness and conceptualized this process in phases of "disengaging from the street". The phases below are described in the order as presented in Karabanow (2008); the phases are not linear, and it often takes repeated attempts to exit homelessness.

Contemplation

During this phase, the emerging adult becomes disenchanted with homelessness. Emerging adults become bored with the daily struggles of survival; many become worn out by the toll of hardships associated with homelessness, a desire for something more stable, and feelings that they were finally ready to start the process of exiting homelessness (Karabanow, 2008).

Motivation to Change

This phase is characterized by courage to initiate changes that move toward exiting homelessness. Emerging adults face an unknown process of disengagement, so hope, courage, motivation, and desire are paramount to moving through this process. Motivation can be heightened by increased responsibilities (e.g., being a parent) and is enhanced by support from family/caregivers or friends and a willingness to ask for help (Karabanow, 2008).

Securing Help

Emerging adults exiting homelessness might seek housing stability, engage with formal institutions (e.g., returning to school), and often utilize service provisions such as shelters, drop-in clinics, and outreach programs (Karabanow, 2008). Through these services, youth are often provided with a safe and caring environment within which they can start to navigate questions about self-identity as they look at the factors contributing to their homelessness and motivation to change.

Transitioning from Homelessness to Housed

This is the most active and difficult stage in the process of exiting homelessness and requires reducing ties with the homeless community, leaving physical areas in which the emerging adults have survived thus far, and incorporating into mainstream society (Karabanow, 2008). Yet continued reliance on street connections to supplement income and maintain trusted relationships is likely to occur. Establishing new relationships off the streets is instrumental to the success of this phase, even though emerging adults often express feelings of loneliness as they transition from a state of homelessness (Karabanow, 2008).

Changing Routine

Changes in employment, housing, education, and establishing new connections necessitate a change in daily routine when exiting homelessness. Emotional and cognitive shifts occur as youth feel increased self-esteem, self-confidence, and consistency. Employment is integral to this phase as it indicated a shift in lifestyle (Karabanow, 2008).

"Successful Exiting"

Emerging adults viewed success in terms of emotional, spiritual, and situational changes that promote directionality, control, and stability, not simply whether one has a secure dwelling. This distinction is important because youth might be at risk of re-entering homelessness (e.g., precarity state outlined in Chapter 1) if proper supports are not in place even after secure housing has been obtained. Housing, employment, and/or education are important for successful exiting, but are conceptualized in the larger sense of stability and belonging (Karabanow, 2008). The presence of someone (e.g., service provider, friend) who could "be there" throughout the transition promoted successful exiting (Karabanow, 2008).

EA and the Process of Disengaging from Homelessness

The goal of EA is to navigate the transition from adolescence to full adulthood, where individuals seek to establish independence, explore identity, and gain stability in various areas like education, career, and relationships. For those disengaging from homelessness, the process involves breaking free from the cycle of instability, securing stable housing, gaining access to education and employment, and building a support system. It requires addressing both immediate needs (e.g., safety, basic resources) and long-term goals (e.g., personal growth, financial independence). The aim is to create a pathway toward permanent stability, emotional well-being, and a fulfilling adulthood free from the constraints of homelessness. The following section describes the processes of disengagement from homelessness during EA.

Identity Exploration

During this phase of development, love, work, and worldviews come to define one's identity (Arnett, 2000). Karabanow et al. (2016) found that homeless youth experienced identity exploration like mainstream youth, yet they also wrestle with trauma unlike anything experienced by mainstream youth and survive/exist within a lived experience of marginalization (Karabanow et al., 2016). The stigma of being homeless can be detrimental to identity (McNaughton, 2008); internalization of the negative stereotypical characteristics can promote behavior that aligns with these stereotypes (Barker, 2016). This marginalization can leave homeless youth feeling uncared for and abandoned by family and service providers (Karabanow et al., 2016). Homeless youth share similar identity explorations to those in the mainstream culture, but from a place of disadvantage and feelings of being alone, making it difficult to enter the process of disengaging from homelessness.

A Time of Instability

Instability is characteristic of EA because this cohort often changes plans (Arnett, 2007). Yet the nature of instability experienced by homeless youth is different from mainstream youth. Youth who are homeless have often experienced childhood trauma (Karabanow et al., 2025), which is inherently destabilizing. Higher ACE scores and lower SES are associated with greater perceived instability during EA (Davis et al., 2018; Landberg et al., 2019). Instability experienced as part of the process of entering, engaging with, and exiting homelessness can inadvertently direct individuals to aspire to internalize such instability from which they would like to escape (Barker, 2016). This internalized instability and history of hardship may make this period of instability experienced by emerging adults different from the experiences of their non-homeless peers (Karabanow et al., 2016).

The nature of instability experienced by emerging adults who are homeless can make it difficult to enter the phases of disengaging with homelessness. Specifically, when emerging adults who are homeless feel that they are the only person they can count on (Karabanow et al., 2016), it makes it difficult to secure help. Additionally, if emerging adults who are homeless have internalized instability and are from equity-deserving groups (Barker, 2016, p. 201), this perceived social stigma can promote low self-esteem, feelings of being trapped, and guilt around being homeless (Kidd, 2007), all of which might negatively affect contemplation and motivation to exit homelessness. Internalized feelings of instability can impair changing routines because routines require stability. Emerging adults who are homeless can also feel a sense of disempowerment (Karabanow et al., 2016), which might make the prospect of disengagement from homelessness seem insurmountable.

Self-Focused Time

Mainstream emerging adults focus on their own wants and needs as they explore academics, careers, and relationships (Arnett, 2007). Yet this self-focused time is experienced differently for those who take on the burden of adulthood prematurely (Karabanow et al., 2016). Emerging adults who are homeless are forced into adult responsibilities but are still considered youth within the mainstream culture (Karabanow et al., 2016). Stability afforded by secure housing can elicit feelings of being unprepared for the responsibilities of adulthood (Karabanow et al., 2016), which often stems from their traumatic upbringing (Karabanow et al., 2016). While securing help is a component of disengaging from homelessness (Karabanow, 2008), homeless youth survive the streets, find secure housing, and engage with service providers largely on their own (Karabanow et al., 2016). These findings indicate that the self-focus that is characteristic of mainstream EA is not experienced by emerging adults who are homeless with as much freedom and opportunity as their mainstream counterparts.

A Time of In-Between

A characteristic of EA is a feeling of being in between adolescence and adulthood (Arnett, 2007). Markers of adulthood are financial independence, responsibility for one's actions, and independent decision making (Arnett, 2007). The time of in-between for homeless youth was characterized by fundamental changes in their view of self (Karabanow et al., 2016), which correlates with many of the processes of disengagement described by Karabanow (2008). Youth felt they were ready to exit from homelessness, obtain housing, engage in employment and/or education, change their daily routines, and redefine their sense of self, yet progress was precarious. Housing might improve physical health, but physical impacts of being homeless (e.g., HIV, back pain) interfered with obtained stability (Karabanow et al., 2016). There was little room for error while disengaging from homelessness and mistakes jeopardized stability (Karabanow et al., 2016). This sense of fragility to stability makes the prospect of returning to the streets ever-present (Karabanow et al., 2016).

There was also a sense of in-between in relation to peer and familial support as youth transition from homelessness. Street youth often develop relationships and families within the street culture (Smith, 2008), yet distancing from these relationships is integral to leaving homelessness (Karabanow, 2008), even in the absence of bridging relationships in the mainstream culture. The time of in-between for youth who are experiencing homelessness is in relation to their proximity to the streets, support, and stability.

A Time of Possibility

EA is a time of positive expectations and hope for the future (Arnett, 2000), a sentiment that is also expressed by youth experiencing homelessness. Despite their hardships, youth experiencing homelessness felt hope and determination for their future (Karabanow et al., 2016). Securing help (both health and social support) was integral to this imagining, as was supportive, accessible housing that provided leeway for developmentally appropriate mistakes (Karabanow et al., 2016). Changing daily routines to incorporate aspects that promote positive changes for the future not only helps with transitioning from homelessness but also redefines a sense of self (Karabanow et al., 2016).

Conclusion

Emerging adults who experience homelessness navigate this developmental period while surviving the changes and risks associated with being unhoused. The intersection of these challenges means that emerging adults experiencing homelessness are often caught in a cycle that makes it difficult to transition into stable adulthood. Addressing these issues requires comprehensive solutions that include stable housing, access to education and employment opportunities, mental health care, and social support networks. Support should be developmentally informed and supported by research and policy efforts to better understand these experiences and build in the supports needed for this population to thrive.

References

Ararso, Y., Beharie, N.N., Scheidell, J.D., Schatz, D., Quinn, K., Doran, K.M., Khan, M.R. (2021) The joint effect of childhood abuse and homelessness on substance use in adulthood. *Substance Use & Misuse* 56, 660–667. https://doi.org/10.1080/10826084.2021.1887249

Arnett, J. (2000) Emerging adulthood: A theory of development from the late teens through the twenties. *The American Psychologist* 55, 469–480. https://doi.org/10.1037//0003-066X.55.5.469

Arnett, J., Žukauskienė, R., Sugimura, K. (2014) The new life stage of emerging adulthood at ages 18–29 years: Implications for mental health. *The Lancet Psychiatry* 1, 569–576. https://doi.org/10.1016/S2215-0366(14)00080-7

Arnett, J.J. (2007) Emerging adulthood: What is it, and what is it good for? *Child Development Perspectives* 1, 68–73. https://doi.org/10.1111/j.1750-8606.2007.00016.x

Arnett, J.J. (2004) *Emerging adulthood: The winding road from the late teens through the twenties, Emerging adulthood: The winding road from the late teens through the twenties*. New York: Oxford University Press.

Bakken, K. (2023) Employment barriers in homeless young adults and youth. *Canadian Journal of Family and Youth/Le Journal Canadien de Famille et de la Jeunesse* 15, 161–169.

Barker, J. (2016) A habitus of instability: Youth homelessness and instability. *Journal of Youth Studies* 19, 665–683. https://doi.org/10.1080/13676261.2015.1098772

Bender, K., Yang, J., Ferguson, K., Thompson, S. (2015) Experiences and needs of homeless youth with a history of foster care. *Children and Youth Services Review* 55, 222–231. https://doi.org/10.1016/j.childyouth.2015.06.007

Bowen, E., Ball, A., Jones, A.S., Miller, B. (2021) Toward many emerging adulthoods: A theory-based examination of the features of emerging adulthood for cross-systems youth. *Emerging Adulthood* 9, 189–201. https://doi.org/10.1177/2167696821989123

Budescu, M., Sisselman-Borgia, A., Torino, G.C. (2021) Experience of homelessness discrimination among emerging adults: A qualitative and quantitative analysis. *Emerging Adulthood* 9, 690–701. https://doi.org/10.1177/2167696819845751

Coates, J. and McKenzie-Mohr, S. (2010) Out of the frying pan, into the fire: Trauma in the lives of homeless youth prior to and during homelessness. *The Journal of Sociology & Social Welfare* 37, 65–96. https://doi.org/10.15453/0191-5096.3561

Davies, B.R., Allen, N.B. (2017) Trauma and homelessness in youth: Psychopathology and intervention. *Clinical Psychology Review* 54, 17–28. https://doi.org/10.1016/j.cpr.2017.03.005

Davis, J.P., Dumas, T.M., Roberts, B.W. (2018) Adverse childhood experiences and development in emerging adulthood. *Emerging Adulthood* 6, 223–234. https://doi.org/10.1177/2167696817725608

Dawson-Rose, C., Shehadeh, D., Hao, J., Barnard, J., Khoddam-Khorasani, L. (Ladi), Leonard, A., Clark, K., Kersey, E., Mousseau, H., Frank, J., Miller, A., Carrico, A., Schustack, A., Cuca, Y.P. (2020) Trauma, substance use, and mental health symptoms in transitional age youth experiencing homelessness. *Public Health Nursing* 37, 363–370. https://doi.org/10.1111/phn.12727

Eriksson, P.L., Wängqvist, M., Carlsson, J., Frisén, A. (2020) Identity development in early adulthood. *Developmental Psychology* 56, 1968–1983. https://doi.org/10.1037/dev0001093

Gaetz, S., Donaldson, J., Richter, T., Gulliver, T. (2013) *The State of Homelessness in Canada 2013*. Toronto: Canadian Homelessness Research Network Press.

Gaetz, S., O'Grady, B., Kidd, S., Schwan, K. (2016) *Without a Home: The National Youth Homelessness Survey*. Toronto: Canadian Observatory on Homelessness Press.

Government of Canada (2022) Housing, infrastructure and Communities Canada - Homelessness data snapshot: The National Shelter Study 2022 update [WWW Document]. *Canada.ca*. https://housing-infrastructure.canada.ca/homelessness-sans-abri/reports-rapports/data-shelter-2022-donnees-refuge-eng.html

Government of Canada (2020) Housing, infrastructure and communities Canada - Homelessness data snapshot: Youth homelessness in Canada [WWW Document]. *Canada.ca*. https://housing-infrastructure.canada.ca/homelessness-sans-abri/reports-rapports/youth-homelessness-2024-itinerance-jeunes-eng.html

Karabanow, J. (2008) Getting off the street: Exploring the processes of young people's street exits. *American Behavioral Scientist* 51, 772–788. https://doi.org/10.1177/0002764207311987

Karabanow, J. (2006) Becoming a street youth: Uncovering the stages to street life. *Journal of Human Behavior in the Social Environment* 13, 49–72.

Karabanow, J. (2004) Making organizations work: Exploring characteristics of anti-oppressive organizational structures in street youth shelters. *Journal of Social Work* 4, 47–60. https://doi.org/10.1177/1468017304042420

Karabanow, J., Hopkins, S., Kisely, S., Parker, J., Hughes, J., Gahagan, J., Campbell, L.A. (2007) Can you be healthy on the street? Exploring the health experiences of Halifax street youth. *Canadian Journal of Urban Research* 16, 12–32.

Karabanow, J., Kidd, S., Frederick, T., Hughes, J. (2018) *Homeless Youth and the Search for Stability*. Wilfrid Laurier Univ. Press.

Karabanow, J., Kidd, S., Frederick, T., Hughes, J. (2016) Toward housing stability: Exiting homelessness as an emerging adult. *The Journal of Sociology & Social Welfare* 43, 121.

Karabanow, J., Titterness, A., Hughes, J., Wu, H., Good, S. (2025) The trauma of youth homelessness: Youth on the street. In *Reframing Trauma Through Social Justice: Resisting the Politics of Mainstream Trauma Discourse*. Routledge, pp. 161–179. https://doi.org/10.4324/9781003379591-10

Kidd, S.A. (2007) Youth homelessness and social stigma. *Journal of Youth and Adolescence* 36, 291–299. https://doi.org/10.1007/s10964-006-9100-3

Kim, Y., Bender, K., Ferguson, K.M., Begun, S., DiNitto, D.M. (2018) Trauma and posttraumatic stress disorder among homeless young adults: The importance of victimization experiences in childhood and once homeless. *Journal of Emotional and Behavioral Disorders* 26, 131–142. https://doi.org/10.1177/1063426617710239

Labelle, R., Berthiaume, C., Daigle, M., Breton, J.-J., Houle, J. (2020) Mental health, suicidal behaviour, and primary healthcare among homeless youth. *Canadian Journal of Community Mental Health* 39, 25–38. https://doi.org/10.7870/cjcmh-2020-029

Landberg, M., Lee, B., Noack, P. (2019) What alters the experience of emerging adulthood? How the experience of emerging adulthood differs according to socioeconomic status and critical life events. *Emerging Adulthood* 7, 208–222. https://doi.org/10.1177/2167696819831793

Malenfant, J., Schwan, K., French, D., Gaetz, S., Redman, M. (2020) *Preventing Youth Homelessness in the Canadian Education System: Young People Speak Out*. Toronto, ON: Canadian Observatory on Homelessness Press.

Martijn, C., Sharpe, L. (2006) Pathways to youth homelessness. *Social Science & Medicine* 62, 1–12. https://doi.org/10.1016/j.socscimed.2005.05.007

McNaughton, C. (2008) *Transitions Through Homelessness*. London: Palgrave Macmillan UK. https://doi.org/10.1057/9780230227347

O'Connor, M., Sanson, A., Hawkins, M.T., Letcher, P., Toumbourou, J.W., Smart, D., Vassallo, S., Olsson, C.A. (2011) Predictors of positive development in emerging adulthood. *Journal of Youth and Adolescence* 40, 860–874. https://doi.org/10.1007/s10964-010-9593-7

Pitcher, C., Saewyc, E., Browne, A., Rodney, P. (2019) Access to primary health care services for youth experiencing homelessness: "you shouldn't need a health card to be healthy". *Witness: The Canadian Journal of Critical Nursing Discourse* 1, 73–92.

Schwan, K., Gaetz, S., French, D., Redman, M., Thistle, J.A., Dej, E. (2018) *What Would It Take? Youth across Canada Speak Out on Youth Homelessness Prevention*. Canadian Observatory on Homelessness Press.

Smith, H. (2008) Searching for kinship: The creation of street families among homeless youth. *American Behavioral Scientist* 51, 756–771. https://doi.org/10.1177/0002764207311986

Syed, M., Seiffge-Krenke, I. (2013) Personality development from adolescence to emerging adulthood: Linking trajectories of ego development to the family context and identity formation. *Journal of Personality and Social Psychology* 104, 371–384. https://doi.org/10.1037/a0030070

Tucker, J.S., Davis, J.P., Perez, L.G., Klein, D.J., D'Amico, E.J. (2022) Late adolescent predictors of homelessness and food insecurity during emerging adulthood. *Journal of Adolescent Health* 70, 736–742. https://doi.org/10.1016/j.jadohealth.2021.10.035

Wenzel, S., Holloway, I., Golinelli, D., Ewing, B., Bowman, R., Tucker, J. (2012) Social networks of homeless youth in emerging adulthood. *Journal of Youth and Adolescence* 41, 561–571. https://doi.org/10.1007/s10964-011-9709-8

Wood, D., Crapnell, T., Lau, L., Bennett, A., Lotstein, D., Ferris, M., Kuo, A. (2018) Emerging adulthood as a critical stage in the life course. In *Handbook of Life Course Health Development*, edited by N. Halfon, C. B. Forrest, R. M. Lerner, E. M. Faustman. Cham: Springer International Publishing, pp. 123–143. https://doi.org/10.1007/978-3-319-47143-3_7

22

KEY SOCIAL LOCATIONS RELEVANT TO HOMELESSNESS PREVENTION

Global South Perspectives

Regina Celia Fiorati, Carla Regina Silva and Larissa Soares de Melo

This chapter examines how public policies for the homeless population are structured in one country in the Global South—Brazil. We focus on housing policies, as well as the daily implementation of the National Policy for the Homeless Population in a colonized country marked by neoliberal-aligned governments that perpetuate vast, naturalized social inequalities. After describing this context, we provide an overview of three distinct and interrelated projects aimed at taking an emancipatory approach to the problem of homelessness through university outreach projects using the arts and mutual aid approaches to improving the health of the homeless population.

How this Chapter Guides Practice, Research, and Policy in Homelessness Prevention

Knowledge of homelessness, and how it is managed at community and population levels in the Global South, is essential for understanding ways of addressing homelessness across the globe. Framed within a public policy perspective aimed at eradicating hunger and poverty, strategies identified in this chapter advocate for guaranteed access to housing, employment, income, and education while prioritizing equity in the Global South. The analysis presented in this chapter employs intersectional frameworks to examine groups most affected by systemic inequities, contextualized through markers of social inequality. The analysis presented in this chapter, and the application of this approach described, can inform researchers, practitioners, and policymakers on approaches that are uniquely attuned to a Global South perspective.

DOI: 10.4324/9781003541332-26

Introduction

In Brazil, policy for the homeless population is primarily structured through the intersection of the Unified Social Assistance System (SUAS) and the Unified Health System (SUS), with specific services for this demographic. These services operate independently yet with interdependent workflows to ensure cohesive care. Historically, the National Social Assistance Policy (2004), as noted by Santos, Côrtes, and Margarites (2022), has been influenced since the colonial era by religiously rooted charitable and paternalistic practices—values that distort the very conception of public policy as a citizenship right and a state obligation to address social inequalities. This dynamic remains an ongoing paradigm shift (Costa, 2024). Public investment in Social Assistance policy still lags behind other governmental priorities, reflected in unstable budgets and a lack of integrated planning to address structural vulnerabilities (Koga, 2006).

This fragility is exacerbated by neoliberal, religious, and politically negotiated management under SUAS, often instrumentalized for electoral gains, perpetuating colonial-era paternalism. Within this context, the National Policy for the Homeless Population (2009) operates in a community-oriented manner, yet is influenced by institutional constraints, where housing rights are theorized but underdeveloped, contributing to Brazil's persistent housing deficit.

Homeless Population Assistance Policy in Brazil: Guidelines, Legal Frameworks, and Challenges

Public policies grounded in universality, equity, and social participation, integrating SUAS and SUS actions, are outlined in the 2009 National Policy (Brazil, 2011). Assistance strategies to reduce street homelessness are centralized in SUAS, which coordinates community care through collective and individual approaches (Brazil, 2009). The SUAS network includes the Specialised Reference Centre for the Homeless Population (*Centro POP*), offering daytime services (e.g., bathing, meals, laundry, social interaction) and referrals to sectoral policies via multidisciplinary teams, which offer specialized services to this population and integrate with the Medium Complexity Social Protection of the specified public policy (Brazil, 2011). The Centro POP's objective is to provide daytime services to individuals experiencing homelessness, serving as a consistent space for daily living activities (AVDs) such as bathing, food, laundry, social interaction, and referrals to sectoral policies and/or specific services, based on the individual needs of those being assisted, through individualized follow-up by health and social care providers such as social workers, psychologists, occupational therapists, and others (Brazil, 2011).

Among the referrals from the Centro POP, there is the possibility of directing individuals to institutional shelter services, depending on the local network's structure and availability of vacancies. This care strategy integrates with the high complexity social protection of the SUAS (also known as the Ministry of Development and Social Assistance, Family and Fight Against Hunger) and includes the following modalities: institutional shelter, transitional housing, and shelter services in residential facilities, each with its own entry point and typification that guides internal operation, team composition, and objectives according to the stage of care the individual is experiencing. However, all services operate 24 hours a day with multidisciplinary teams working in organized shifts (Brazil, 2014). As in many countries across the globe, institutional shelter services are considered the main response of the Brazilian state to the care of the homeless population. However, this predominance highlights the structural limitations of public policies in the country, with which there is a historical and unresolved housing deficit that prioritizes emergency solutions over permanent housing strategies. This model is insufficient to keep up with the exponential growth of the homeless population, perpetuating cycles of social vulnerability for many Brazilian people.

Services in Brazil for unhoused persons include institutional shelter services (24/7 care under High-Complexity Social Protection), yet these reflect systemic limitations. For example, there are only 26,000 shelter beds in the country (Ministério do Desenvolvimento e Assistência Social, Família e Combate à Fome, 2023) for an estimated 281,000 homeless individuals (IPEA, 2023). This inadequate number of shelter beds to meet demand represents an emergency response that perpetuates cycles of vulnerability for people who are unhoused, rather than alleviating homelessness and the health consequences with which it is associated. This is further compounded by the fact that such organizations are frequently managed by religious entities, with rules and regulations that institutionalize persons experiencing homelessness (Teixeira, 2021). Notably, Brazil has implemented only three Housing First initiatives: Projeto Ruas (Belo Horizonte), Cáritas Brasileira (Curitiba), and Braços Abertos (São Paulo, discontinued in 2017). This lack of uptake of a known evidence-based intervention, coupled with the lack of emergency shelter beds across an entire country, is a reminder of a state that is failing to adequately meet the needs of this population.

Strategies for Participation in Daily Life and Emancipatory Cultural Production

The experiences reported here show the life stories of human groups in high social vulnerability generated by the neoliberal and neocolonialist capitalist system (Palacios, 2017; Pino Morán et al., 2015; Silva et al.,

2018). Three hegemonic forces sustain exclusion: neoliberal capitalism, colonialism, and heteropatriarchy (Polanco & Morrison, 2019; Núñez, 2019; Silvestrini et al., 2019). Neoliberalism, as Harvey (2008) notes, enshrines private property and free markets, exacerbating hierarchies and violence (Fanon, 1963). Homeless individuals face systemic regulation, medialization, and penalization (Wacquant, 2009), necessitating access to public policies, community support, and dignified living conditions. Neoliberalism, through its mechanism of neocolonial power, introduces, through the State, a policy of managing bodies and identities, putting, in many contexts, the signs of an insidious colonialism, continuing to perpetuate and maintain genocide, epistemicide, and feminicide (Segato, 2016; (Dardot & Laval, 2016). It is necessary to consider what Frantz Fanon (1963, p. 47) defines as "violence in its raw state", that is, colonial capitalist violence. This is a situation that is imposed on people who live on the streets, because it is only those who most suffer the effects of the social inequalities imposed by neoliberal capitalism and its neocolonialism.

There is no specific data on the mortality rate of the homeless population in Brazil. There are reports that some municipalities produce, and/or data cross-referencing is also carried out independently by specific cities, which characterize local quantitative and qualitative data. The most recent data specified is from the City of São Paulo, with a record of 1,200 deaths of homeless people in the capital between 2022 and 2023, with violence and the use of substances such as crack and fentanyl being the main causes of death. However, it is important to emphasize that in addition to the lack of standardized records, there is also underreporting of the contexts of deaths (São Paulo, 2023).

It is necessary to establish approaches that are ethically and politically committed to the social changes and transformation that are undeniably present in contemporary times. Reflecting on "leaving the streets" is both urgent and essential, and economic conditions play a crucial role in resolving this issue. However, being in a safe home is not merely about fulfilling a dream or residing in a house—it encompasses numerous actions, strategies, relationships, habits, rules, and forms of coexistence that cannot be addressed solely through economic means. Thus, community work is essential for providing comprehensive care for individuals with experiences of homelessness, enabling them to first recognize themselves (either for the first time or once again) as human beings, endowed with rights, citizens capable of forming bonds and relationships, whose presence is powerful, creative, and capable of contributing to the wider community.

From this reflective theoretical perspective, the integrated teaching, research, and university extension projects developed by the Human Activities and Occupational Therapy (AHTO) group at the Federal

University of São Carlos (Brazil) since 2015 serve as examples of practices that are ethically and politically committed to homeless people and their multisectoral demands, while also promoting the education of occupational therapists engaged with/in social transformation. Since 2015, the AHTO has maintained close ties with the Municipal Social Assistance Secretariat of the City Council and the Centro Pop service, developing various integrated projects in collaboration with the team and users of this service each year. All work is conducted in partnership with other sectors, including education, health, employment, arts and culture, and social assistance.

Art and Mutual Aid Strategies for Emancipation

In this section, we present three projects aimed at taking an emancipatory approach using arts and mutual aid to illustrate ways of raising consciousness around experiences of homelessness in Brazil in which AHTO was deeply involved: (1) "Mais um Corre", (2) Images of the Streets, and (3) Building Bridges. All of this work was developed from a community-based, critical, cultural, and decolonial perspective. Each of these projects has aimed to provide homeless people with spaces of belonging, fostering and strengthening social support networks and ties that encourage meaningful actions, creativity, and experimentation. These initiatives seek to help individuals build life projects and develop a new perception of themselves, based on their strengths, abilities, and aspirations. Integrated teaching, research, and outreach projects have been incorporated and have presented different approaches each year, yet they share common principles and structure. These include weekly, flexible, and open activity workshops, incorporating a broad range of initiatives supported by an artistic, community-based, sensitive, reflective, and critical approach.

Project 1: "Mais um Corre"

The project aimed to use art and culture to create spaces for creativity and empowerment among homeless people. It encouraged the development of skills and opportunities by recognizing and disseminating cultural capital, as well as promoting the exhibition of artistic work created by individuals with experiences of homelessness through travelling exhibitions. This project employed strategies to foster artistic and cultural creations, drawing upon the unique aesthetics of the works produced by artists. Additionally, it promoted a critical perspective of the social perceptions of this population by society, and the complexity of life on the streets (Silva et al., 2018). The cultural project was carried out between 2015 and 2018. The exhibition was presented in various cities, in educational and cultural spaces such as theatres, libraries, cultural centres, conferences, public squares, schools, and museums. It comprises works created using different techniques, including photography, audiovisual productions, painting, collage, modelling, and installations, organized into the following sections: Identity, Memories, Networks, Dreams, and Trajectories.

In this project, two street artists, a poet, and a circus performer participated. They collaborate as part of the interdisciplinary team and perform for the general public who visited the exhibition. During the course of this project, our team offered a guided tour in which the processes and meanings behind the artworks and aesthetics that make up the exhibition are presented, alongside live performances by the artists, who recite their own poetry and present circus acts featuring juggling and clowning. The artists are integrated into the team and receive artistic fees, depending on each educational or cultural space. This recognition of their work helps to shift their sense of self-worth and promote their emancipation, in addition to providing financial support. Moreover, it fosters social and cultural appreciation of their efforts. This requires an authorial creative process, dedication, concentration, creativity, expression, and recognition. In other words, it demands a balanced combination of well-being, emotions, technique, responsibility, self-esteem, and context. See Figures 22.1–22.3 for pictures representing various elements of this exhibition.

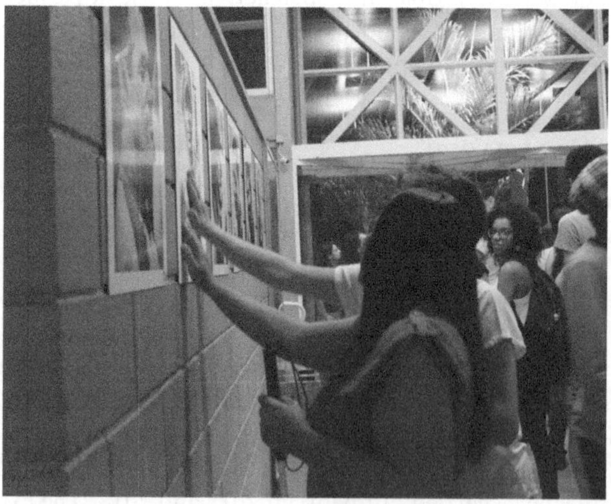

FIGURE 22.1 Public interacting with photographic works

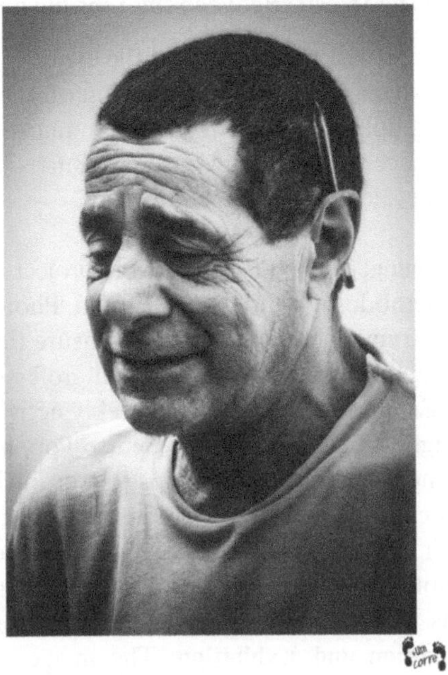

FIGURE 22.2 Photography shown at the exhibition

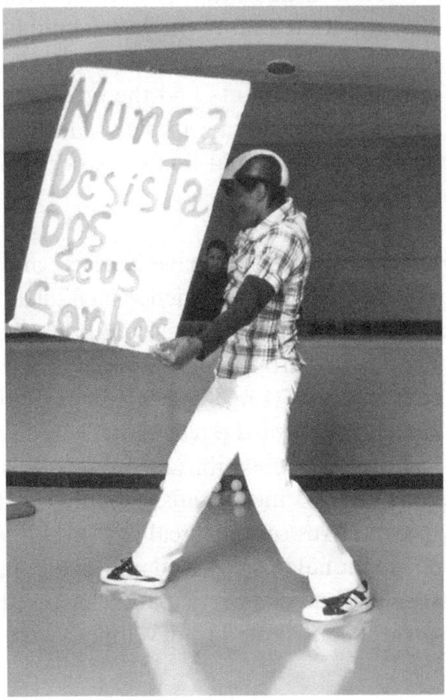

FIGURE 22.3 Circus artist during a performance

Project 2: Images of the Streets: Between the Sensible and the Invisible

The objective of this project was to expand the expression, agency, empowerment, and social participation of people living on the streets. To achieve this, we used photography as a means of communication and expression, based on the photovoice methodology (Wang & Burris, 1997).

The project was developed in four stages:

1 **Planning and Training**: During this stage, the project team was trained in the photovoice methodology and its application. Photography classes and camera-handling training were provided to ensure that the project team could teach participants in a more skilled and professional manner.
2 **Workshops and Exhibition Preparation**: Weekly activity workshops were conducted for eight months in 2017 at Centro Pop, involving 30 regular participants. In these workshops, participants were invited to walk around the city and visit cultural spaces, exhibitions, and parks, capturing photographs from their own perspectives and everyday experiences. They then selected their photographs and wrote captions, expressing their demands, desires, creations, and, most importantly, their personal viewpoints.
3 **Project Dissemination and Exhibition**: The images and captions were grouped into ten categories based on similarity, expression, and content. A selection of the five most representative images from each category was printed and displayed in a dedicated exhibition, fostering appreciation, exchange, and dissemination among the general public.
4 **Data Analysis and Evaluation of Actions and Strategies**: Evaluation meetings were held with all participants and the project team. A final report was produced, and part of the data was analysed in a Final Degree Thesis (TFG), written by an occupational therapy student who completed her professional internship.

This project enabled participants to engage in active and conscious expression through images and text. The experience facilitated the recognition of both collective and individual strengths and qualities, the discovery of aesthetic and artistic expression through photography, and the exercise of citizenship and social participation (Engelen et al., 2021). Notably, many of the venues visited had previously denied participants entry due to the stigma of homelessness. The photographic exhibition provided visibility and a platform for dialogue for homeless individuals, encouraging the wider community to adopt new perspectives on their realities. In this way, the guidelines related to culture, occupational therapy, and photovoice facilitated the social inclusion and participation of participants involved in the project. Furthermore, this project contributed to developing participants' awareness

"Olha minha selfie aí!"
Izaac Martins da Silva
Cerrado UFSCar – São Carlos – Novembro/2017

FIGURE 22.4 "Look at my Selfie"

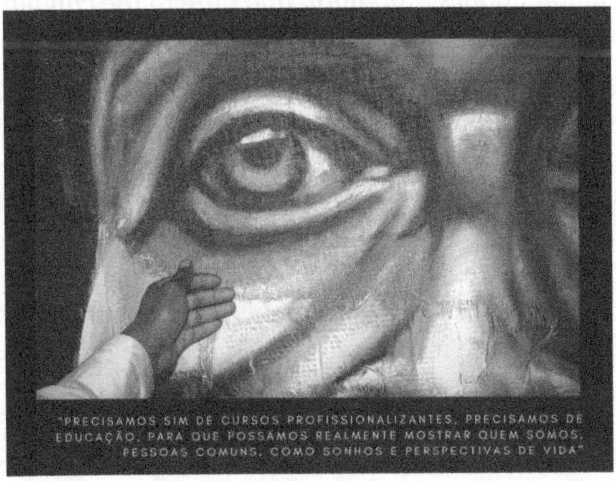
"PRECISAMOS SIM DE CURSOS PROFISSIONALIZANTES, PRECISAMOS DE EDUCAÇÃO, PARA QUE POSSAMOS REALMENTE MOSTRAR QUEM SOMOS, PESSOAS COMUNS, COMO SONHOS E PERSPECTIVAS DE VIDA"

FIGURE 22.5 Self-representation

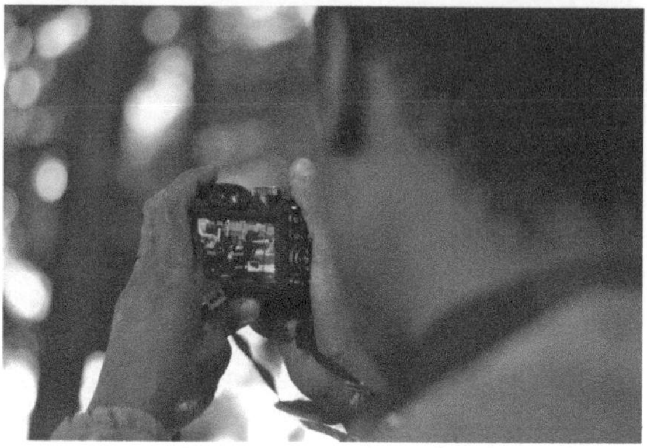

FIGURE 22.6 A participant focusing their camera while taking photographs

of citizenship, social and human rights, and cultural accessibility. See Figures 22.4–22.6 that illustrate the products and process of this project.

Project 3: Building Bridges—Attention and Care to the Population in Street Situations

The third project we highlight in this chapter was developed by the University of São Paulo in Ribeirão Preto, Brazil. The project, called "*Building Bridges: Attention and Care for the Homeless Population*", was a multidisciplinary university extension initiative involving undergraduate students from occupational therapy, medicine, nursing, psychology, pharmacy, and dentistry. It is a health-related project that operates within the framework of "*Consultório na Rua*" (Street Clinic), a Brazilian public service under Primary Health Care (APS). This service involves a mobile health team that reaches out to homeless individuals, providing care where they are and referring them to other health services through the intranet of the SUS, with a focus on harm reduction. The "Pontes" Project works in conjunction with SUS and can also direct individuals to additional health services within the SUS Health Care Network. The project provides care on weekends in public squares and other locations where homeless individuals take shelter and live, offering medical, therapeutic, occupational, dental, and other services through volunteer health professionals and faculty members who supervise the students involved. Care is provided both inside tents and through mobile assistance. Through its academic coordination, the project holds a seat on the *Municipal Intersectoral Committee on Public Policies for the Homeless Population of Ribeirão Preto*, São Paulo, Brazil. Within this forum, advocacy efforts focus

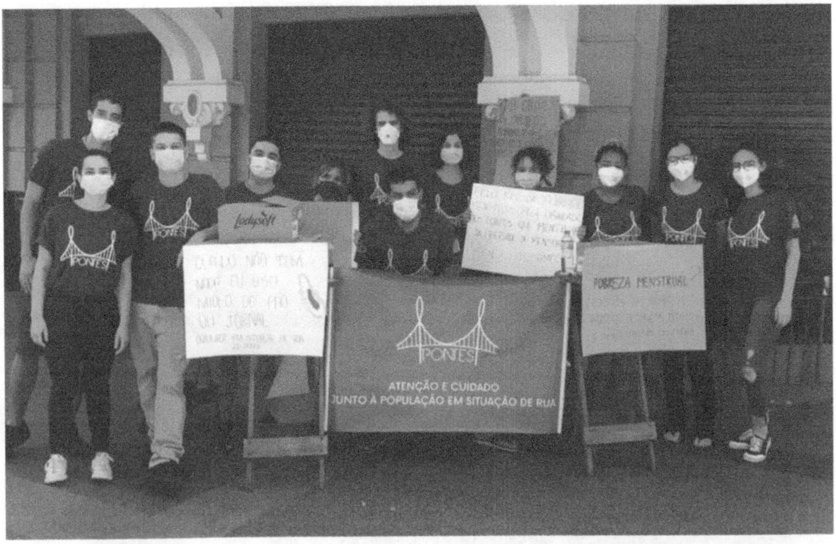

FIGURE 22.7 Interdisciplinary team of students from the Bridges Project

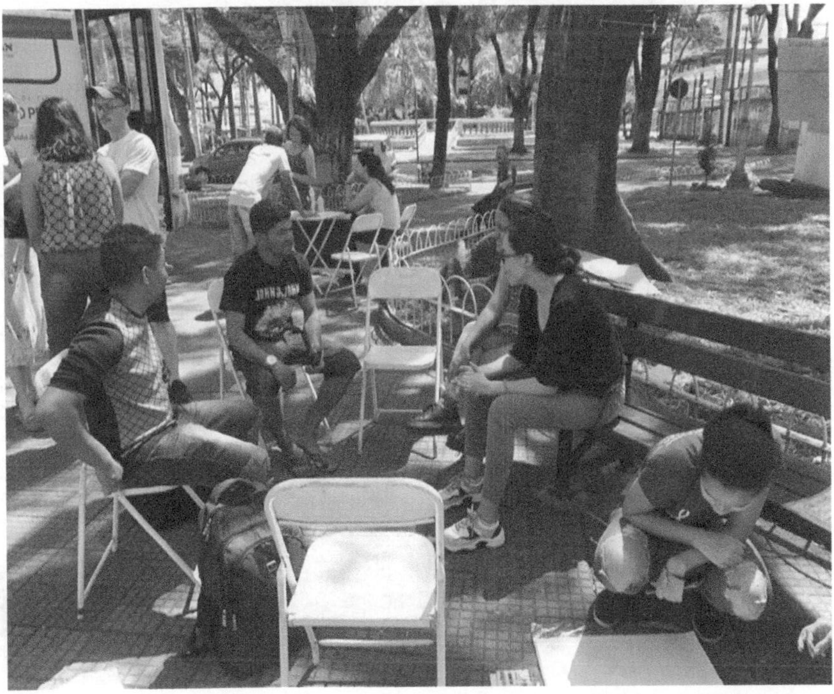

FIGURE 22.8 Group dynamics of students with homeless people (daily life on the streets)

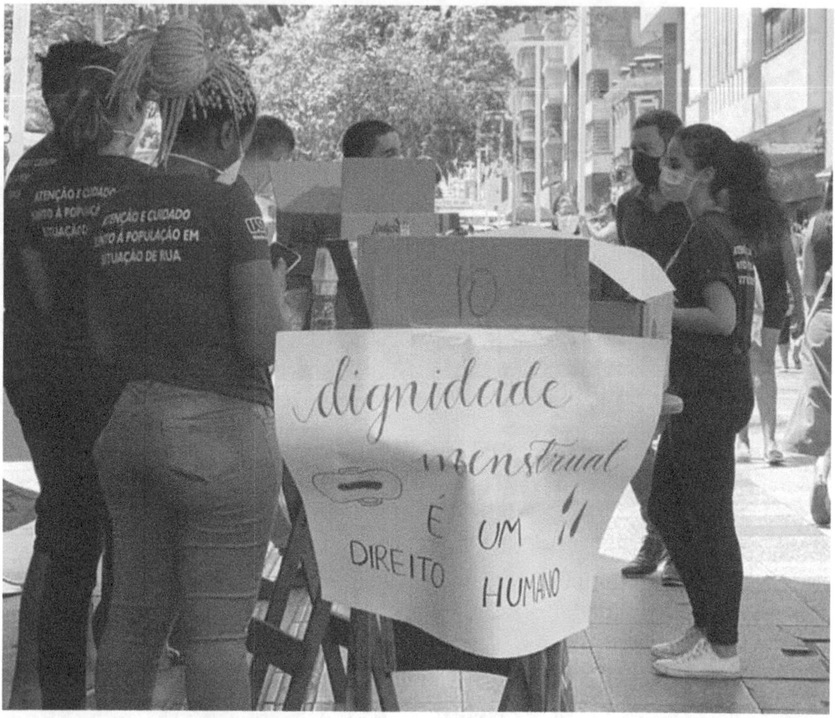

FIGURE 22.9 Students distributing sanitary pads in a menstrual dignity campaign for homeless women

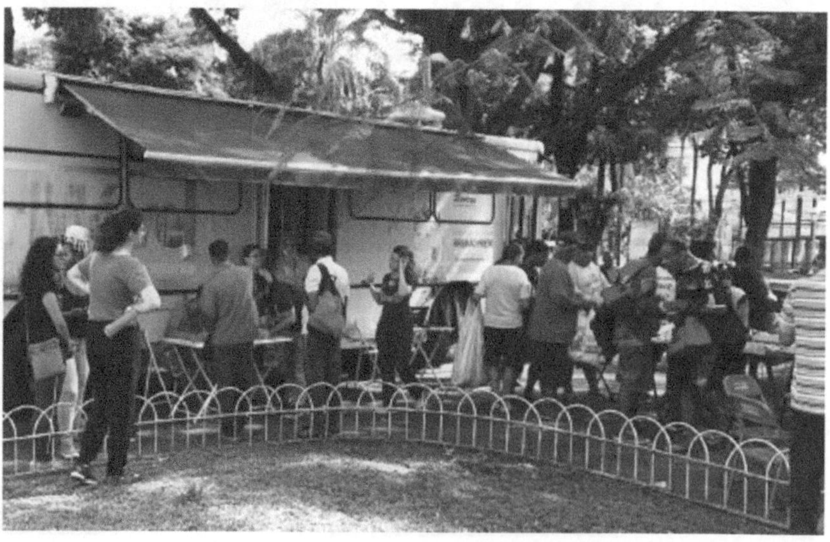

FIGURE 22.10 Truck equipped with a medical office

on establishing effective housing policy, moving beyond the current approach based on institutional shelters. The committee also promotes housing policies aligned with the Housing First approach. See Figures 22.7–22.10, which depict photographs of these initiatives in action.

Conclusion

In Brazil, the push for an effective public housing policy—one that surpasses the outdated institutional shelter model rooted in philanthropic social assistance, charity, and guardianship—is still in its early stages. This stagnation hinders efforts towards self-determination and emancipation for the homeless population. The principles guiding housing projects based on the model remain limited and are largely dependent on the attitudes and political will of local governments or initiatives from Civil Society Organizations, Non-Governmental Organizations, and Universities. The primary challenge lies in expanding movements that advocate for the creation and implementation of such policies.

References

Brazil (2009) *Decree No. 7,053 of December 23, 2009. National Policy for the Homeless Population, Official Gazette of the Union.*

Brazil. Ministry of Social Development (2011) *Technical Guidelines: Specialized Reference Center for Homeless Population - Centro POP*. Brasília: MDS. (SUAS and Homeless Population Series, v.3).

Brazil. National Social Assistance Council (2014) *National Typification of Social Assistance Services*. Reprint. Brasília: CNAS.

Brazil. Institute of Applied Economic Research (2023) *Estimate of the homeless population in Brazil (2022–2023)*. Technical Note No. 87. Brasília: IPEA. Available at: [https://www.ipea.gov.br/portal/images/stories/PDFs/nota_tecnica/230323_nt_87_dirur_poprua.pdf] (Accessed: 29 March 2025).

Costa, R.C.S. (2024) *Affluent displacements for the right to citizenship and distributive social protection in the Unified Social Assistance System*. PhD Thesis. São Paulo: Pontifical Catholic University of São Paulo.

Dardot, P. & Laval, C. (2016) *The new way of the world: On neoliberal society*. London: Verso. (English translation of original French work).

Engelen, A-M., Silva, C. R., Zango, I. M., Cloete, L. G., Schiller, S., Kagwiza, J. N., Hengelaar, R., Celik, Z. (2021) Community development in occupational therapy education: learning from global experiences. In *Teaching and learning practices that promote sustainable development and active citizenship*, ed. 1. Hershey: IGIGlobal, v.1, pp. 276–305.

Fanon, F. (1963) *The wretched of the earth*. New York: Grove Press. (English translation of original French work).

Harvey, D. (2005) *A brief history of neoliberalism*. Oxford: Oxford University Press.

Koga, D. (2006) 'Social assistance policy in Brazil', in *Popular participation in public policies: Space for building Brazilian democracy*, edited by Albuquerque, M.C., São Paulo: Instituto Pólis, pp. 49–64.

Ministério do Desenvolvimento e Assistência Social, Família e Combate à Fome. (2023) *Censo SUAS 2022: levantamento nacional de informações da Assistência Social*. https://aplicacoes.mds.gov.br/sagi/censuas/v2/relatorios.php

Núñez, C.M.V. (2019) 'Southern occupational therapies: A proposal for understanding', *Brazilian Journal of Occupational Therapy*, 27(3), pp. 671–680. Available at: https://doi.org/10.4322/2526-8910.ctoarf1859

Palacios, M. (2017) Reflexiones sobre las prácticas comunitarias: aproximación a una Terapia Ocupacional del Sur. *Revista Ocupación Humana*, 17(1), 73–88.

Polanco Cerón, N. & Morrison, R. (2019) 'Patriarchy, hegemonic masculinity and occupations: Processes of perpetuation of sexism. Argentine Journal of Occupational Therapy. [Patriarcado, masculinidad hegemónica y ocupaciones: procesos de perpetuación del sexismo]'. *Revista Argentina de Terapia Ocupacional*, 5(1), 75–84.

Pino Morán, J. A., Ceballos, M., & Sepúlveda, R. (2015) Terapia Ocupacional comunitaria crítica. Diálogos y reflexiones para iniciar una propuesta colectiva. *TOG (A Coruña)*, 12(22). http://www.revistatog.com/num22/pdfs/colab3.pdf

Santos, P.R., Côrtes, S.V. & Margarites, G.C. (2022) 'From guardianship to citizenship', *Society and State*, 37(1), pp. 245–270.

Segato, R.L. (2016) *The war against women*. New York: Palgrave Macmillan. (English translation of original Spanish work).

Silva, C.R., et al. (2018) 'Creative strategies and the homeless population', *Brazilian Journal of Occupational Therapy*, 26(2), pp. 489–500. Available at: https://doi.org/10.4322/2526-8910.ctoRE1128

Silvestrini, M. S., Silva, C. R., & Prado, A. C. da S. A. (2019) Terapia ocupacional e cultura: dimensões ético-políticas e resistências. *Cadernos Brasileiros De Terapia Ocupacional*, *27*(4), 929–940. https://doi.org/10.4322/2526-8910.ctoARF1727

Teixeira, S. (2021) *Social assistance and human rights*. São Paulo: XYZ Editora.

Wacquant, L. (2009) *Punishing the poor: The neoliberal government of social insecurity*. Durham: Duke University Press.

Wang, C. & Burris, M.A. (1997) 'Photovoice: Concept, methodology, and use for participatory needs assessment', *Health Education & Behavior*, 24(3), pp. 369–387.

CONCLUSION

Carrie Anne Marshall, Rebecca Gewurtz and Skye Barbic

Homelessness is a pressing global issue, and one that will take significant and dedicated efforts to address. In this book, we presented the Bridging the Transition Framework, with chapters written by authors representing a range of backgrounds, lived experiences, and health and social care disciplines. Each component of the framework was presented, with evidence-informed recommendations for approaches that can be used with individuals and families, communities and populations. Individuals who have experienced homelessness for prolonged periods or over several episodes present with high degrees of complexity and in a structural context that can make leaving homelessness permanently a seemingly insurmountable challenge. Preventing homelessness in this population requires an interdisciplinary approach, and one that acknowledges not only individual factors, but also how community structures and policies implemented across populations contribute to ongoing homelessness. The Bridging the Transition Framework offers a way of seeing the problem of homelessness through the lens of function and participation, and draws attention to potential solutions at individual, community, and population levels. By coming together as persons with lived experience, researchers, health and social care providers, policymakers, and advocates, we believe that it is possible to prevent and end homelessness. As a global community, it is more important than ever before to work together to contribute to the development, implementation and evaluation of solutions, and demand thoughtful action, political will, and persistence to address this international crisis. Homelessness is not an intractable problem, impossible to solve, or something to be managed. It is a serious social problem that we can effectively address by working together within and across communities so that everyone has a safe and adequate place to live and thrive.

DOI: 10.4324/9781003541332-27

INDEX

Pages in *italics* refer to figures and pages in **bold** refer to tables.

For Product Safety Concerns and Information please contact our EU representative GPSR@taylorandfrancis.com Taylor & Francis Verlag GmbH, Kaufingerstraße 24, 80331 München, Germany